Taking SIDES

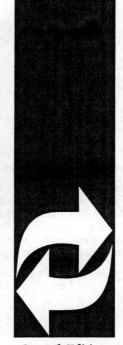

Clashing Views on Controversial Bioethical Issues

Seventh Edition

Edited, Selected, and with Introductions by

Carol Levine

Dushkin/McGraw-Hill
A Division of The McGraw-Hill Companies

For Hannah, Amy, and Asher

Photo Acknowledgments

Part 1 Middlesex Memorial Hospital
Part 2 Digital Stock
Part 3 Ted Croner
Part 4 Middlesex Memorial Hospital
Part 5 WHO/Photo by E. Rice
Part 6 WHO/Photo by J. Mohr
Part 7 UN Photo 148868/John Isaac

Cover Art Acknowledgment

Charles Vitelli

Manufactured in the United States of America

Seventh Edition

10 9 8 7 6 5 4 3 2 1

Library of Congress Cataloging-in-Publication Data

Main entry under title:
    Taking sides: clashing views on controversial bioethical issues/edited, selected, and with introductions by Carol Levine.—7th ed.
    Includes bibliographical references and index.
    1. Bioethics. I. Levine, Carol, *comp.*

174.957′4
0-697-37535-8
ISSN: 1091-8809

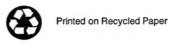 Printed on Recycled Paper

PREFACE

This is a book about choices—hard and tragic choices. The choices are hard not only because they often involve life and death but also because there are convincing arguments on both sides of the issues. An ethical dilemma, by definition, is one that poses a conflict not between good and evil but between one good principle and another that is equally good. The choices are hard because the decisions that are made—by individuals, groups, and public policymakers—will influence the kind of society we have today and the one we will have in the future.

Although the views expressed in the selections in this volume are strong —even passionate—they are also subtle, concerned with the nuances of the particular debate. *How* one argues matters in bioethics; you will see and have to weigh the significance of varying rhetorical styles and appeals throughout this volume.

Although there are no easy answers to any of the issues in the book, the questions will be answered in some fashion—partly by individual choices and partly by decisions that are made by professionals and government. We must make them the best answers possible, and that can only be done by informed and thoughtful consideration. This book, then, can serve as a beginning for what ideally will become an ongoing process of examination and reflection.

Changes to this edition   Although many popular issues remain from the previous edition, the basic structure of the book has been changed for the first time since the third edition. There are now seven parts: Medical Decision Making; Death and Dying; Choices in Reproduction; Children and Bioethics; Genetics; Human and Animal Experimentation; and Bioethics and Resource Allocation. There are also seven completely new issues: *Is Informed Consent Still Central to Medical Ethics?* (Issue 1); *Can Family Interests Ethically Outweigh Patient Autonomy?* (Issue 2); *Are Some Advance Directives Too Risky for Patients?* (Issue 4); *Should Physicians Be Allowed to Assist in Patient Suicide?* (Issue 5); *Do Parents Harm Their Children When They Refuse Medical Treatment on Religious Grounds?* (Issue 12); *Should Parents Always Be Told of Genetic-Testing Availability?* (Issue 15); and *Should Patient-Centered Medical Ethics Govern Managed Care?* (Issue 19). In addition, the NO selection has been replaced in Issue 8 *(Should Courts Be Permitted to Order Women to Use Long-Acting Contraceptives?)* to bring the debate up to date. In all, there are 15 new selections. Part introductions, issue introductions, and postscripts have been revised as necessary. Also, when applicable, I have provided Internet site addresses (URLs) in the postscripts that should prove useful as starting points for further research.

i

A word to the instructor   An *Instructor's Manual With Test Questions* (multiple-choice and essay) is available through the publisher, and a general guidebook, *Using Taking Sides in the Classroom*, which discusses methods and techniques for using the pro/con approach in any classroom setting, is also available. An on-line version of *Using Taking Sides in the Classroom* and a correspondence service for Taking Sides adopters can be found at www.cybsol.com/usingtakingsides/.

Taking Sides: Clashing Views on Controversial Bioethical Issues is only one title in the Taking Sides series; the others are listed on the back cover. If you are interested in seeing the table of contents for any of the other titles, please visit the Taking Sides Web site at http://www.dushkin.com/takingsides/.

Acknowledgments   I received helpful comments and suggestions from the many users of *Taking Sides* across the United States and Canada. Their suggestions have enhanced the quality of this edition of the book and are reflected in the new selections and issues.

Special thanks go to those who responded with specific suggestions for the seventh edition:

James G. Anderson
Purdue University

Thomas E. Brown
Atlantic Community
    College

Joan M. Chapdelaine
Salve Regina College

Persis C. Coleman
Rollins College

Cheryl Slaughter Ellis
Middle Tennessee State
    University

Samuel D. Fohr
University of
    Pittsburgh–Bradford

Beverly Hawkins
Widener University

James C. Marker
University of
    Wisconsin–Green Bay

Steven McCullagh
Kennesaw State College

David Mowry
Ohio University

John Mpi
St. Peters College

Barry Nobel
Lane Community College

Betty Odello
Los Angeles Pierce College

William Puffenberger
Elizabethtown College

Paul Rowgo
Barry University

Mark Sheldon
Indiana University–
    Northwest

Natalie C. Shiras
Fairfield University

Edward Stevens
Regis College

Eileen Whitney
Clark College

For this edition, Dillan Siegler was an invaluable researcher, commentator, critic, and one-person support system. She also prepared the *Instructor's Manual*. Both of us have benefited immeasurably from Ben Munisteri's and Lauri Posner's careful work on previous editions. Marna Howarth of the Hastings Center staff responded to inquiries efficiently, promptly, and with great good humor. For their assistance in previous editions, which gave me a solid base from which to proceed, I want to thank Paul Homer, Eric Feldman, and Arthur Caplan. I would particularly like to thank Daniel Callahan, director of the Hastings Center, and Willard Gaylin, both now retired, for their early encouragement in this project.

Carol Levine

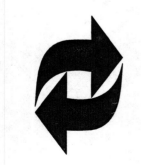

CONTENTS IN BRIEF

CONTENTS

Physician Robert M. Arnold and professor of psychiatry and sociology Charles
W. Lidz assert that informed consent in clinical care is an essential process
that promotes good communication and patient autonomy despite the obstacles of implementation. Professor of medical ethics Robert M. Veatch argues
that informed consent is a transitional concept that is useful only for moving
toward a more radical framework in which physicians and patients are paired
on the basis of shared deep social, moral, and institutional values.

John Hardwig, an associate professor of medical ethics, argues that the prevalent ethic of patient autonomy ignores family interests in medical treatment
decisions. He maintains that physicians should recognize these interests as
legitimate. Bioethicist Jeffrey Blustein maintains that although families can be
an important resource in helping patients make better decisions about their
care, the ultimate decision-making authority should remain with the patient.

Nursing professor Inge B. Corless asserts that restricting the practice of HIV-infected health care workers rather than implementing universal protections to prevent infection actually puts patients at greater risk of infection. Philosopher Carson Strong argues that physicians infected with HIV should be restricted from certain procedures, particularly those involving an open wound.

Psychiatrist Christopher James Ryan argues that advance directives that refuse active treatment in situations when a patient's incompetence is potentially reversible should be abolished because healthy people are likely to underestimate their desire for treatment should they become ill. Geriatricians Steven Luttrell and Ann Sommerville assert that respect for the principle of autonomy requires that individuals be permitted to make risky choices about their own lives and that ignoring autonomous choices made by competent adults reinstates the outmoded notion of medical paternalism.

Physician Timothy E. Quill discusses the case of his patient "Diane" in arguing that in some cases, physicians' indirect assistance in suicide honors patients' choices and prevents severe suffering. Psychiatrist Herbert Hendin asserts that individual cases presented to justify legalizing physician-assisted suicide fail to deal with the underlying medical failures to control pain, create an illusion of control over death, and do not acknowledge the likelihood that the practice will kill thousands of patients inappropriately.

Physician Bernard C. Meyer argues that physicians who adhere to a rigid
formula of truth telling fail to appreciate the differences in patients' readiness
to hear and understand the information. Philosopher Sissela Bok argues that
the harm resulting from disclosure is less than physicians may think and is
outweighed by the benefits.

Physician Steven H. Miles maintains that physicians' duty to follow patients'
wishes ends when the requests are inconsistent with what medical care can
reasonably be expected to achieve. Philosopher Felicia Ackerman contends
that decisions involving personal values, such as those regarding quality of
life, should be made by the patient or family, not by the physician.

Jim Persels, editor in chief of the *Southern Illinois University Law Journal,* contends that the use of long-acting but reversible contraceptive technologies as
requirements for probation for women convicted of child abuse or drug use
serves to guard the unborn while simultaneously limiting the intrusion on the
individual's privacy rights and the state's burden of supervision. Law professor Rebecca Dresser argues that sentencing women to use contraceptives
is unjust because it has a disproportionately coercive effect on women, espe-

cially low-income minority women, with a very small likelihood of reducing child abuse and neglect.

Philosopher Bonnie Steinbock argues for a pro-choice position based on the moral status of the fetus and the pregnant woman's moral right to bodily self-determination. Psychologist Sidney Callahan asserts that pregnant women have a moral obligation to carry their fetuses to term.

Pediatrician and county health commissioner Mark S. Rapoport argues that the knowledge that a baby may be HIV-infected benefits the baby's health. Pediatrician Alan R. Fleischman argues that mandatory testing is detrimental to the development of the trusting relationship that is essential for providing services to both mother and child.

Pediatric surgeon Michael R. Harrison asserts that anencephalic newborns should be treated as brain-dead rather than as brain-absent so that their organs can be transplanted. Philosopher John D. Arras and pediatric neurologist Shlomo Shinnar argue that the current definition of brain death reflects sound public policy and good ethics.

Philosopher Ruth Macklin argues that Jehovah's Witness parents forfeit their
rights to control their children when their refusal to permit blood transfusion
—even when it is based on religious conviction—will result in the death of or
severe harm to the children. Professor of philosophy Mark Sheldon assesses
the case of Jehovah's Witness parents who refuse to allow their children to
undergo blood transfusions and concludes that they cannot be said to be truly
harming or neglecting their children. Rather, they are placing their children's
spiritual interests above worldly ones.

Professor of history and philosophy of science Evelyn Fox Keller warns that
the Human Genome Project's beneficent focus on "disease-causing genes"
may lead to the abuse of inherently ambiguous standards of normality. Professor of humanities Daniel J. Kevles and professor of biology Leroy Hood
maintain that a resurgence of negative eugenics as a result of this project is
highly unlikely.

The American Council of Life Insurance and the Health Insurance Association of America assert that denying insurers access to genetic test results could lead to higher premiums for most policyholders. Thomas H. Murray, a professor of biomedical ethics, warns that genetic tests will likely be used by insurance companies to increase the price of or even deny people access to health insurance.

Mary Z. Pelias, attorney and professor of genetics, argues that parental autonomy and family privacy should govern decisions about whether or not to test children for genetic predispositions to disease and that physicians and genetic counselors have an obligation to disclose full information. Law professor Diane E. Hoffmann and pediatrician Eric A. Wulfsberg assert that caution and restraint should govern decisions on testing for genetic predispositions in children and that safeguards should be adopted to diminish the potentially negative effects of testing and to protect children's best interests.

Jerod M. Loeb and his colleagues, representing the American Medical Society's Group on Science and Technology, assert that concern for animals cannot impede the development of methods to improve the welfare of humans. Philosopher Tom Regan argues that those who support animal research fail to show proper respect for animals' inherent value.

Bioethicist Douglas K. Martin argues that the option to donate fetal tissue for
therapeutic use may influence some women to choose abortion. Bioethicists
Dorothy E. Vawter and Karen G. Gervais contend that knowledge of the
option to donate tissue is not an incentive for a woman to abort a fetus she
would otherwise carry to term.

Philosopher Daniel Callahan believes that people who have lived a full natural life span should be offered care that relieves suffering but not expensive
life-prolonging technologies. Sociologist Amitai Etzioni argues that rationing
health care for the elderly would invite restrictions on health care for other
groups.

Physician Ezekiel J. Emanuel and attorney Nancy Neveloff Dubler argue that
the expansion of managed care and the imposition of significant cost controls could undermine critical aspects of the physician-patient relationship,
including freedom of choice, careful assessments of physician competence,
time available for communication, and continuity of care. Attorney Michael
J. Malinowski contends that medical ethics can no longer be focused on indi-

vidual patients and physicians but must develop a social conscience, which means recognizing that costs matter, that not everyone can have access to everything, and that resources must be rationed fairly and openly.

Attorney Lori B. Andrews believes that donors, recipients, and society will benefit from a market in body parts so long as owners retain control over their bodies. Ethicist Thomas H. Murray argues that the gift relationship should govern the transfer of body parts.

INTRODUCTION

Medicine and Moral Arguments

Carol Levine

In the fall of 1975, a 21-year-old woman lay in a New Jersey hospital—as she had for months—in a coma, the victim of a toxic combination of barbiturates and alcohol. Doctors agreed that her brain was irreversibly damaged and that she would never recover. Her parents, after anguished consultation with their priest, asked the doctors and hospital to disconnect the respirator that was artificially maintaining their daughter's life. When the doctors and hospital refused, the parents petitioned the court to be made her legal guardian so that they could authorize the withdrawal of treatment. After hearing all the arguments, the court sided with the parents, and the respirator was removed. Contrary to everyone's expectations, however, the young woman did not die but began to breathe on her own (perhaps because, in anticipation of the court order, the nursing staff had gradually weaned her from total dependence on the respirator). She lived for 10 years until her death in June 1985—comatose, lying in a fetal position, and fed with tubes—in a New Jersey nursing home.

The young woman's name was Karen Ann Quinlan, and her case brought national attention to the thorny ethical questions raised by modern medical technology: When, if ever, should life-sustaining technology be withdrawn? Is the sanctity of life an absolute value? What kinds of treatment are really beneficial to a patient in a "chronic vegetative state" like Karen's? And, perhaps the most troubling question, who shall decide? These and similar questions are at the heart of the growing field of biomedical ethics or (as it is usually called) *bioethics*.

Ethical dilemmas in medicine are, of course, nothing new. They have been recognized and discussed in Western medicine since a small group of physicians—led by Hippocrates—on the Isle of Cos in Greece, around the fourth century B.C., subscribed to a code of practice that newly graduated physicians still swear to uphold today. But unlike earlier times, when physicians and scientists had only limited abilities to change the course of disease, today they can intervene in profound ways in the most fundamental processes of life and death. Moreover, ethical dilemmas in medicine are no longer considered the sole province of professionals. Professional codes of ethics, to be sure, offer some guidance, but they are usually unclear and ambiguous about what to do in specific situations. More important, these codes assume that whatever decision is to be made is up to the professional, not the patient. Today, to an ever-greater degree, laypeople—patients, families, lawyers, clergy, and others—want to and have become involved in ethical decision making not only in individual cases, such as the Quinlan case, but also in large societal decisions, such as how to allocate scarce medical resources, including high-technology machinery, newborn intensive care units, and the expertise of physicians. While questions about the physician-patient relationship and individual cases are still prominent in bioethics (see, for example, the issues on truth telling and assisting dying patients in suicide), today the field covers a broad range of other decisions as well, such as the harvesting and transplantation of organs, equity in access to health care, and the future of animal experimentation.

This involvement is part of broader social trends: a general disenchantment with the authority of all professionals and, hence, a greater readiness to challenge the traditional belief that "doctor knows best"; the growth of various civil rights movements among women, the aged, and minorities—of which the patients' rights movement is a spin-off; the enormous size and complexity of the health care delivery system, in which patients and families often feel alienated from the professional; the increasing cost of medical care, much of it at public expense; and the growth of the "medical model," in which conditions that used to be considered outside the scope of physicians' control, such as alcoholism and behavioral problems, have come to be considered diseases.

Bioethics began in the 1950s as an intellectual movement among a small group of physicians and theologians who started to examine the questions raised by the new medical technologies that were starting to emerge as the result of the heavy expenditure of public funds in medical research after World War II. They were soon joined by a number of philosophers who had become disillusioned with what they saw as the arid abstractions of much analytic philosophy at the time and by lawyers who sought to find principles in the law that would guide ethical decision making or, if such principles were not there, to develop them by case law and legislation or regulation. Although these four disciplines—medicine, theology, philosophy, and law—still dominate the field, today bioethics is an interdisciplinary effort, with political scientists, economists, sociologists, anthropologists, nurses, allied health professionals, policymakers, psychologists, and others contributing their special perspectives to the ongoing debates.

The issues discussed in this volume attest to the wide range of bioethical dilemmas, their complexity, and the passion they arouse. But if bioethics today is at the frontiers of scientific knowledge, it is also a field with ancient roots. It goes back to the most basic questions of human life: What is right? What is wrong? How should people act toward others? And why?

While the *bio* part of *bioethics* gives the field its urgency and immediacy, we should not forget that the root word is *ethics*.

APPLYING ETHICS TO MEDICAL DILEMMAS

To see where bioethics fits into the larger framework of academic inquiry, some definitions are in order. First, *morality* is the general term for an individual's or a society's standards of conduct, both actual and ideal, and of the character traits that determine whether people are considered "good" or "bad." The scientific study of morality is called *descriptive ethics*; a scientist —generally an anthropologist, sociologist, or historian—can describe in empirical terms what the moral beliefs, judgments, or actions of individuals or societies are and what reasons are given for the way they act or what they believe. The philosophical study of morality, on the other hand, approaches the subject of morality in one of two different ways: either as an analysis of the concepts, terms, and methods of reasoning (*metaethics*) or as an analysis of what those standards or moral judgments ought to be (*normative ethics*). Metaethics deals with meanings of moral terms and logic; normative ethics, with which the issues in this volume are concerned, reflects on the kinds of actions and principles that will promote moral behavior.

Because normative ethics accepts the idea that some acts and character traits are more moral than others (and that some are immoral), it rejects the rather popular idea that ethics is relative. Because different societies have different moral codes and values, ethical relativists have argued that there can be no universal moral judgments: What is right or wrong depends on who does it and where, and whether or not society approves. Although it is certainly true that moral values are embedded in a social, cultural, and political context, it is also true that certain moral judgments are universal. We think it is wrong, for example, to sell people into slavery—whether or not a certain society approved or even whether or not a person wanted to be a slave. People may not agree about what these universal moral values are or ought to be, but it is hard to deny that some such values exist.

The other relativistic view rejected by normative ethics is the notion that whatever feels good *is* good. In this view, ethics is a matter of personal preference, weightier than one's choice of which automobile to buy, but not much different in kind. Different people, having different feelings, can arrive at equally valid moral judgments, according to the relativistic view. Just as we should not disregard cultural factors, we should not overlook the role of emotion and personal experience in arriving at moral judgments. But to give emotion ultimate authority would be to consign reason and rationality —the bases of moral argument—to the ethical trash heap. At the very least, it would be impossible to develop a just policy concerning the care of vulnerable persons, like the mentally retarded or newborns, who depend solely on the vagaries of individual caretakers.

Thus, if normative ethics is one branch of philosophy, bioethics is one branch of normative ethics; it is normative ethics applied to the practice of medicine and science. There are other branches—business ethics, legal ethics, journalism ethics, and military ethics, for example. One common term for the entire grouping is *applied and professional ethics*, because these ethics deal with the ethical standards of the members of a particular profession and how they are applied in the professionals' dealings with each other and the rest of society. Bioethics is based on the belief that some solutions to the dilemmas that arise in medicine and science are more moral than others and that these solutions can be determined by moral reasoning and reflection.

ETHICAL THEORIES

If the practitioners of bioethics do not rely solely on cultural norms and emotions, what are their sources of determining what is right or wrong? The most comprehensive source is a theory of ethics—a broad set of moral principles (or perhaps just one overriding principle) that is used in measuring human conduct. Divine law is one such source, of course, but even in the Western religious traditions of bioethics (both the Jewish and Catholic religions have rich and comprehensive commentaries on ethical issues, and the Protestant religion has a less cohesive but still important tradition) the law of God is interpreted in terms of human moral principles. A theory of ethics must be acceptable to many groups, not just the followers of one religious tradition. Most writers outside the religious traditions (and some within them) have looked to one of three major traditions in ethics: teleological theories, deontological theories, and natural law theories.

Teleological Theories

Teleological theories are based on the idea that the end or purpose (from the Greek *telos,* or end) of the action determines its rightness or wrongness. The most prominent teleological theory is *utilitarianism.* In its simplest formulation, an act is moral if it brings more good consequences than bad ones. Utilitarian theories are derived from the works of two English philosophers: Jeremy Bentham (1748–1832) and John Stuart Mill (1806–1873). Rejecting the absolutist religious morality of his time, Bentham proposed that "utility"— the greatest good for the greatest number—should guide the actions of human beings. Invoking the hedonistic philosophy of Epicurean Greeks, Bentham said that pleasure (*hedon* in Greek) is good and pain is bad. Therefore, actions are right if they promote more pleasure than pain and wrong if they promote more pain than pleasure. Mill found the highest utility in "happiness," rather than pleasure. (Mill's philosophy is echoed in the Declaration of Independence's espousal of "life, liberty, and the pursuit of happiness.") Other utilitarians have looked to a range of utilities, or goods (including friendship, love, devotion, and the like) that they believe ought to be weighed in the balance—the utilitarian calculus.

Utilitarianism has a pragmatic appeal. It is flexible, and it seems impartial. However, its critics point out that utilitarianism can be used to justify suppression of individual rights for the good of society ("the ends justify the means") and that it is difficult to quantify and compare "utilities," however they are defined.

Utilitarianism, in its many forms, has had a powerful influence on bioethical discussion, partly because it is the closest to the case-by-case risk/benefit ratio that physicians use in clinical decision making. Joseph Fletcher, a Protestant theologian who was one of the pioneers in bioethics in the 1950s, developed utilitarian theories that he called *situation ethics.* He argued that a true Christian morality does not blindly follow moral rules but acts from love and sensitivity to the particular situation and the needs of those involved. He has enthusiastically supported most modern technologies on the grounds that they lead to good ends.

Writers in this volume who use utilitarian theories to arrive at their moral judgments are Michael R. Harrison, who supports the use of anencephalic infants—babies born without brains—as organ donors; Bernard C. Meyer, who defends withholding the truth from dying patients on the grounds that it leads to better consequences than truth telling; and Jerod M. Loeb and his colleagues, who defend animal experimentation.

Deontological Theories

The second major type of ethical theory is *deontological* (from the Greek *deon*, or duty). The rightness or wrongness of an act, these theories hold, should be judged on whether or not it conforms to a moral principle or rule, not on whether it leads to good or bad consequences. The primary exponent of a deontological theory was Immanuel Kant (1724–1804), a German philosopher. Kant declared that there is an ultimate norm, or supreme duty, which he called the "Moral Law." He held that an act is moral only if it springs from a "good will," the only thing that is good without qualification.

We must do good things, said Kant, because we have a duty to do them, not because they result in good consequences or because they give us pleasure (although that can happen as well). Kant constructed a formal "Categorical Imperative," the ultimate test of morality: "I ought never to act except in such a way that I can also will that my maxim should become universal law." Recognizing that this formulation was far from clear, Kant said the same thing in three other ways. He explained that a moral rule must be one that can serve as a guide for everyone's conduct; it must be one that permits people to treat each other as ends in themselves, not solely as means to another's ends; and it must be one that each person can impose on himself by his own will, not one that is solely imposed by the state, one's parents, or God. Kant's Categorical Imperative, in the simplest terms, says that all persons have equal moral worth and that no rule can be moral unless all people can apply it autonomously to all other human beings. Although on its own Kant's Categorical Imperative is merely a formal statement with no moral content at all, he gave some examples of what he meant: "Do not commit suicide," and "Help others in distress."

Kantian ethics is criticized by many who note that Kant gives little guidance on what to do when ethical principles conflict, as they often do. Moreover, they say, his emphasis on autonomous decision making and individual will neglects the social and communal context in which people live and make decisions. It leads to isolation and unreality. These criticisms notwithstanding, Kantian ethics has stimulated much current thinking in bioethics. In this volume, the idea that certain actions are in and of themselves right or wrong underlies, for example, Sissela Bok's appeal to truth telling; Mary Z. Pelias's support of physicians' always disclosing the availability of genetic testing to parents; and Thomas H. Murray's rejection of the idea of a market in body parts.

Two modern deontological theorists are philosophers John Rawls and Robert M. Veatch. In *A Theory of Justice* (1971), Rawls places the highest value on equitable distribution of society's resources. He believes that society has a fundamental obligation to correct the inequalities of historical circumstance and natural endowment of its least well off members. According to this theory, some action is good only if it benefits the least well off. (It can also benefit others, but that is secondary.) His social justice theory has influenced bioethical writings concerning the allocation of scarce resources.

Veatch has applied Rawlsian principles to medical ethics. In his book *A Theory of Medical Ethics* (1981), he offers a model of social contract among professionals, patients, and society that emphasizes mutual respect and responsibilities. This contract model will, he hopes, avoid the narrowness of professional codes of ethics and the generalities and ambiguities of more broadly based ethical theories. In Issue 1 of this volume, Veatch challenges current concepts of informed consent as outmoded.

Natural Law Theory

The third strain of ethical theory that is prominent in bioethics is *natural law theory*, first developed by St. Thomas Aquinas (1223–1274). According to this theory, actions are morally right if they accord with our nature as human beings. The attribute that is distinctively human is the ability to reason and to exercise intelligence. Thus, argues this theory, we can know the good, which is objective and can be learned through reason. References to natural law theory are prominent in the works of Catholic theologians and writers; they see natural law as ultimately derived from God but knowable through the efforts of human beings. The influence of natural law theory can be seen in this volume in Sidney Callahan's pro-life feminist opposition to abortion.

Theory of Virtue

The *theory of virtue*, another ethical theory with deep roots in the Aristotelian tradition, has recently been revived in bioethics. This theory stresses not the morality of any particular actions or rules but the disposition of individuals to act morally, to be virtuous. In its modern version, its primary exponent is Alasdair MacIntyre, whose book *After Virtue* (1980) urges a return to the Aristotelian model. Gregory Pence has applied the theory of virtue directly to medicine in *Ethical Options in Medicine* (1980); he lists temperance in personal life, compassion for the suffering patient, professional competence, justice, honesty, courage, and practical judgment as the virtues that are most desirable in physicians. Although this theory has not yet been as fully developed in bioethics as the utilitarian or deontological theories, it is likely to have particular appeal for physicians—many of whom have resisted formal ethics education on the grounds that moral character is the critical factor and that one can best learn to be a moral physician by emulating one's mentors.

Although various authors, in this volume and elsewhere, appeal in rather direct ways to either utilitarian or deontological theories, often the various types are combined. One may argue both that a particular action is immoral in and of itself and that it will have bad consequences (some commentators say even Kant used this argument). In fact, probably no single ethical theory is adequate to deal with all the ramifications of the issues. In that case we can turn to a middle level of ethical discussion. Between the abstractions of ethical theories (Kant's Categorical Imperative) and the specifics of moral judgments (always obtain informed consent from a patient) is a range of concepts—ethical principles—that can be applied to particular cases.

ETHICAL PRINCIPLES

In its four years of deliberation, the National Commission for the Protection of Human Subjects of Biomedical and Behavioral Research grappled with some of the most difficult issues facing researchers and society: When, if ever, is it ethical to do research on fetuses, on children, or on people in mental institutions? This commission—which was composed of people from various religious backgrounds, professions, and social strata—was finally able to agree on specific recommendations on these questions, but only after they had finished their work did the commissioners try to determine what ethical principles they had used in reaching a consensus. In their Belmont Report (1978), named after the conference center where they met to discuss this question, the commissioners outlined what they considered to be the three most important ethical principles (respect for persons, beneficence, and justice) that should govern the conduct of research with human beings. These three principles, they believed, are generally accepted in our cultural tradition and can serve as basic justifications for the many particular ethical prescriptions and evaluations of human action. Because of the principles' general acceptance and widespread applicability, they are at the basis of most bioethical discussion. Although philosophers argue about whether other principles—preventing harm to others or loyalty, for example—ought to be accorded equal weight with these three or should be included under another umbrella, they agree that these principles are fundamental.

Respect for Persons
Respect for persons incorporates at least two basic ethical convictions, according to the Belmont Report. Individuals should be treated as autonomous agents, and persons with diminished autonomy are entitled to protection. The derivation from Kant is clear. Because human beings have the capacity for rational action and moral choice, they have a value independent of anything that they can do or provide to others. Therefore, they should be treated in a way that respects their independent choices and judgments. Respecting autonomy means giving weight to autonomous persons' considered opinions and choices, and refraining from interfering with their choices unless

those choices are clearly detrimental to others. However, since the capacity for autonomy varies with age, mental disability, or other circumstances, those people whose autonomy is diminished must be protected—but only in ways that serve their interests and do not interfere with the level of autonomy that they do possess.

Two important moral rules are derived from the ethical principle of respect for persons: informed consent and truth telling. Persons can exercise autonomy only when they have been fully informed about the range of options open to them, and the process of informed consent is generally considered to include the elements of information, comprehension, and voluntariness. Thus, a person can give informed consent to some medical procedure only if he or she has full information about the risks and benefits, understands them, and agrees voluntarily—that is, without being coerced or pressured into agreement. Although the principle of informed consent has become an accepted moral rule (and a legal one as well), it is difficult—some say impossible—to achieve in a real-world setting. It can easily be turned into a legalistic parody or avoided altogether. But as a moral ideal it serves to balance the unequal power of the physician and patient.

Another important moral ideal derived from the principle of respect for persons is truth telling. It held a high place in Kant's theory. In his essay "The Supposed Right to Tell Lies from Benevolent Motives," he wrote: "If, then, we define a lie merely as an intentionally false declaration towards another man, we need not add that it must injure another...; for it always injures another; if not another individual, yet mankind generally.... To be truthful in all declarations is therefore a sacred and conditional command of reasons, and not to be limited by any other expediency."

Other important moral rules that are derived from the principle of respect for persons are confidentiality and privacy.

Beneficence

Most physicians would probably consider beneficence (from the Latin *bene*, or good) the most basic ethical principle. In the Hippocratic Oath it is used this way: "I will apply dietetic measures for the benefit of the sick according to my ability and judgment; I will keep them from harm and injustice." And further on, "Whatever houses I may visit, I will comfort and benefit the sick, remaining free of all intentional injustice." The phrase *Primum non nocere* (First, do no harm) is another well-known version of this idea, but it appears to be a much later, Latinized version—not from the Hippocratic period.

Philosopher William Frankena has outlined four elements included in the principle of beneficence: (1) One ought not to inflict evil or harm; (2) one ought to prevent evil or harm; (3) one ought to remove evil or harm; and (4) one ought to do or promote good. Frankena arranged these elements in hierarchical order, so that the first takes precedence over the second, and so on. In this scheme, it is more important to avoid doing evil or harm than to do good. But in the Belmont Report, beneficence is understood as an obligation—

first, to do no harm, and second, to maximize possible benefits and minimize possible harms.

The principle of beneficence is at the basis of Timothy E. Quill's support of allowing physicians to assist some patients in suicide and of Christopher James Ryan's concerns that some advance directives are too risky for patients.

Justice

The third ethical principle that is generally accepted is justice, which means "what is fair" or "what is deserved." An injustice occurs when some benefit to which a person is entitled is denied without good reason or when some burden is imposed unduly, according to the Belmont Report. Another way of interpreting the principle is to say that equals should be treated equally. However, some distinctions—such as age, experience, competence, physical condition, and the like—can justify unequal treatment. Those who appeal to the principle of justice are most concerned about which distinctions can be made legitimately and which ones cannot (see the issue on gender bias in medicine and research).

One important derivative of the principle of justice is the recent emphasis on "rights" in bioethics. Given the successes in the 1960s and 1970s of civil rights movements in the courts and political arena, it is easy to understand the appeal of "rights talk." An emphasis on individual rights is part of the American tradition, in a way that emphasis on the "common good" is not. The language of rights has been prominent in the abortion debate, for instance, where the "right to life" has been pitted against the "right to privacy" or the "right to control one's body." The "right to health care" is a potent rallying cry, though it is one that is difficult to enforce legally. Although claims to rights may be effective in marshaling political support and in emphasizing moral ideals, those rights may not be the most effective way to solve ethical dilemmas. Our society, as philosopher Ruth Macklin has pointed out, has not yet agreed on a theory of justice in health care that will determine who has what kinds of rights and—the other side of the coin—who has the obligation to fulfill them.

WHEN PRINCIPLES CONFLICT

These three fundamental ethical principles—respect for persons, beneficence, and justice—all carry weight in ethical decision making. But what happens when they conflict? That is what this book is all about.

On each side of the issues included in this volume are writers who appeal, explicitly or implicitly, to one or more of these principles. For example, in Issue 8, Jim Persels sees beneficence as paramount and would approve under some circumstances involuntary implantation of long-acting contraceptives as a way to prevent child abuse. Rebecca Dresser sees such a policy as an intrusion into the autonomy of the individual and as having no predictable benefit to the child.

Some of the issues are concerned with how to interpret a particular principle: Whether, for example, it is more or less beneficent to allow a physician to assist in suicide, or whether patients can best be protected from HIV transmission in a health care setting by putting restrictions on HIV-infected practitioners or by using a voluntary system of education on infection control.

Will it ever be possible to resolve such fundamental divisions—those that are not merely matters of procedure or interpretation but of fundamental differences in principle? Lest the situation seem hopeless, consider that some consensus does seem to have been reached on questions that seemed equally tangled a few decades ago. The idea that government should play a role in regulating human subjects research was hotly debated, but it is now generally accepted (at least if the research is medical, not social or behavioral in nature, and is federally funded). And the appropriateness of using the criteria of brain death for determining the death of a person (and the possibility of subsequent removal of their organs for transplantation) has largely been accepted and written into state laws. The idea that a hopelessly ill patient has the legal and moral right to refuse treatment that will only postpone dying is also well established (though it is often hard to exercise because hospitals and physicians continue to resist it). Finally, nearly everyone now agrees that health care is distributed unjustly in the United States—a radical idea only a few years ago. There is, of course, sharp disagreement about whose responsibility it is to rectify the situation—the government's or the private sector's.

In the 12 years since the first edition of this book was published, the dominance of principles as the foundation of bioethics has been challenged. Several philosophers have pointed out, as already noted, that the "mid-level" principles are not grounded in a unified moral theory. Other writers have described the philosophical mode of argument as too arid and abstract, and they have called for the inclusion of other forms of discourse, such as public policy, emotion-based reasoning, and narrative or "storytelling."

Besides the virtue theory, already described, two other candidates have their defenders. The ethics of caring has been presented as an alternative to traditional bioethics reasoning. Women, it is claimed, embody an ethic of caring, which is itself a prime aim of healing relationships. An ethic of caring would focus on relationships rather than autonomy, on reconciliation rather than winning an argument, and on nurturing rather than imposing dominance. While the absence of caring relationships is clearly a problem in modern health care, this view has been severely criticized by many, including women, as failing to provide a sufficient basis for replacing ethical principles.

Another mode of analysis that is being revived is casuistry. Although associated with the Middle Ages and religious thinking, casuistry is simply a way of reaching consensus on principles by focusing on concrete cases—the clearest ones first, and then the harder ones. The casuist reaches principles from the bottom up, rather than deciding cases from the top (principles first) down.

A final form of analysis is clinical ethics. Its practitioners focus on the clinical realities of moral choices as they emerge in ordinary health care. It is not antithetical to principles but brings abstractions back to reality by measuring proposed solutions against the real world in which doctors and patients live and work.

Edmund Pellegrino, a distinguished physician and ethicist, has seen many changes in the 50 years he has been involved in medicine. Looking toward the future, he does not see the death of principles, but he does foresee some changes. "Physicians and other health workers must become familiar with shifts in contemporary moral philosophy," he says, "if they are to maintain a hand in restructuring the ethics of their profession." But clinicians, too, must change, to "provide a reality check on the nihilism and skepticism of contemporary philosophy. Medical ethics is too ancient and too essential... to be left entirely to the fortuitous currents of philosophical fashion or the unsupported assertion of clinicians."

Although there is consensus in some areas, in others there is only controversy. This book will introduce you to some of the ongoing debates. Whether or not we will be able to move beyond opposing views to a realm of moral consensus will depend on society's willingness to struggle with these issues and to make the hard choices that are required.

PART 1

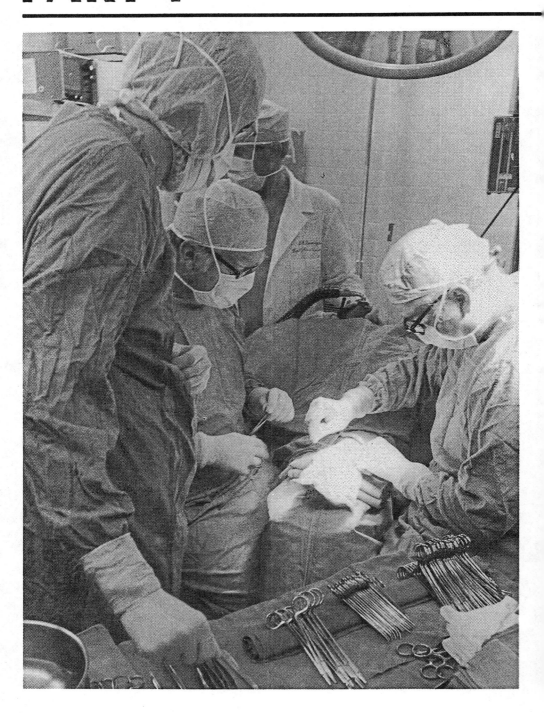

Medical Decision Making

In earlier times medical decision making was of concern only to physicians. With their presumed greater knowledge and with patients' best interests at heart, they were entrusted with making life-and-death, as well as critical, decisions. Ironically, although physicians had greater power in those times than they do today, they also had less ability to treat. As medicine has grown more technologically and scientifically sophisticated, the range of people who have an interest in making decisions—and, in some cases, a right to do so—among the medical options has grown. Law and ethics have reaffirmed the status of the patient as the primary decision maker. Nevertheless, many ambiguous and troubling situations remain in implementing patients' wishes. It is not even clear that patients have the moral right to make arbitrary decisions about aspects of their care, especially when their preferences impinge on the rights of others, such as family members, physicians, and other patients. This section explores some of the issues that arise when making medical decisions.

■ Is Informed Consent Still Central to
    Medical Ethics?

■ Can Family Interests Ethically Outweigh
    Patient Autonomy?

■ Should HIV-Infected Surgeons Be
    Allowed to Operate?

ISSUE 1

Is Informed Consent Still Central to Medical Ethics?

YES: Robert M. Arnold and Charles W. Lidz, from "Informed Consent: Clinical Aspects of Consent in Health Care," in Warren T. Reich, ed., *Encyclopedia of Bioethics, vol. 3,* rev. ed. (Simon & Schuster, 1995)

NO: Robert M. Veatch, from "Abandoning Informed Consent," *Hastings Center Report* (March–April 1995)

ISSUE SUMMARY

YES: Physician Robert M. Arnold and professor of psychiatry and sociology Charles W. Lidz assert that informed consent in clinical care is an essential process that promotes good communication and patient autonomy despite the obstacles of implementation.

NO: Professor of medical ethics Robert M. Veatch argues that informed consent is a transitional concept that is useful only for moving toward a more radical framework in which physicians and patients are paired on the basis of shared deep social, moral, and institutional values.

Informed consent is undoubtedly one of the best-known and, arguably, one of the least-implemented concepts in modern medicine. Although much of modern medical ethics has ancient roots, the idea of informed consent is relatively recent. Until the mid-twentieth century most medical ethics were firmly based on the obligations of physicians to act for the benefit of their patients but not to inform or consult with them in making decisions. On the contrary, information was supposed to be managed carefully in order to protect patients from bad news and to keep them hopeful.

The first "Code of Medical Ethics" of the American Medical Association relied heavily on the work of Thomas Percival, a British physician whose book *Medical Ethics* (1803) played a crucial role in the field for more than a century. Percival believed that the patient's right to the truth was less important than the physician's obligation to benefit the patient. Deception, in the interest of doing good, was thus justified. The patient's consent to treatment, informed or otherwise, is not mentioned in early codes of medical ethics, although on a practical level doctors had to have a patient's permission to perform most procedures.

The modern concept of informed consent came to medical ethics through the courts. The earliest influential decision was *Schloendorff v. New York Hospi-*

tal (1914), in which the court ruled that a patient's right to "self-determination" obligated a physician to obtain consent. This case laid the basis for further litigation. The most influential series of decisions occurred in the 1950s and 1960s, when rulings went beyond the obligation to obtain consent to include an explicit duty to disclose information relevant to the patient who is making a decision about consent. The term *informed consent* first appeared in *Salgo v. Leland Stanford, Jr., University Board of Trustees* (1957).

While the earlier cases had been based on the patient's right to be free from unwanted bodily intrusion (legally, "battery"), the court in *Natanson v. Kline* (1960) held that physicians who withheld information while obtaining consent were guilty of negligence. Imposing a legal duty on physicians to inform their patients of the risks, benefits, and alternatives to treatment exposed them to the risk of malpractice suits. Another factor that influenced the ascendance of informed consent in medical treatment were parallel discussions about the ethics of research involving human subjects. Voluntary consent to participate in research was a cornerstone of the Nuremberg Code of 1947, which was issued after the trials of Nazi physicians who had performed lethal experiments on nonconsenting prisoners.

Nevertheless, traditions die hard, and little change was seen in actual practice until the resurgence of interest in medical ethics in the 1970s. In 1972 the case of *Canterbury v. Spence* established a far-reaching patient-centered disclosure standard. The ruling stated, "The patient's right of self-decision can be effectively exercised only if the patient possesses enough information to enable an intelligent choice. . . . Social policy does not accept the paternalistic view that the physician may remain silent because divulgence might prompt the patient to forego needed therapy." In the 1980s and 1990s court cases have focused on individuals who lack the competence to provide informed consent, such as comatose patients, children, and mentally ill persons.

Although the physician's duty to obtain informed consent and the patient's right to information are now firmly established in law and grounded in the ethical principle of respect for persons, medical practice varies considerably. In Warren T. Reich, ed., *Encyclopedia of Bioethics* (1995), Tom L. Beauchamp and Ruth R. Faden, philosophers who have studied informed consent extensively, assert, "The overwhelming impression from the empirical literature and from reported clinical experience is that the actual process of soliciting informed consent often falls short of a serious show of respect for the decisional authority of patients."

The following selections illustrate two views of the future of informed consent. Robert M. Arnold and Charles W. Lidz reassert the importance of informed consent and offer ways in which the process can be improved in the clinical setting, despite the many obstacles. Robert M. Veatch argues that the concept of informed consent is inherently inadequate because clinicians can never assess fully, and thus can never recommend, what might be in the patient's best interests.

3

YES

Robert M. Arnold and
Charles W. Lidz

INFORMED CONSENT: CLINICAL ASPECTS OF CONSENT IN HEALTH CARE

Health-care decision making is an everyday event, not only for doctors and patients but also for nurses, psychologists, social workers, emergency medical technicians, dentists, and other health professionals. Since the 1960s, however, the cultural ideal of how those decisions should be made has changed considerably. The concept that medical decision making should rely exclusively on the physician's expertise has been replaced by a model in which health-care professionals share information and discuss alternatives with patients who then make the ultimate decisions about treatment. This article reviews the origins in the United States of this ideal in the doctrine of informed consent, discusses various arguments against its use in clinical decision making, and describes a model for effectively incorporating it into clinical practice with competent patients.

The concept of informed consent gained its initial support as part of the general societal trend toward broadening access to decision making during the 1960s. Thus, the initial support for informed consent came from legal and philosophic circles rather than from health-care professionals. In the legal arena, informed consent has been used to develop minimal standards for doctor-patient interactions and clinical decision making (Appelbaum et al., 1987). Although there are some differences by jurisdiction, widely accepted legal standards require that health-care professionals inform patients of the risks, benefits, and alternatives of all proposed treatments and then allow the patient to choose among acceptable therapeutic alternatives. In academia, informed consent has served as a cornerstone for the development of the discipline of bioethics. Based on the importance of autonomy in moral discourse, philosophers have argued that health-care professionals are obligated to engage patients in discussions regarding the goals of therapy and the alternatives for reaching those goals and that patients are the final decision makers regarding all therapeutic decisions.

There also has been some support for informed consent within academic medicine, but there seems to be little enthusiasm for it in routine medical

From Robert M. Arnold and Charles W. Lidz, "Informed Consent: Clinical Aspects of Consent in Health Care," in Warren T. Reich, ed., *Encyclopedia of Bioethics, vol. 3*, rev. ed. (Simon & Schuster, 1995), pp. 1250–1256. Copyright © 1995 by Warren T. Reich. Reprinted by permission of Macmillan Reference USA, a division of Simon & Schuster. References omitted.

practice (Lidz et al., 1984). Physicians typically think of informed consent as a legal requirement for a signed piece of paper that is at best a waste of time and at worst a bureaucratic, legalistic interference with their care for patients. Rather than seeing informed consent as a process that promotes good communication and patient autonomy, many health-care professionals view informed consent as a complex, legally prescribed recitation of risks and benefits that only frightens or confuses patients. There are various objections to informed consent that clinicians often make, and it will be useful to review those objections here.

OBJECTIONS TO INFORMED CONSENT

Consent cannot be truly "informed." Many practicing clinicians report that their patients are unable to understand the complex medical information necessary for a fully rational weighing of alternative treatments. There is considerable research support for this view. A variety of studies document that patients recall only a small percentage of the information that professionals present to them (Meisel and Roth, 1981); that they are not as good decision makers when they are sick as at other times (Sherlock, 1986); and that they often make decisions based on medically trivial factors. Informed consent thus appears either to promote uninformed, and thus suboptimal, decisions or to encourage patients to blindly accept health-care professionals' recommendations. In either case informed consent appears to be a charade, and a dangerous one at that.

That patients often do have difficulty understanding important aspects of medical decisions does not mean that health-care professionals are the best decision makers about the patient's treatment. Knowledge about medical facts is not enough. Wise house buyers will have a structural engineer check over an old house, but few would be willing to allow the engineer to choose their house for them. Just as structural engineers cannot decide which house a family should buy because they lack knowledge about the family's pattern of living, personal tastes, and potential family growth, health-care professionals cannot scientifically deduce the best treatment for a specific patient simply from the medical facts. Because what matters to individuals about their health depends on their lifestyles, past experiences, and values, choosing the "optimal therapy" is not a purely "objective" matter. Thus, patients and health-care professionals both contribute essential knowledge to the decision-making process—patients bring their knowledge of their personal situation, goals, and values, and health-care professionals bring their expertise on the nature of the problem and the technology that may be used to meet the patient's goals.

Informed-consent disclosures, even if they are well done, may not lead to what clinicians might consider optimal decisions. Most people make major life decisions, such as whom to marry and which occupation to take up, based on faulty or incomplete information. Patients' lack of understanding of medical information in choosing treatment is probably no worse than their lack of information in choosing a spouse, nor are medical decisions more important than spousal choice. Respecting patient autonomy means allowing individuals to make their own decisions even if the health-care professional disagrees with them. Informed-consent disclosures can improve patient decisions, but they cannot be expected to lead to perfect decisions.

Moreover, although sick persons have some defects in their rational abilities, so do health-care professionals. There are no data that demonstrate that health-care professionals' reasoning abilities are better than patients. In fact, some of the most famous research on the difficulties individuals have with the rational use of probabilistic data involves physicians (Dawson and Ackes, 1987). Health professionals must be careful not to be to pessimistic about patients' ability to become informed decision makers. Patients may not be able to become as technically well-informed as professionals, but they clearly can understand and make decisions based on relevant information. A recent study, for example, showed that patients' decisions regarding life-sustaining treatment changed when they were given accurate information about the therapy's chance of success (Murphy et al., 1994).

Most important, the difficulty of educating sick persons does not justify unilateral decision making. Rather, it places a special obligation on health-care professionals to communicate clearly with patients. Using technical jargon, trying to give all of the available information in one visit, and not asking what the patient wants to know is a recipe for confusing even the most intelligent patient. A growing literature, for example, discusses the problems patients have understanding uncertainty about treatment outcomes and suggests ways to help patients deal with such uncertainty (Katz, 1984). Health-care professionals also need to become more familiar with different cultural patterns of communication in order to talk with patients from different cultural backgrounds. For ex-

ample, although a simple, factual discussion of depression and its treatment may be acceptable to most middle-class Americans, it would be seen as inappropriate by a first-generation Vietnamese male (Hahn, 1982), whose culture discourages viewing depression as a disease. There is no reason, in principle, why a person who daily makes decisions at home and work cannot, with help, understand the medical data sufficiently to become involved in medical decisions. Health-care professionals must learn how best to present that help.

Patients do not wish to be involved in decision making. Many health-care professionals believe that it is unfair to force patients to make decisions regarding their medical care. After all, they argue, patients pay their health-care professionals to make medical decisions. The empirical literature partially supports the view that patients want professionals to make treatment decisions for them (Steele et al., 1987). For example, in a study of male patients' preferences about medical decision making regarding hypertension, only 53 percent wanted to participate at all in the decision-making process.

There is no reason to force patients to be involved in decisions if they do not want to be. However, unless the health professional asks, he or she cannot know how involved a patient wants to be. Indeed, patients may not always want to be involved in decision making, since many have been socialized into believing that "the doctor knows best." This is particularly true for poorer patients. Studies have shown that physicians wrongly assume that because patients with fewer socioeconomic resources ask fewer questions, they do not want as much information. These patients may in fact want just as much information, but they have been socialized into a different way of interacting with health-care professionals (Waitzkin, 1984).

Patients may choose to allow someone else to make the decision for them. However, when a patient asks, "What would you do if you were me?" the underlying question may be, "As an expert in biomedicine, what alternative do you think will best maximize my values or interest?" If this is the case, the health-care professional should respond by making a recommendation and justifying it in terms of the patient's values or interests. More frequently, the patient is asking, "If you had this disease, what therapy would you choose?" This question presumes that the professional and patient have the same values, needs, and problems, something that is often not true. Health-care professionals should respond by pointing this out and by emphasizing the importance of the patients' values in the decision-making process.

Although many patients do not want to be actively involved in decision making, they almost always want more information concerning their illness than the health-care professional gives them. Health-care professionals should not assume that just because patients do not wish to choose their therapy, they do not want information. Patients may desire information so as to increase compliance or make modifications in other areas of their lives, as well as to make medical decisions.

There are harmful effects of informing patients. Health-care professionals often justify withholding information from patients because of their belief that informing patients would be psychologically damaging and therefore contrary to the principle of nonmaleficence. Many health-care professionals, however, over-estimate potential psychological harm and neglect the positive effects of full disclosure (Faden et al., 1986). Moreover, bad news can often be communicated in a way that ameliorates the psychological effects of the disclosure (Quill and Townsend, 1991). Truth-telling must be distinguished from "truth dumping." Explanation of the care that can be provided, and empathic attention to the patient's fears and uncertainties can often prevent or mitigate otherwise more painful news.

Informed consent takes too much time. Respecting autonomy and promoting patient well-being, the values served through informed consent, are fundamental to good medicine. However, adhering to the ideals of medical practice takes time, time to help patients understand their illness and work through their emotional reactions to stressful information; to discuss each party's preconceptions and to clarify the therapeutic goals; to decide on a treatment plan; and to elicit questions about diagnosis and treatment.

In U.S. health care, time is money. As many commentators have noted, physicians are less well reimbursed for talking to patients than for performing invasive tests. This may discourage doctors from spending enough time discussing treatment options with patients. Changes in physician reimbursement, such as the Relative-Value Based Scale, which are designed to increase reimbursement for cognitive skills, including the time it takes to discuss diagnosis and treatment with patients, will encourage physicians to discuss patients' preferences with them. The ultimate justification for spending time to facilitate patient decisions, however, is the same as that for spending any time in medical care: that patients will be better cared for.

CLINICAL APPROACHES TO INFORMED CONSENT

Many of the problems in implementing informed consent result at least in part from the way informed consent has been implemented in clinical practice. Informed consent has become synonymous with the "consent form," a legal invention with a legitimate role in documenting that informed consent has taken place, but hardly a substitute for the discussion process leading to informed consent (Andrews, 1984).

A pro forma approach: An event model of informed consent. In many clinical settings, consent begins when "it is time to get consent," typically just prior to the administration of treatment. The process of getting the patients' consent consists of the recitation by a physician or nurse of the list of material risks and benefits and a request that the patient sign for the proposed treatment. This "conversation" is a very limited one that emphasizes the transfer of information from the physician or nurse to the patient. This procedure does meet the minimal legal requirements for informed consent efficiently. However, it does not meet the higher ethical goal of informed consent, which is to empower patients by educating and involving them in their treatment plans. Instead, it imposes an almost empty ritual on an unchanged relationship between health-care provider and patient (Katz, 1984).

The procedure just described assumes that care involves a series of discrete, circumscribed decisions. In fact, much of clinical medicine consists of a series of frequent, interwoven decisions that must be repeatedly reconsidered as more information becomes available. When "it is time to get consent," there may be nothing left to decide. Consider the operative consent form obtained the evening prior to an operation. After patients have discussed with their families whether to be admitted to the hospital, rearranged their work and child-care schedules for admission, and undergone a long and painful diagnostic workup, the decision to have surgery seems preordained. The evening before the operation, patients do not seriously evaluate the operation's risks and benefits; consent is pro forma. No wonder some health-care professionals feel that "consent" is a waste of time and energy.

The event model for gathering informed consent falls far short of meeting the ethical goal of ensuring patient participation in the decision-making process. Rather than engaging the patient as an active participant in the decision-making process, the patient's role is too agree to or veto the health-care professionals' recommendations. Little attempt is made to elicit patient preferences and to consider how treatment might address them.

A dialogical approach: The process model of informed consent. Fortunately, it is possible to fulfill legal requirements for informed consent while maximizing active patient participation in the clinical setting. An alternative to the event model described above, which sees informed consent as an aberration from clinical practice, the process model attempts to integrate informed consent into all aspects of clinical care (Appelbaum et al., 1987). The process model of informed consent assumes that each party has something to contribute to the decision-making process. The physician brings technical knowledge and experience in treating patients with similar problems. Patients bring knowledge about their life circumstances and the ability to assess the effect that treatment may have on them. Open discussion makes it possible for the patient and the physician to examine critically their views and to determine what might be optimal treatment.

The process model also recognizes that medical care rarely involves only one decision, made at a single point in time. Decisions about care frequently begin with the suspicion that something is wrong and that treatment may be necessary, and end only when the patient leaves follow-up care. Decisions involve diagnostic as well as therapeutic interventions. Some decisions are made in one visit, while others occur over a prolonged period of time. Although some interactions between health-care professional and patient involve explicit decisions, decisions are made at each interaction, even if the decision is only to continue treatment. The process model also recognizes that various health-care professionals may play a role in making sure that the patients' consent is informed. For example, a woman deciding on various breast cancer treatments may talk with an oncologist and a surgeon about the risks of various treatments, with a nurse about the side effects of medication, with a social worker about financial issues in treatment, and with a patient-support group about her husband's reaction to a possible mastectomy.

Ideally, then, informed consent involves shared decision making over a period of time, that is, a dialogue throughout the course of the patient's relationship with various health-care professionals. Such a dialogue aims to facilitate patient participation and to strengthen the therapeutic alliance.

TASKS INVOLVED IN INFORMED CONSENT

Consent is a series of interrelated tasks. First, the patient and professional must agree on the problem that will be the focus of their work together (Eisenthal and Lazare, 1976). Most nonemergency consultations involve complex negotiations between health-care professional and patient regarding the definition of the patient's problem. The patient may see the problem as a routine physical examination for a work release, the need for advice, or the investigation of a physical symptom. If professionals are to respond effectively to the patients' goals, they must find out the reason for the visit. Whereas physicians typically focus on biomedical information and its implications, patients typically view the problem in the context of their social situation (Fisher and Todd, 1983). The differences between the patient's perceptions of the problem and the professional's must be explicitly worked through since agreement regarding the focus of the interactions lead to increased patient satisfaction and compliance with further treatment plans (Meichenbaum and Turk, 1987).

Even when the professional and patient have agreed on what the problem is, substantial misunderstanding may arise regarding the treatment goals. The patient may expect the medically impossible, or may expect outcomes based on knowledge of life circumstances about which the physician is unaware. Since assessing the risks and benefits of any treatment option depends on therapeutic goals, the professional and patient must agree on the goals the therapy aims to accomplish.

Finding out what the patient wants is more complicated than merely inquiring, "What do you want?" A patient typically does not come to the professional with well-developed preferences regarding medical therapy except "to get better," with little understanding of what this may involve. As a patient's knowledge and perspective change over the course of an illness, so too may the patient's views regarding the therapeutic goals.

Because clinicians provide much of the medical information needed to ensure that the patient's preferences are grounded in medical possibility, health-care professionals play a significant role in how a patient's preferences evolve. It is important that they understand that patients may reasonably hold different goals from those their practitioners hold. This as particularly true when they come from different economic strata. For example, a physician's emphasis on the most medically sophisticated care may pale in the light of the patient's financial problems. Therapeutic goals, like the definition of the problem, require ongoing clarification and negotiation.

After agreeing upon the problem and the therapeutic goals, the health-care professional and the patient must choose the best way to achieve them. If patients have been involved in the prior two steps, the decision about a treatment plan will more likely reflect their values than if they are merely asked to assent to the clinician's strategy.

Health-care professionals often ask how much information they must supply to ensure that the patient is an informed participant in the decision-making process (Mazur, 1986). There is a more important question: Has the information been provided in a manner that the patient can understand? While the law only requires that health-care professionals inform patients, morally valid consent requires that patients understand the information conveyed. Ensuring patient understanding requires attention to the quality as well as the quantity of information presented (Faden, 1977).

A great deal of empirical data has been collected concerning problems with consent forms. These forms have been criticized, for example, as being unintelligible because of their length and use of technical language (Appelbaum et al., 1987). Health-care professionals thus need to be aware of, and facile in using, a variety of methods to increase patients' comprehension of information; these include verbal techniques, written information, or interactive videodiscs (Stanley et al., 1984).

Still, the question of how much information to present remains. The legal standards regarding information disclosure —what a reasonable patient would find essential to making a decision or what a reasonably prudent physician would disclose—are not particularly helpful. Howard Brody has suggested two important features: (1) The physician must disclose the basis on which the proposed treatment or the alternative possible treatments have been chosen; and (2) the patient must be encouraged to ask questions, suggested by the disclosure about the physician's reasoning, and the questions need to be answered to the patient's satisfaction (Brody, 1989). Health-care professionals must also inform patients when controversy exists about the various therapeutic options. Similarly, patients should also be told the degree to which the recommendation is based on established scientific evidence versus personal experience or educated guesses.

Two other factors will influence the amount of information that should be given: the importance of the decision, given the patient's situation and goals, and the amount of consensus within the health-care professions regarding the agreed-upon therapy. For example, a low-risk intervention, such as giving influenza vaccines to elderly patients, offers a clear-cut benefit with minimal risk. In this case, the professional should describe the intervention and recommend it because of its benefits. A detailed description of the infrequent risks is not needed unless the patient asks or is known to be skeptical of medical interventions. Interventions that present greater risks or a less clear-cut risk–benefit ratio require a longer description—for example, the decision to administer AZT to an HIV (human immunodeficiency virus)-positive, asymptomatic woman with a CD4 count of 400. In neither case is a discussion of pathophysiology or biochemistry necessary. It must be emphasized that there is no formula for deciding how much a patient needs to be told. The amount of information necessary will depend on the patient's individual situation, values, and goals.

Finally, an adequate decision-making process requires continual updating of information, monitoring of expectations, and evaluation of the patient's progress in reaching the chosen or revised goals.

Thus the final step in informed consent is follow-up. This step is particularly important for patients with chronic diseases in which modifications of the treatment plan are often necessary.

The process model of informed consent just described has many advantages. Because it assumes many short conversations over time rather than one long interaction, it can be more easily integrated into the professional's ambulatory practice than the event model; it allows patients to be much more involved in decision making and ensures that treatment is more consistent with their values. Furthermore, the continual monitoring of patients' understanding of their disease, the treatment, and its progress is likely to reduce misunderstandings and increase their investment in, and adherence to, the treatment plan. Thus, the process model of informed consent is likely to promote both patient autonomy and well-being.

There are situations in which this approach is not very helpful. Some health-care professionals, anesthesiologists or emergency medical technicians, for example, are not likely to have ongoing relationships with patients. In emergencies, there is not time for a decision to develop through a series of short conversations. In these cases, informed consent may more closely approximate the event model. However, since most medical care is delivered by primary-care practitioners in an ambulatory setting, the process model of informed consent is more helpful.

NO

Robert M. Veatch

ABANDONING INFORMED CONSENT

Consent has emerged as a concept central to modern medical ethics. Often the term is used with a modifier, such as *informed* or *voluntary* or *full*, as in loosely used phrases like "fully informed and voluntary consent." In some form or another, modern ethics in health care could hardly function without the notion of consent.

While we might occasionally encounter an old-guard retrograde longing for the day when physicians did not have to go through the process of getting consent, by and large consent is now taken as a given, at least at the level of theory. To be sure, we know that actual consent is not obtained in all cases and even when consent is obtained, it may not be adequately informed or autonomous. For purposes of this discussion, we shall not worry about the deviations from the ideal; rather the focus will be on whether consent ought to be the goal.

This consensus in favor of consent may turn out to be all too facile. *Consent* may be what can be called a transition concept, one that appears on the scene as an apparently progressive innovation, but after a period of experience turns out to be only useful as a transition to a more thoroughly revisionary conceptual framework.

This paper will defend the thesis that consent is merely a transitional concept. While it emerged in the field as a liberal, innovative idea, its time may have passed and newer, more enlightened formulations may be needed. Consent means approval or agreement with the actions or opinions of another; terms such as *acquiescence* and *condoning* appear in the dictionary definitions. In medicine, the physician or other health care provider will, after reviewing the facts of the case and attempting to determine what is in the best interest of the patient, propose a course of action for the patient's concurrence. While a few decades ago it might have been considered both radical and innovative to seek the patient's acquiescence in the professional's clinical judgment, by now that may not be nearly enough. It is increasingly clear if one studies the theory of clinical decisionmaking that there is no longer any basis for presuming that the clinician can even guess at what is in the overall best interest of the patient. If that is true, then a model in which the clinician

From Robert M. Veatch, "Abandoning Informed Consent," *Hastings Center Report*, vol. 25, no. 2 (March–April 1995). Copyright © 1995 by The Hastings Center. Reprinted by permission.

guesses at what he or she believes is best for the patient, pausing only to elicit the patient's concurrence, will no longer be sufficient. Increasingly we will have to go beyond patient consent to a model in which plausible options are presented (perhaps with the professional's recommendation regarding a personal preference among them, based on the professional's personally held beliefs and values), but with no rational or "professional" basis for even guessing at which one might truly be in the patient's best interest....

Modern medicine has reluctantly made room for the consent doctrine and has recognized, at least in theory, the right of patients to consent and refuse consent to certain kinds of treatment. Usually explicit consent is reserved for these more complex and exotic decisions. It is still common to hear people distinguish between treatments for which consent is required and those for which it is not. Surely it would be better to speak of those for which consent must be explicit and others that still require consent even though the consent can be implied or presumed. For example, many would probably say that routine blood drawings of modest amounts of blood can be done without consent. This would more appropriately be described as being done without explicit consent and with no specific information needing to be transmitted. The mere extending of the arm should count as an adequate consent.

Likewise, when a physician writes a prescription, he or she is supposed to review the alternatives and choose the best medication, select a brand name or generic equivalent, choose a route of administration, a dosage level, and length of use of the medication. The patient may signal "consent" simply by accepting the prescription and getting it filled at the local pharmacy.

Up until now no one has seriously questioned the adequacy, from the left, of an approach that permits explicit consent for special and complex treatment, including research and surgery, and implicit or presumed consent for more routine procedures. More careful analysis reveals that, in fact, the consent model buys into more of the traditional, authoritarian understanding of clinical decisionmaking than many people realize. As in the days prior to the development of the consent doctrine, the clinician is still supposed to draw on his or her medical knowledge to determine what he or she believes is in the best interest of the patient and propose that course of treatment. Terms such as "doctor's orders" may have been replaced by more appropriate images, but the physician is still expected to determine what is "medically indicated," the "treatment of choice," or what in the "clinical judgment" of the practitioner is best for the patient. The clinician then proposes that course, subject only to the qualification that through either word or action, the patient signals approval of the physician-determined plan.

CONSENT AND THE THEORY OF THE GOOD

Current work on the theory of medical decisionmaking and in axiology [the study of the theory of the good] makes increasingly clear that this pattern no longer makes sense. It still rests on the outdated presumption that the clinician's moral responsibility is to do what is best for the patient, according to his or her ability and judgment, and that there is some reason to hope that the clinician can determine what is in the patient's best interest. The idea in medical ethics of doing what is best for the patient has achieved the status of an unquestioned platitude, but like many platitudes, it may not stand the test of more careful examination. On several levels the problems are beginning to show.

The Best Interest Standard in Surrogate Decisions. The "best interest standard" has become the standard for surrogate decisionmaking in cases in which the wishes of the patient are not known and substituted judgment based on the patient's beliefs and values is not possible. But the best interest standard, if taken literally, is terribly implausible. In fact, no decisionmaker is held to it in practice.

Two problems arise. First, since such judgments are increasingly recognized to be terribly complex and subjective, it is now widely accepted that the surrogate need not choose literally what is best. It would be extremely difficult to determine whether the absolute best choice has been made. Surely, the opinion of the attending physician cannot serve as a definitive standard. A privately appointed, parochial ethics committee might be better, but still surely is not definitive. If every surrogate decision were taken to court, we still would not have an absolute assurance that the best choice had been made.

Fortunately, we generally do not hold parents and other surrogates to a literal best interest standard when they make decisions for their wards. We expect, tolerate, even encourage a reasonable range of discretion. That is why it makes sense to replace the best interest standard with a "standard of reasonableness"

or what could be called a "reasonable interest standard."[1]

There is a second reason why the best interest standard is inappropriate for surrogate decisions. Often surrogates have legitimate moral obligations to people other than the patient. Parents, for example, are pledged to serve the welfare of their other children. When best interests conflict, it is logically impossible to fulfill simultaneously the best interest standard for more than one child at the same time. Surely, all that is expected is that a reasonable balance of the conflicting interests be pursued.

Problems With Best Interest in Clinician Judgments. Although the problems with the best interest standard in surrogate decisions are more immediately apparent, a more fundamental and important problem with best interest arises when clinicians are held to the best interest standard in an ethic of patient care. For a clinician to guess at what is the best course for the patient, three assumptions must be true regarding a theory of the good. First, the clinician must be expected to determine what will best serve the patient's medical or health interest; second, the clinician must be expected to determine how to trade off health interests with other interests; and third, the clinician must be expected to determine how the patient should relate the pursuit of her best interest to other moral goals and responsibilities, including serving the interests of others and fulfilling any moral duties she may have that happen to conflict with her interest. An examination of the theories of the good and the morally right will reveal that it is terribly implausible to expect a typical clinician to be able to perform any one of these tasks completely correctly, let alone all three of them. If the clinician cannot be expected to guess at what serves the well-being of the patient and determine when patient well-being should be subordinated to other moral requirements, then there is no way that he or she can be expected to propose a course of treatment to which the patient would offer mere consent.

... [W]e can understand what promotes the good for persons better by asking what the elements are that contribute to one's well-being. Another way of putting the question would be to ask in what areas one's limited amount of personal resources—time, money, energy, and material—ought to be invested in order to maximize well-being.

The Main Elements of Well-Being. Several elements can be identified. These would surely include some concern with medicine or what could be called one's organic well-being. Closely related, but distinct, would be psychological well-being. It would be a terrible distortion to assume that well-being involved only the organic and psychological, however. Reasonable persons would devote considerable attention and resources to other elements, including the social, legal, occupational, religious, aesthetic, and other components that together make up one's total well-being. There is no reason to assume that each of these components is the same size. By trading off emphasis on different components one should be able to increase or decrease the size of the whole. Well-being is not a zero-sum game.

The problem is central to the concern about the concept of consent. It is unrealistic to expect experts in any one component to be able to speak knowledgeably about well-being in its other components. If this is true, then it makes no sense to expect them to come up with a proposed intervention that will promote the total well-being of the individual....

WHY EXPERTS SHOULD NOT PROPOSE A COURSE FOR PATIENT CONSENT

It should now be clear why it makes no sense to continue to rely on consent as the mode of transaction between professionals and their clients. In order for a physician to make an initial estimate of which treatment best served the patient's interest, he or she would first have to develop a definitive theory of the relationship among various medical goods and pick the course that best served the patient's medical good. Then the clinician would have to estimate correctly the proper relationship between the patient's medical good and all other components of the good so that the patient's overall well-being was served.

Even if this could be done, there is a final problem. In virtually any moral theory the well-being of the individual is only one element. Plausible consequentialist theories (such as utilitarianism) also insist that the good of other parties be taken into account. Plausible nonconsequentialist theories, including Kantian theories, natural law theories, much of biblical ethics, and all other deontological theories, hold that knowing what will be in the best interests of persons does not necessarily settle the question of the right thing to do. Many patients may purposely want to consider options that do not maximize their well-being. A patient may acknowledge, for example, that his well-being would be served if he lived longer, but choose to sacrifice his interests to conserve resources for his offspring. A pregnant woman might conclude, for another example, that her interests would be served if she had an abortion, but that such a course would still be morally wrong. Both of these people would rationally not choose the course of action that admittedly maximized their personal well-being. Even if physicians can figure out what maximizes medical well-being and how medical well-being should be related to other elements of well-being, that still does not necessarily lead to the course that is right, all things considered. To know what is "good medicine" and what should be recommended for the patient's assessment and consent, one needs to know how to answer all three of these questions. There is no basis for assuming that physicians have any special expertise in answering any of them....

CHOICE: THE LIBERAL ALTERNATIVE

If consent is no longer adequate as a mechanism for assuring that the patient's beliefs and values will help shape decisions about what a patient ought to do, what are the alternatives? Adherents to medical ethical systems that emphasize autonomy may prefer the concept of choice to that of consent. In this alternative the patient would be presented with a list of plausible treatment options, together with a summary of the potential benefits and risks of each. It is important to emphasize that choice is conceptually different from consent and potentially could replace consent as the basis for patient involvement in health care decisions.

This "liberal" solution, however, faces serious, probably insurmountable problems. First, if the choices that are plausible for the patient are contingent on the beliefs and values of the patient, then the professional cannot be sure that all plausible options are being presented unless he or she has knowledge of the patient's beliefs and values—knowledge that we have argued is normally unavailable. Second, some options (for example, suicide) may be so offensive to some practitioners that they ought not to present them. Third, it is increasingly recognized that even the description of the "facts" necessarily must incorporate certain value judgments, such that even the clinician of good will cannot give a value-free account of the likely outcomes of the alternatives. In short, while the choice alternative may go part of the way toward giving the patient more active control, it is naive to believe it will be able to solve the problems with the consent model.

PAIRING BASED ON "DEEP VALUES"

There is another alternative worth considering. If a clinician is skilled and passionately committed to maximizing the patient's welfare, and knows the belief and value structure and socioeconomic and cultural position of the patient quite well, there would be some more reason to hope for a good guess. Unfortunately, not only is that an ever-vanishing possibility, even knowing the value system of the patient well probably would not be sufficient. The value choices that go into a judgment about what is best for another are so complex and subtle that merely knowing the other's values and trying to empathize will probably not be enough. There is ample evidence that unconscious value distortions will not only influence the clinician's judgment about what is best, but even influence the very interpretation of the scientific data.

There might be more hope if the patient were to choose her cadre of well-being experts (lawyers, accountants, physicians) on the basis of their "deep" value systems. That way when unconscious bias and distortion occur, as inevitably they must, they will tip the decision in the direction of the patient's own system.

I say "deep" value system because I want to make clear that I am not referring to the cursory assessment of the professional's personality, demeanor and short-term tastes. That would hardly suffice. If, however, there were alignments, "value pairings," based on the most fundamental worldviews of the lay person and professional, then there would be some hope. This probably would mean picking providers on the basis of their religious and political affiliations, philosophical and social inclinations, and other deeply penetrating worldviews. To the extent that the provider and patient were of the same mind set, then there is some reason that the technically competent clinician could guess fairly well what would serve the patient's interest.

The difficulty in establishing a convergence of deep values cannot be underestimated. Surely it would not be sufficient, for instance, to pair providers and patients on the basis of their institutional religious affiliations. Not all members of a religious denomination think alike. But there is reason to hope that people can establish an affinity of deep value orientations, at least for certain types of medical services. For example, certain institutionalized health care delivery systems are now organizing around identifiable value frameworks, recruiting professional and administrative staff on the basis of commitment to that value framework, and then announcing that framework to the public so as to attract only those patients who share the basic value commitment of the institution. A hospice is organized around such a constellation of values. It recruits staff committed to those values and attracts patients who share that commitment. When hospice-based health care providers present options to patients they should admit that they do not present all possible options. (They do not propose an aggressive oncology protocol, for instance; most would not present physician-assisted suicide or active mercy killing.) They should also admit that when they explain options and their potential benefits and harms they do so in ways that incorporate a tone of voice or body language that reflects their value judgments. Patients, however, need be less concerned about this value encroachment than if they were discussing options with a provider who was deeply, instinctively committed to maximally aggressive life preservation. There will be biases, but they will be less corrupting of the patient's own perspective.

Other delivery systems are beginning to organize around deep value orientations: feminist health centers, holistic health clinics, and the National Institutes of Health Clinical Center all announce at least their general value orientations to potential patients.

Providing an institutional framework for pairing based on deep value convergence in more routine health care may be more difficult, but not impossible. HMOs could be organized by social and religious groups that could formally articulate certain value commitments. A Catholic HMO, like a Catholic hospital, could articulate to potential members not only a set of values pertaining to obstetrical and gynecological issues, but also a framework for deciding which treatments are morally expendable as disproportionally burdensome. A liberal Protestant health care system would announce a different framework; a libertarian secular system still another. A truly Protestant health care system, for example, would probably reflect the belief that the lay person is capable of having control over the "text." The medical record, accordingly, would plausibly be placed in the patient's hands just as the Bible is.

Such value pairings will obviously not be a total matching, but they should at least place provider and patient in the same general camp. Moreover, organizing health care delivery on the basis of explicit value pairings would put both provider and patient on notice that values are a necessary and essential part of health care decisionmaking, a part that cannot be avoided and cannot be handled adequately by merely obtaining the consent of the patient to a randomly assigned provider's guess about what would be best.

With such an arrangement the problems that arise with use of consent for the normal random pairing of lay people and professionals is mitigated. The clinician has a more plausible basis for guessing what would serve the interests of the patient and, more importantly, will let a system of beliefs and values influence the presentation of medical information in a way that is more defensible. To be sure, such deep value pairing will not eliminate the problem of the necessary influence of beliefs and values on communication of medical facts, but it will structure the communication so that the inevitable influence will resemble the influence that the patient would have brought to the data were he or she to become an authority in medical science.

Barring such radical adjustment in the basis for lay-professional pairings, there is no reason to believe that the process of consent will significantly advance the lay person's role in the medical decisionmaking process. The concept of consent will have to be replaced with a more radical, robust notion of active patient participation in the choice among plausible alternatives—either by getting much greater information to the patient or by actively selecting the professional on the basis of convergence of "deep" value systems.

REFERENCES

1. Robert M. Veatch, "Limits of Guardian Treatment Refusal: A Reasonableness Standard," *American Journal of Law & Medicine* 9, no. 4 (Winter 1984): 427–68; Robert M. Veatch, *Death, Dying, and the Biological Revolution*, rev. ed. (New Haven: Yale University Press, 1989).

POSTSCRIPT

Is Informed Consent Still Central to Medical Ethics?

The Patient Self-Determination Act, a federal law that went into effect in 1991, requires health care institutions to advise patients about their right to accept or refuse medical care and to offer them an opportunity to create an advance directive indicating their medical choices should they become incompetent. Nevertheless, there is considerable evidence that patients and their designated health care proxies are not brought into decision making at the end of life in a timely and effective way. There are also some limits on what kinds of information must be provided to patients. In the 1993 case of *Arato v. Avedon*, the California Supreme Court supported information sharing and patient-centered decision making but ruled that doctors need not supply explicit statistical information about life expectancy to patients. See George J. Annas, "Informed Consent, Cancer, and Truth in Prognosis," *The New England Journal of Medicine* (January 20, 1994).

Nonetheless, the concept of informed consent, from Western political and ethical theories that place a high value on individual self-determination, remains a central principle in the United States. Cultural groups who have different traditions may not share this value. Two articles in a recent issue of the *Journal of the American Medical Association* (September 13, 1995)—"Western Bioethics on the Navajo Reservation," by Joseph A. Carrese and Lorna A. Rhodes, and "Ethnicity and Attitudes Toward Patient Autonomy," by Leslie J. Blackhall—suggest that disclosing negative information and involving patients in decision making may be contrary to the beliefs of certain ethnic populations.

The most comprehensive account of informed consent is *A History and Theory of Informed Consent* by Ruth L. Faden, Tom L. Beauchamp, and Nancy M. P. King (Oxford University Press, 1986). Another useful volume, particularly in terms of psychiatric treatment, is *Informed Consent: Legal Theory and Clinical Practice* by Paul S. Appelbaum, Charles W. Lidz, and Alan Meisel (Oxford University Press, 1987). Jay Katz's *The Silent World of Doctor and Patient* (Free Press, 1984) is an insightful discussion of the reasons physicians may be reluctant to disclose information to their patients. And Christine Laine and Frank Davidoff describe the evolution from physician-based medicine in "Patient-Centered Medicine," *Journal of the American Medical Association* (January 10, 1996). For more sources on informed consent and other biomedical ethics issues, see the following Web site of the Medical College of Wisconsin: http://www.mcw.edu/bioethics/. This site contains a bioethics literature database that is regularly updated.

ISSUE 2

Can Family Interests Ethically Outweigh Patient Autonomy?

YES: John Hardwig, from "What About the Family?" *Hastings Center Report* (March/April 1990)

NO: Jeffrey Blustein, from "The Family in Medical Decisionmaking," *Hastings Center Report* (May–June 1993)

ISSUE SUMMARY

YES: John Hardwig, an associate professor of medical ethics, argues that the prevalent ethic of patient autonomy ignores family interests in medical treatment decisions. He maintains that physicians should recognize these interests as legitimate.

NO: Bioethicist Jeffrey Blustein maintains that although families can be an important resource in helping patients make better decisions about their care, the ultimate decision-making authority should remain with the patient.

In law and ethics, parents are considered the rightful decision makers for their minor children. Although controversies still arise, no other institution or individual has been identified as having a more legitimate claim to the right to make decisions regarding a minor's welfare. Similarly, when medical decisions need to be made for an incompetent adult, physicians often consult with family members to determine the course of action that seems most appropriate, given the patient's condition and the family's values and history.

Apart from these significant exceptions (which consume a major portion of the biomedical ethics literature), the family has until very recently been viewed primarily as a source of emotional support for the patient and an endorser of physician recommendations. The competent patient's right to make an autonomous decision remains a central ethical principle. Health care providers seldom involve family members directly in making decisions or in choosing among various treatment alternatives, even though many medical decisions have an enormous impact on the family. For example, the decision to care for a seriously ill person at home, rather than in a nursing home, has a major effect on those who will be expected to participate in the care and to give up their privacy and space. If the treatment decision involves heavy expenses that are not covered by insurance or a government program, the life goals of other family members—such as a college education for children—may be jeopardized. In some cases, the family may lose a home or members may be forced to leave their jobs or to stop participating in important activities in order to provide care.

As cost-containment efforts rapidly continue to push medical care from its institutional base (in hospitals and nursing homes) to outpatient clinics, community-based services, and the home, these issues are likely to arise with greater frequency. Home care now involves high-technology equipment, such as intravenous chemotherapy, total parenteral nutrition (tube feeding through the stomach), and other invasive procedures. More than 7 million Americans (the majority of which are women) are currently providing home-based care to a relative or friend who is chronically ill, disabled, or elderly. Most family members want to care for their loved ones, but the "informal" care they provide is neither paid for nor reimbursed by insurance.

The dynamic and ever-changing concept of "family" is a further complication. Today, the medical, legal, and social systems in the United States recognize the nuclear family (comprised of a mother, a father, and minor children) as prototypical, but the reality in which many Americans live is quite different. There are divorced and remarried families; extended, intergenerational families; families of affiliation, such as gay and lesbian couples; and families of loosely related kin and friends. While self-defined families include many people outside traditional definitions, the options for participating in medical decision making or representing a particular person's interests remain narrow unless an individual has been legally designated as a health care proxy.

The multiple structures of family also mean that there is no single strategy for resolving conflicts among family members or between family members and health care providers. Differing perspectives may create disagreement even among well-intentioned family members, and, in more extreme circumstances, a family member may advocate a certain path of action for reasons that seem suspect (for instance, a large inheritance may be involved or there may be evidence of abuse or neglect). Sometimes, a representative of the hospital ethics committee is helpful in guiding discussions and resolving conflicts, but in other instances, the courts have to get involved to exclude someone who is unsuitable to participate in making decisions.

The two selections that follow explore the ramifications of including family members as decision makers in the care of a competent patient. John Hardwig asserts that in many cases family members have a greater interest than the patient in which treatment option is chosen and that in those cases the interests of family members ought to override those of the patient. Jeffrey Blustein declares that the locus of decisional authority should remain with the patient.

YES   John Hardwig

WHAT ABOUT THE FAMILY?

We are beginning to recognize that the prevalent ethic of patient autonomy simply will not do. Since demands for health care are virtually unlimited, giving autonomous patients the care they want will bankrupt our health care system. We can no longer simply buy our way out of difficult questions of justice by expanding the health care pie until there is enough to satisfy the wants and needs of everyone. The requirements of justice and the needs of other patients must temper the claims of autonomous patients.

But if the legitimate claims of other patients and other (non-medical) interests of society are beginning to be recognized, another question is still largely ignored: To what extent can the patient's family legitimately be asked or required to sacrifice their interests so that the patient can have the treatment he or she wants?

This question is not only almost universally ignored, it is generally implicitly dismissed, silenced before it can even be raised. This tacit dismissal results from a fundamental assumption of medical ethics: medical treatment ought always to serve the interests of the patient. This, of course, implies that the interests of family members should be irrelevant to medical treatment decisions or at least ought never to take precedence over the interests of the patient. All questions about fairness to the interests of family members are thus precluded, regardless of the merit or importance of the interests that will have to be sacrificed if the patient is to receive optimal treatment.

Yet there is a whole range of cases in which important interests of family members are dramatically affected by decisions about the patient's treatment; medical decisions often should be made with those interests in mind. Indeed, in many cases family members have a greater interest than the patient in which treatment option is exercised. In such cases, the interests of family members often ought to *override* those of the patient.

The problem of family interests cannot be resolved by considering other members of the family as "patients," thereby redefining the problem as one of conflicting interests among *patients*. Other members of the family are not always ill, and even if ill, they still may not be patients. Nor will it do to define the whole family as one patient. Granted, the slogan "the patient is the family" was coined partly to draw attention to precisely the issues I wish to raise, but the idea that the whole family is one patient is too monolithic. The conflicts of interests, beliefs, and values among family members are often too real and run too deep to treat all members as "the patient." Thus, if I am correct, it is sometimes the moral thing to do for a physician to sacrifice the interests of her patient to those of nonpatients—specifically, to those of the other members of the patient's family.

But what is the "family"? As I will use it here, it will mean roughly "those who are close to the patient." "Family" so defined will often include close friends and companions. It may also exclude some with blood or marriage ties to the patient. "Closeness" does not, however, always mean care and abiding affection, nor need it be a positive experience—one can hate, resent, fear, or despise a mother or brother with an intensity not often directed toward strangers, acquaintances, or associates. But there are cases where even a hateful or resentful family member's interests ought to be considered.

This use of "family" gives rise to very sensitive ethical—and legal—issues in the case of legal relatives with no emotional ties to the patient that I cannot pursue here. I can only say that I do not mean to suggest that the interests of legal relatives who are not emotionally close to the patient are always to be ignored. They will sometimes have an important financial interest in the treatment even if they are not emotionally close to the patient. But blood and marriage ties can become so thin that they become *merely* legal relationships. (Consider, for example, "couples" who have long since parted but who have never gotten a divorce, or cases in which the next of kin cannot be bothered with making proxy decisions.) Obviously, there are many important questions about just whose interests are to be considered in which treatment decisions and to what extent.

CONNECTED INTERESTS

There is no way to detach the lives of patients from the lives of those who are close to them. Indeed, the intertwining of lives is part of the very meaning of closeness. Consequently, there will be a broad spectrum of cases in which the treatment options will have dramatic and different impacts on the patient's family.

I believe there are many, many such cases. To save the life of a newborn with serious defects is often dramatically to affect the rest of the parents' lives and, if they have other children, may seriously compromise the quality of their lives, as well... The husband of a woman with Alzheimer's disease may well have a life totally dominated for ten years or more by caring for an increasingly foreign and estranged wife... The choice between aggressive and palliative care or, for that matter, the difference between either kind of care and suicide in the case of a father with terminal cancer or AIDS may have a dramatic emotional and financial impact on his wife and children... Less dramatically, the choice between two medications, one of which has the side effect of impotence, may radically alter the life a couple has together... The drug of choice for controlling high blood pressure may be too expensive (that is, requires too many sacrifices) for many families with incomes just above the ceiling for Medicaid...

Because the lives of those who are close are not separable, to be close is to no longer have a life entirely your own to live entirely as you choose. To be part of a family is to be morally required to make decisions on the basis of thinking about what is best for all concerned, not simply what is best for yourself. In healthy families, characterized by genuine care, one wants to make decisions on this basis, and many people do so quite naturally and automatically. My own grandfather committed suicide after his heart attack as a final gift to his wife—he had plenty of life insurance but not nearly enough health insurance, and he feared that she would be left homeless and destitute if he lingered on in an incapacitated state. Even if one is not so inclined, however, it is irresponsible and wrong to exclude or to fail to consider the interests of those who are close. Only when the lives of family members will not be importantly affected can one rightly make exclusively or even predominantly self-regarding decisions.

Although "what is best for all concerned" sounds utilitarian, my position does not imply that the right course of action results simply from a calculation of what is best for all. No, the seriously ill may have a right to special consideration, and the family of an ill person may have a duty to make sacrifices to respond to a member's illness. It is one thing to claim that the ill deserve special consideration; it is quite another to maintain that they deserve exclusive or even overriding consideration. Surely we must admit that there are limits to the right to special treatment by virtue of illness. Otherwise, everyone would be morally required to sacrifice all other goods to better care for the ill. We must also recognize that patients too have moral obligations, obligations to try to protect the lives of their families from destruction resulting from their illnesses.

Thus, unless serious illness excuses one from all moral responsibility—and I don't see how it could—it is an oversimplification to say of a patient who is part of a family that "it's his life" or "after all, it's his medical treatment," as if his life and his treatment could be successfully isolated from the lives of the other members of his family. It is more accurate to say "it's their lives" or "after all, they're all going to have to live with his treatment." Then the really serious moral questions are not *whether* the interests of family members are relevant to decisions about a patient's medical treatment or *whether* their interests should be included in his deliberations or in deliberations about him, but how far family and friends can be asked to support and sustain the patient. What sacrifices can they be morally required to make for his health care? How far can they reasonably be asked to compromise the quality of their lives so that he will receive the care that would improve the quality of his life? To what extent can he reasonably expect them to put their lives "on hold" to preoccupy themselves with his illness to the extent necessary to care for him?

THE ANOMALY OF MEDICAL DECISIONMAKING

The way we analyze medical treatment decisions by or for patients is plainly anomalous to the way we think about other important decisions family members make. I am a husband, a father, and still a son, and no one would argue that I should or even responsibly could decide to take a sabbatical, another job, or even a weekend trip *solely* on the basis of what

I want for myself. Why should decisions about my medical treatment be different? Why should we have even *thought* that medical treatment decisions might be different?

Is it because medical decisions, uniquely, involve life and death matters? Most medical decisions, however, are not matters of life and death, and we as a society risk or shorten the lives of other people—through our toxic waste disposal decisions, for example—quite apart from considerations of whether that is what they want for themselves.

Have we been misled by a preoccupation with the biophysical model of disease? Perhaps it has tempted us to think of illness and hence also of treatment as something that takes place *within* the body of the patient. What happens in my body does not—barring contagion—affect my wife's body, yet it usually does affect her.

Have we tacitly desired to simplify the practice and the ethics of medicine by considering only the *medical* or health-related consequences of treatment decisions? Perhaps, but it is obvious that we need a broader vision of and sensitivity to *all* the consequences of action, at least among those who are not simply technicians following orders from above. Generals need to consider more than military consequences, businessmen more than economic consequences, teachers more than educational consequences, lawyers more than legal consequences.

Does the weakness and vulnerability of serious illness imply that the ill need such protection that we should serve only their interests? Those who are sick may indeed need special protection, but this can only mean that we must take special care to see that the interests of the ill are duly considered. It does not follow that their interests are to be served exclusively or even that their interests must always predominate. Moreover, we must remember that in terms of the dynamics of the family, the patient is not always the weakest member, the member most in need of protection.

Does it make *historical*, if not logical, sense to view the wishes and interests of the patient as always overriding? Historically, illnesses were generally of much shorter duration; patients got better quickly or died quickly. Moreover, the costs of the medical care available were small enough that rarely was one's future mortgaged to the costs of the care of family members. Although this was once truer than it is today, there have always been significant exceptions to these generalizations.

None of these considerations adequately explains why the interests of the patient's family have been thought to be appropriately excluded from consideration. At the very least, those who believe that medical treatment decisions are morally anomalous to other important decisions owe us a better account of how and why this is so.

LIMITS OF PUBLIC POLICY

It might be thought that the problem of family interests *is* a problem only because our society does not shelter families from the negative effects of medical decisions. If, for example, we adopted a comprehensive system of national health insurance and also a system of public insurance to guarantee the incomes of families, then my sons' chances at a college education and the quality of the rest of their lives might not have to be sacrificed were I to receive optimal medical care.

However, it is worth pointing out that we are still moving primarily in the *opposite* direction. Instead of designing policies that would increasingly shelter family members from the adverse impact of serious and prolonged illnesses, we are still attempting to shift the burden of care to family members in our efforts to contain medical costs. A social system that would safeguard families from the impact of serious illness is nowhere in sight in this country. And we must not do medical ethics as if it were.

It is perhaps even more important to recognize that the lives of family members could not be sheltered from all the important ramifications of medical treatment decisions by *any* set of public policies. In any society in which people get close to each other and care deeply for each other, treatment decisions about one will often and *irremediably* affect more than one. If a newborn has been saved by aggressive treatment but is severely handicapped, the parents may simply not be emotionally capable of abandoning the child to institutional care. A man whose wife is suffering from multiple sclerosis may simply not be willing or able to go on with his own life until he sees her through to the end. A woman whose husband is being maintained in a vegetative state may not feel free to marry or even to see other men again, regardless of what some revised law might say about her marital status.

Nor could we desire a society in which friends and family would quickly lose their concern as soon as continuing to care began to diminish the quality of their own lives. For we would then have alliances for better but not for worse, in health, but not in sickness, until death appears on the horizon. And we would all be poorer for that. A man who can leave his wife the day after she learns she has cancer, on the grounds that he has his own life to live, is to be deplored. The emotional inability or principled refusal to separate ourselves and our lives from the lives of ill or dying members of our families is *not* an unfortunate fact about the structure of our emotions. It is a desirable feature, not to be changed even if it could be; not to be changed even if the resulting intertwining of lives debars us from making exclusively self-regarding treatment decisions when we are ill.

Our present individualistic medical ethics is isolating and destructive. For by implicitly suggesting that patients make "their own" treatment decisions on a self-regarding basis and supporting those who do so, such an ethics encourages each of us to see our lives as simply our own. We may yet turn ourselves into beings who are ultimately alone.

FIDELITY OR FAIRNESS?

Fidelity to the interests of the patient has been a cornerstone of both traditional codes and contemporary theories of medical ethics. The two competing paradigms of medical ethics—the "benevolence" model and the "patient autonomy" model—are simply different ways of construing such fidelity. Both must be rejected or radically modified. The admission that treatment decisions often affect more than just the patient thus forces major changes on both the theoretical and the practical level. Obviously, I can only begin to explore the needed changes here.

Instead of starting with our usual assumption that physicians are to serve the interests of the patient, we must build our theories on a very different assumption: The medical and nonmedical interests of both the patient and other members of the patient's family are to be considered. It is only in the special case of patients without family that we can simply follow the patient's wishes or pursue the patient's interests. In fact, I would argue that we must build our theory of medical ethics on the presumption of equality: the interests of patients and family members are morally to be weighed equally; medical and nonmedical interests of the same magnitude deserve equal consideration in making treatment decisions. Like any other moral presumption, this one can, perhaps, be defeated in some cases. But the burden of proof will always be on those who would advocate special consideration for any family member's interests, including those of the ill.

Even where the presumption of equality is not defeated, life, health, and freedom from pain and handicapping conditions are extremely important goods for virtually everyone. They are thus very important considerations in all treatment decisions. In the majority of cases, the patient's interest in optimal health and longer life may well be strong enough to outweigh the conflicting interests of other members of the family. But even then, some departure from the treatment plan that would maximize the patient's interests may well be justified to harmonize best the interests of all concerned or to require significantly smaller sacrifices by other family members. That the patient's interests may often outweigh the conflicting interests of others in treatment decisions is no justification for failing to recognize that an attempt to balance or harmonize different, conflicting interests is often morally required. Nor does it justify overlooking the morally crucial cases in which the interests of other members of the family ought to override the interests of the patient. Changing our basic assumption about how treatment decisions are to be made means reconceptualizing the ethical roles of both physician and patient, since our understanding of both has been built on the presumption of patient primacy, rather than fairness to all concerned. Recognizing the moral relevance of the interests of family members thus reveals a dilemma for our understanding of what it is to be a physician: Should we retain a fiduciary ethic in which the physician is to serve the interests of her patient? Or should the physician attempt to weigh and balance all the interests of all concerned? I do not yet know just how to resolve this dilemma. All I can do here is try to envision the options.

If we retain the traditional ethic of fidelity to the interests of the patient, the physician should excuse herself from making treatment decisions that will affect the lives of the family on grounds of a moral conflict of interest, for she is a one-sided advocate. A lawyer for one of the parties cannot also serve as judge in the case. Thus, it would be unfair if a physician conceived as having a fiduciary relationship to her patient were to make treatment decisions that would adversely affect the lives of the patient's family. Indeed, a physician conceived as a patient advocate should not even *advise* patients or family members about which course of treatment should be chosen. As advocate, she can speak only to what course of treatment would be best for the patient, and must remain silent about what's best for the rest of the family or what should be done in light of everyone's interests.

Physicians might instead renounce their fiduciary relationship with their patients. On this view, physicians would no longer be agents of their patients and would not strive to be advocates for their patients' interests. Instead, the physician would aspire to be an impartial advisor who would stand knowledgeably but sympathetically outside all the many conflicting interests of those affected by the treatment options, and who would strive to discern the treatment that would best harmonize or balance the interests of all concerned.

Although this second option contradicts the Hippocratic Oath and most other codes of medical ethics, it is not, perhaps, as foreign as it may at first seem. Traditionally, many family physicians—especially small-town physicians who knew patients and their families well—attempted to attend to both medical and nonmedical interests of all concerned. Many contemporary physicians still make decisions in this way. But we do not yet have an ethical theory that explains and justifies what they are doing.

Nevertheless, we may well question the physician's ability to act as an impartial ethical observer. Increasingly, physicians do not know their patients, much less their patients' families. Moreover, we may doubt physicians' abilities to weigh evenhandedly medical and nonmedical interests. Physicians are trained to be especially responsive to medical interests and we may well want them to remain that way. Physicians also tend to be deeply involved with the interests of their patients, and it may be impossible or undesirable to break this tie to enable physicians to be more impartial advisors. Finally, when someone retains the services of a physician, it seems reasonable that she be able to expect that physician to be *her* agent, pursuing *her* interests, not those of her family.

AUTONOMY AND ADVOCACY

We must also rethink our conception of the patient. On one hand, if we continue to stress patient autonomy, we must recognize that this implies that patients have moral responsibilities. If, on the other hand, we do not want to burden patients with weighty moral responsibilities, we must abandon the ethic of patient autonomy.

Recognizing that moral responsibilities come with patient autonomy will require basic changes in the accepted meanings of both "autonomy" and "advocacy." Because medical ethics has ignored patient responsibilities, we have come to interpret "autonomy" in a sense very different from [German philosopher Immanuel] Kant's original use of the term. It has come to mean simply the patient's freedom or right to choose the treatment he believes is best for himself. But as Kant knew well, there are many situations in which people can achieve autonomy and moral well-being only by sacrificing other important dimensions of their well-being, including health, happiness, even life itself. For autonomy is the *responsible* use of freedom and is therefore diminished whenever one ignores, evades, or slights one's responsibilities. Human dignity, Kant concluded, consists in our ability to refuse to compromise our autonomy to achieve the kinds of lives (or treatments) we want for ourselves.

If, then, I am morally empowered to make decisions about "my" medical treatment, I am also morally required to shoulder the responsibility of making very difficult moral decisions. The right course of action for me to take will not always be the one that promotes my own interests.

Some patients, motivated by a deep and abiding concern for the well-being of their families, will undoubtedly consider the interests of other family members. For these patients, the interests of their family are *part* of their interests. But not all patients will feel this way. And the interests of family members are not relevant *if* and *because* the patient wants to consider them; they are not relevant because they are *part* of the patient's interests. They are relevant *whether or not* the patient is inclined to consider them. Indeed, the *ethics* of patient decisions is most poignantly highlighted precisely when the patient is inclined to decide without considering the impact of his decision on the lives of the rest of his family.

Confronting patients with tough ethical choices may be part and parcel of treating them with respect as fully competent adults. We don't, after all, think it's right to stand silently by while other (healthy) adults ignore or shirk their moral responsibilities. If, however, we believe that most patients, gripped as they often are by the emotional crisis of serious illness, are not up to shouldering the responsibility of such decisions or should not be burdened with it, then I think we must simply abandon the ethic of patient autonomy. Patient autonomy would then be appropriate only when the various treatment options will affect only the patient's life.

The responsibilities of patients imply that there is often a conflict between patient autonomy and the patient's interests (even as those interests are defined by the patient). And we will have to rethink our understanding of patient advocacy in light of this conflict: Does the patient advocate try to promote the patient's (self-defined) *interests*? Or does she promote the patient's *autonomy* even at the expense of those interests? Responsible patient advocates can hardly encourage patients to shirk their moral responsibilities. But can we really expect health care providers to promote patient autonomy when that means encouraging their patients to sacrifice health, happiness, sometimes even life itself?

If we could give an affirmative answer to this last question, we would obviously thereby create a third option for reinterpreting the role of the physician: The physician could maintain her traditional role as patient advocate without being morally required to refrain from making treatment decisions whenever interests of the patient's family are also at stake *if* patient advocacy were understood as promoting patient autonomy *and* patient autonomy were understood as the responsible use of freedom, not simply the right to choose the treatment one wants.

Much more attention needs to be paid to all of these issues. However, it should be clear that absolutely central features of our theories of medical ethics—our understanding of physician and patient, and thus of patient advocacy as well as patient dignity, and patient autonomy—have presupposed that the interests of family members should be irrelevant or should always take a back seat to the interests of the patient. Basic conceptual shifts are required once we acknowledge that this assumption is not warranted.

WHO SHOULD DECIDE?

Such basic conceptual shifts will necessarily have ramifications that will be felt throughout the field of medical ethics, for a host of new and very different issues are raised by the inclusion of family interests. Discussions of privacy and confidentiality, of withholding/withdrawing treatment, and of surrogate decisionmaking will all have to be reconsidered in light of the interests of the family. Many individual treatment decisions will also be affected, becoming much more complicated than they already are. Here, I will only offer a few remarks about treatment decisions, organized around the central issue of who should decide.

There are at least five answers to the question of who should make treatment decisions in cases where important interests of other family members are also at stake: the patient, the family, the physician, an ethics committee, or the courts. The physician's role in treatment decisions has already been discussed. Resort to either the courts or to ethics committees for treatment decisions is too cumbersome and time-consuming for any but the most troubling cases. So I will focus here on the contrast between the patient and the family as appropriate decisionmakers. It is worth noting, though, that we need not arrive at one, uniform answer to cover all cases. On the contrary, each of the five options will undoubtedly have its place, depending on the particulars of the case at hand.

Should we still think of a patient as having the right to make decisions about "his" treatment? As we have seen, patient autonomy implies patient responsibilities. What, then, if the patient seems to be ignoring the impact of his treatment on his family? At the very least, responsible physicians must caution such patients against simply opting for treatments because they want them. Instead, physicians must speak of responsibilities and obligations. They must raise considerations of the quality of many lives, not just that of the patient. They must explain the distinction

between making a decision and making it in a self-regarding manner. Thus, it will often be appropriate to make plain to patients the consequences of treatment decisions for their families and to urge them to consider these consequences in reaching a decision. And sometimes, no doubt, it will be appropriate for family members to present their cases to the patient in the hope that his decisions would be shaped by their appeals.

Nonetheless, we sometimes permit people to make bad or irresponsible decisions and *excuse* those decisions because of various pressures they were under when they made their choices. Serious illness can undoubtedly be an extenuating circumstance, and perhaps we should allow some patients to make some self-regarding decisions, especially if they insist on doing so and the negative impact of their decisions on others is not too great.

Alternatively, if we doubt that most patients have the ability to make treatment decisions that are really fair to all concerned, or if we are not prepared to accept a policy that would assign patients the responsibility of doing so, we may conclude that they should not be empowered to make treatment decisions in which the lives of their family members will be dramatically affected. Indeed, even if the patient were completely fair in making the decision, the autonomy of other family members would have been systematically undercut by the fact that the patient alone decided.

Thus, we need to consider the autonomy of all members of the family, not just the patient's autonomy. Considerations of fairness and, paradoxically, of autonomy therefore indicate that the *family* should make the treatment decision, with all competent family members whose lives will be affected participating. Many such family conferences undoubtedly already take place. On this view, however, family conferences would often be morally *required*. And these conferences would not be limited to cases involving incompetent patients; cases involving competent patients would also often require family conferences.

Obviously, it would be completely unworkable for a physician to convene a family conference every time a medical decision might have some ramifications on the lives of family members. However, such discussion need not always take place in the presence of the physician; we can recognize that formal family conferences become more important as the impact of treatment decisions on members of the patient's family grows larger. Family conferences may thus be morally *required* only when the lives of family members would be dramatically affected by treatment decisions.

Moreover, family discussion is often morally *desirable* even if not morally required. Desirable, sometimes, even for relatively minor treatment decisions: After the family has moved to a new town, should parents commit themselves to two-hour drives so that their teenage son can continue to be treated for his acne by the dermatologist he knows and whose results he trusts? Or should he seek treatment from a new dermatologist?

Some family conferences about treatment decisions would be characterized throughout by deep affection, mutual understanding, and abiding concern for the interests of others. Other conferences might begin in an atmosphere charged with antagonism, suspicion, and hostility but move toward greater understanding, reconciliation, and harmony within the family. Such conferences would be sig-

nificant goods in themselves, as well as means to ethically better treatment decisions. They would leave all family members better able to go on with their lives.

Still, family conferences cannot be expected always to begin with or move toward affection, mutual understanding, and a concern for all. If we opt for joint treatment decisions when the lives of several are affected, we need to face the fact that family conferences will sometimes be bitter confrontations in which past hostilities, anger, and resentments will surface. Sometimes, too, the conflicts of interest between patient and family, and between one family member and another will be irresolvable, forcing families to invoke the harsh perspective of justice, divisive and antagonistic though that perspective may be. Those who favor family decisions when the whole family is affected will have to face the question of whether we really want to put the patient, already frightened and weakened by his illness, through the conflict and bitter confrontations that family conferences may sometimes precipitate.

We must also recognize that family members may be unable or unwilling to press or even state their own interests before a family member who is ill. Such refusal may be admirable, even heroic; it is sometimes evidence of willingness to go "above and beyond the call of duty," even at great personal cost. But not always. Refusal to press one's own interests can also be a sign of inappropriate guilt, of a crushing sense of responsibility for the well-being of others, of acceptance of an inferior or dominated role within the family, or of lack of a sense of self-worth. All of these may well be mobilized by an illness in the family. Moreover, we must not minimize the power of the medical setting to subordinate nonmedical to medical interests and to emphasize the well-being of the patient at the expense of the well-being of others. Thus, it will often be not just the patient, but also other family members who will need an advocate if a family conference is to reach the decision that best balances the autonomy and interests of all concerned.

NO

Jeffrey Blustein

THE FAMILY IN MEDICAL DECISIONMAKING

Might it be that family members, by virtue of their closeness to the patient, should not only have some special authority to speak on behalf of patients who are incompetent, but should also share decisional authority with patients who are competent?

A recent proposal that speaks to the family's role in medical decisionmaking has been advanced by John Hardwig. In his provocative essay, "What about the Family?"[1] he contemplates far-reaching changes in medical practice based on a critique of our prevailing patient-centered ethos. My discussion of his proposal is chiefly designed to pave the way for what I call a communitarian account of the role of the family in acute care decisionmaking. This account—which, I hasten to add, I do not endorse—has not to my knowledge been taken seriously as a theoretical possibility in the bioethics literature. Since the label "communitarian" is liable to be misunderstood, I should note at the outset that I am not interested in communitarianism as a political theory. Rather, I want to focus on the family as communitarian political writers sometimes think of it, namely, as a model for their conception of the larger society, and on the basis of this understanding of the family, to mount a challenge to the dominant patient-centered ethos that parallels the communitarian critique of liberal political philosophy. This communitarian position resembles Hardwig's proposal in that it does not regard the competent patient as the ultimate decisionmaker, but takes it as morally significant for the attribution of decisional authority that his or her life is intimately intertwined with the lives of close others. However, as we will see, the communitarian account is philosophically more radical than Hardwig's challenge to the dominant patient-centered medical ethos.

My own position is that the locus of decisional authority should remain the individual patient, but I also argue that family members, by virtue of their closeness to and intimate knowledge of the patient are often uniquely well qualified to shore up the patient's vulnerable autonomy and assist him or her in the exercise of autonomous decisionmaking. Families, in other words, can be an important resource for patients in helping them to make better decisions about their care. Recognition of this fact leads to a broader understanding of the duty to respect patient autonomy than currently prevails in acute care medicine.

FAMILY DECISIONMAKING AND COMPETENT PATIENTS

According to Hardwig, even when the patient is a competent adult, it may be quite appropriate to empower the family, to "make the treatment decision, with all competent family members whose lives will be affected participating." ...

Particular choices about treatment can seriously affect the lives of family members in many ways, interfering not only with their own personal projects and individual life styles, but with their commitments to other family members as well. In any case, they are "separate" in the sense that they diverge from and possibly conflict with patient interests: they are not to be understood as interests in the interests of patients. Of course, those who love the patient also have a direct interest in the protection and promotion of the patient's interests, assuming that the patient has interests that can be protected and promoted. Indeed, this is part of the very meaning of love. But for Hardwig, there can be closeness without love, and even when there is love, there will usually be other interests of family members as well. When all of these interests are taken into account, it may turn out that what is best for the family as a whole is not what is best for the individual patient.

These other interests may be, and frequently are, quite legitimate, and treatment decisions should not be judged morally better or worse solely from the patient's perspective. Indeed, departures from optimal patient care may be justified "to harmonize best the interests of all concerned or to require significantly smaller sacrifices by other family members." Moreover, and very importantly, Hardwig expresses misgivings about the effectiveness of exhorting the patient to consider the impact of his or her decision on the lives of the rest of the family. Patients who seem to be ignoring their family's stake in the outcome of their decisionmaking process may sometimes respond appropriately to appeals from the physician or other family members, but many patients will be too self-involved to give the interests of others proper consideration or will use their illness as a kind of trump card to dominate the rest of the family. Because of this, Hardwig maintains, we must consider a more radical measure to ensure adequate protection of legitimate family interests, namely, rejection of the prevalent medical ethos according to which the competent patient is always the decisive moral agent. Under this ethos, it is certainly permissible for family members to offer information, counsel, and suasion to patients who must make treatment decisions. But the authority to make the decisions still resides with the competent patient alone, and this Hardwig finds untenable.[2]

The "ethic of patient autonomy" allows the competent patient, and the patient alone, to set the terms and conditions of care. Patients may be frightened and distracted by illness and hence in no position to give careful thought to the interests of others, but if their decisionmaking capacity is judged sufficient for the decision at hand, their wishes prevail. This troubles Hardwig because it amounts to giving patients permission to neglect or slight their moral responsibilities to other family members. Seriously ill patients tend to be self-absorbed and to make exclusively self-regarding choices about care, and in those cases where "the lives of family members would be dramatically affected by treatment decisions." . . .

Hardwig's proposal for greater family involvement in medical decisionmaking, however, runs up against the problem of patient vulnerability: joint family decisionmaking provides too many opportunities for the exploitation of patient vulnerability: Serious constraints on patient autonomy, such as anxiety depression, fear, and denial, are inherent in the state of being ill.[3] Illness is also frequently disorienting in that patients find themselves thrust into unfamiliar surroundings, unable to pursue customary routines or to enjoy any significant degree of privacy. For these reasons, the ability of patients to assess their medical needs accurately and protect their own interests effectively is limited and precarious. But if those who are ill and those who are healthy already confront each other on an unequal psychological footing, then family conferences, as Hardwig conceives of them, seem especially ill advised. Weakened and confused by their illness, patients are easy prey to manipulation or coercion by other family members and may capitulate to family wishes out of guilt or fear. (Given that Hardwig would allow even hateful or resentful family members to be included in family conferences, this is not an idle worry) Family members will understandably not want to be seen by the physician as opposing the wishes of the patient and so they might exert pressure on the patient to concur with their opinions about treatment. Of course, even as matters now stand, with decisionmaking not generally thought to belong to the family as a whole, what seems like a patient's autonomous choice often only implements the choice of the others for him or her. But joint family decisionmaking is likely only to exacerbate this problem and to make truly independent choice even more dubious.

Hardwig, it should be noted, does acknowledge that a seriously weakened patient may well need an "advocate," or surrogate participant from outside the family, to take part in the joint family decision. However, this hardly resolves all the difficulties his proposal presents. The presence of an outsider in what is supposed to be a deeply personal and private conference might only create (further) hostility and suspicion among family members. And if consensus in the conference cannot be achieved, the rest of the family could simply overrule the patient's proxy participant, just as it could overrule the patient himself.

From a theoretical point of view, we should, I think, agree with Hardwig about the inadequacy of any view that denies or overlooks the essential interplay between rights and responsibilities. But the practical moral problem as I see it is how to design procedures and structures of decisionmaking that achieve an acceptable balance between rights and responsibilities, between the important values of a patient-centered ethos and the legitimate claims of other family members. If alternative approaches to medical decisionmaking are judged in this light, as Hardwig wants them to be, and not solely in terms of over-all happiness or preference satisfaction or the like, then family decisionmaking for competent patients confronts serious moral objections. For indications are that it will often result not in a mutual accommodation of the autonomy and interests of all affected parties, but rather in a serious erosion of patient autonomy and a subordination of patient interests to the competing interests of other family members.

THE COMMUNITARIAN DEFENSE OF FAMILY DECISIONMAKING

I have focused on the problems that non-ideal, less than fully harmonious families pose for Hardwig's proposal. Critics of the patient-as-primary-agent model might instead restrict their attention to those (admittedly infrequent) cases in which patients belong to close-knit and harmonious families, and with this as their conception of the family, offer a defense of family decisionmaking that challenges the patient-centered model in a more radical way than Hardwig does. In ideal families, suspicions, resentments, disagreements, and the like, if they exist, are muted and do not set the tone of family life. But more importantly, it may be claimed, the conception of the person that underlies the theory of patient autonomy is patently inappropriate here. The patient is not, as this theory presupposes, an atomic entity, a free and rational chooser of ends unencumbered by communal and other allegiances. On the contrary, his or her identity is constituted by family relationships, and he or she is united with other family members through common ends and mutual understanding. In these circumstances, the patient is too enmeshed in a network of relations to others to be properly singled out as the one to make treatment decisions.

I call this the communitarian argument for family decisionmaking to distinguish it from the argument from fairness and autonomy did cussed in the previous section. When I refer below to what "communitarians" say about medical decisionmaking, I am not thinking of any particular authors who have advanced this position.[4] Rather, I am suggesting that elements of the communitarian view can be taken out of their political context and that a challenge to the prevailing patient-centered ethos can be constructed on the basis of a communitarian conception of the ideal family. Let us look at this challenge more closely.

In acute care settings, the relationship between patients and physicians is, if not exactly adversarial, at least one in which patients should not normally suppose that they and their physicians are participants in a common enterprise with common values and goals. The values involved in medical decisionmaking are by no means exclusively medical values, but also largely normative ones about which patients and physicians frequently disagree. In these circumstances, physicians may attempt to coerce compliance with their wishes, which they are in an advantageous position to do, or to control patient decisions by selective disclosure or nondisclosure of information. In recognition of normative diversity and in the face of various threats to patient autonomy in the caregiving relationship, we invoke the notion of patients' rights. Rights accord patients a protected space in which to make their own choices and pursue their ends free of inappropriate interference from others. Having rights, patients can confront caregivers with the demand that their (possibly conflicting) ends be respected.

Communitarian critics of the traditional ethos of patient autonomy need not deny that patients' rights and patient self-determination play an important role in the caregiving relationship. But, they note, the patient is not always to be thought of simply as the one who is sick or in need of medical attention.

If the patient belongs to a close-knit and harmonious family, for example, it is the family as a whole whose values and goals may diverge from those of professional caregivers because such a family is a genuine community, not a mere collection of separate individuals with their own private and possibly conflicting interests. Members of a community have common ends, and these are conceived of and valued as common ends by the members. United by common ends and a common identity, the threats that work against the autonomy of some work against the autonomy of all. Moreover, in these cases the patient would not need to be protected from family pressures for inappropriate treatment. Rather, the family would act as advocate for the patient vis-à-vis the physician, and family decision-making would put patients on a much more equal footing with caregivers.

For communitarians the ethics of acute care, focusing as it does on the individual who is the subject of treatment, rests on a conception of the self that is at odds with how persons define and understand themselves in a community. This is a conception for a world of strangers, where the content of each person's good is, to quote Michael Sandel, "largely opaque" to others, where persons have divergent and possibly conflicting plans and interests, and where their capacity for benevolence is extremely limited.[5] But in the community of a close and harmonious family these conditions do not obtain. Rather, the defining features of such a family are mutual sympathy, common ends, a shared identity, love, and spontaneous affection. Of course, it is sheer wishful thinking, and cavalier as well, to assume that all families are like this. Family life may instead be fraught with dissension and interests may diverge and conflict. In these situations questions of justice come to the fore and the importance of individual rights (and individual patient rights) is enhanced. But within the context of a more or less ideal family, the circumstances that make personal autonomy both an appropriate and a pressing concern prevail to a relatively small degree. . . .

The close-knit, harmonious family is a paradigm of community. Here the well-being of one family member does not just have an impact on the well-being of others, for this can happen in families that are no more than associations of individuals (like the ones Hardwig describes). Rather, in families that are genuine communities individuals identify with one another, such that the well-being of one is *part of* the well being of the other. This being so, the communitarian maintains, decisions that importantly affect the well being of one family member are the province of the entire family. To be sure, in the medical cases there is only one family member, the patient, who literally bears the decision in his or her flesh and bones. But this fact alone, it is believed, does not confer upon the patient a unilateral decisionmaking right. The right to make the decision is still a right of the family in ideal circumstance—a group right rather than a right of individuals.

However, since the communitarian argument for family decisionmaking applies only to families that are communities and not to those that are just collections of individuals whose lives affect each other in major ways, its implications for the practice of medicine will not be as significant as those of Hardwig's proposal. Many families, to acknowledge the obvious again, are not ideal. In addition, physicians frequently have only passing acquaintance with the patient's family and no reliable basis for judging the quality of the patient's relationship with other family members. Even if communitarians reveal genuine inadequacies in the prevalent ethos of patient autonomy and patient rights, physicians will often not be in a position to tell whether, in the particular case at hand, the family is harmonious enough to be entrusted with the authority to make decisions for one of its own. On the other hand, physicians will often have enough information to know that the lives of family members will be seriously affected by treatment decisions, and it is on this fact, not on the existence of a harmonious family, that Hardwig premises the case for joint family decisionmaking.

Still, the communitarian critique of the dominant medical ethos of patient autonomy and individual patients' rights raises interesting and important philosophical issues. Practical implications aside, the theoretical challenge it poses deserves a response. In what follows, I will try to indicate why I think this challenge fails.

HOW THE COMMUNITARIAN CHALLENGE FAILS

Even in families that are true communities of love, the harmony that exists among their members may not be so thoroughgoing that invocation of individual decisionmaking rights loses its point. It is not necessary for community that there be complete identity of all ends and unanimity on all matters of value or the good. On the contrary, there is room for significant disagreement about how to rank different components of a common conception of the good, about the proper means and strategies for achieving it, and about whether certain risks are worth taking to achieve common goals. Even if the members of a family are in broad agreement about what is of most importance in life, for example, this does not ensure that they will assess the costs and benefits of particular medical treatments similarly. Indeed, given the diversity of human nature and experience, such disagreements are not just possible but to be expected. Absolute harmony in decisionmaking and thoroughgoing convergence of values are only found in quite extraordinary communities. And this being the case, individual rights can be seen to have an importance the communitarian fails to acknowledge. They are not just claims we fall back on in the unhappy situation where community is lacking or faltering. Additionally, they serve to secure recognition, of the diverse values and ends that persist even in intact and well-functioning communities. This lack of homogeneity is glossed over by talk of family rights.

Individual rights have an important place in community because the existence of community does not eradicate serious disagreement about ends, about the relationship between particular choices and shared ends, and so forth. Individual rights are needed because a significant degree of diversity may exist even in a group united by a common conception of the good....

It may help here to distinguish between having a right and insisting upon or demanding it. The language of demands does seem ill suited to harmonious families. If family members need to insist against one another that they have a right to make their own decisions, then we are probably dealing with a divided and quite antagonistic family. But these observations do not suffice to banish individual rights from harmonious families because the underlying supposition

—that rights must always be linked to demands—is false. Rights can be expressed in different ways, and what is divisive and antagonistic to community is not the concept of rights, but only a certain way of expressing them. In harmonious families, rights are typically expressed "as reminders—gentle or forceful, matter-of-fact or emotional—of legitimate expectations and entitlements,"[6] and as such they play a vital role in the moral lives of families.

The implications of these remarks for a communitarian defense of family medical decisionmaking are clear. Even in extremely close families, patients may have different priorities from their loved ones and assess life choices in disparate ways, and these differences may surface in disagreements about how and even whether patients should be treated. Patients need their own rights regarding choice of treatment not just because family members cannot always be trusted to have the patient's best interests at heart, but because, even in families where trust is not an issue and there is a remarkable measure of agreement on ends and deep mutual affection, other family members may not always concur with the wisdom of the patient's choices. Rights protect patient autonomy and patient interests in these circumstances.

Further, rights for patients would be appropriate and useful even in those quite unusual families where the minimal sort of disagreement just mentioned is absent. For decisions about treatment often have dramatic and far-reaching consequences for the shape, quality, and duration of a patient's life, and individuals have an interest in determining for themselves the course their lives take. The interest in directing how one's life will go

in accordance with one's values and preferences exists whether these values and preferences are uniquely one's own or shared with other family members, and it calls for recognition even when there is no disagreement between patient and family over the correct treatment decision. This is why patients have rights as individuals even under the unlikely conditions of absolute intrafamilial harmony: they protect the interests that patients have in exercising their agency. . . .

FAMILY INVOLVEMENT IN THE PROCESS OF DECISIONMAKING

These responses to the communitarian position do not show that patient choices about treatment always trump the choices of family members, and they do not cut against Hardwig's argument for joint medical decisionmaking by all affected family members. What they show is only that the dominant patient-centered medical ethos cannot be refuted by the sort of all out attack on the notion of individual rights the communitarian launches. To be sure, an adversarial and legalistic conception of individual rights is ill suited to those cases where family relationships are nonadversarial and there are no deep conflicts of interests, preferences, or values among family members. But if this is the basis for the communitarian claim that community renders individual rights (including patient rights) useless or of minor importance, the communitarian betrays a distorted and incomplete understanding of rights.

Should the choices of competent patients trump the choices of family members, except in the rarest of circumstances? "It is an oversimplification to say of a patient who is part of a family," Hardwig notes, that "it's his life" or "after all, it's his medical treatment." Plainly, this by itself hardly shows that patient choices take priority over the choices of others, for when lives are so intertwined that one life cannot be shaped without also shaping the lives of others, it's *their* lives too. Another approach is to argue for a unilateral decisionmaking right for patients on the ground that patients have more to lose than their family members. That is, when we measure the sacrifices that family members must make for a patient's health care and the costs to the patient of not receiving the treatment that, other family members aside, he or she would select, the patient's sacrifices almost always outweigh the family's. Of course, the reverberations of patients' self regarding choices can be so shattering to the lives of other family members that a calculation of relative costs favors the family instead. But familial hardship from this source is usually less of a burden than serious illness, and this difference would be sufficient to establish at least a presumption in favor of patient decisionmaking.

But if the ethos of patient autonomy survives the challenges I have considered in this paper it is nevertheless the case that current medical practice and medical ethics can be faulted for not giving the family a more prominent place in medical decisionmaking for competent patients, and that both family members and patients suffer as a result. For one thing, as we learned from our discussion of Hardwig, because treatment decisions often do have a dramatic impact on family members, procedures need to be devised, short of giving family members a share of decisional authority, that acknowledge the moral weight of their legitimate interests. For another, though patients might well benefit from family involvement in the process of formulating views about med-

ical treatment, under the regime of patient autonomy patients tend to be treated for the most part as if they were solitary decisionmakers, isolated from intimate others.

The ethos of patient autonomy rightly understood takes seriously the impairments of autonomy that affect us when we are ill. Patients are not ideally autonomous agents but anxious, fearful, depressed, often confused, and subject to ill-considered and mistaken ideas. If we are genuinely concerned about ensuring patient self-determination, we will take these factors into account. Here it is necessary to distinguish, as Jay Katz does, between "choices" and "thinking about choices."[7] According to the dominant medical ethos, choices properly belong to the patient alone. At the same time, patients' capacities for reflective thought and effective action are limited and precarious, obliging them to converse and consult with supportive and caring others if they are to make their best choices. Patients' psychological capacities for autonomy can be enhanced by searching conversations with their physicians—the main point of Katz's book—and (I would add) by conversations with other family members.

To explain why this is so, we may turn to a characterization of the family found in Nancy Rhoden's influential law review article, "Litigating Life and Death."[8] Her argument, which focuses on decisionmaking for incompetent patients, finds within family life features that warrant a legal presumption in favor of family choice. Family members are typically the best decisionmakers partly because of their special epistemic qualifications: they ordinarily have deep and detailed knowledge of one another's lives, characters, values, and desires. This knowledge might be based on specific statements made by one family member to another, for the intimacy of family life encourages and is partly constituted by the unguarded disclosure of one's most private thoughts and deepest feelings. But there may be nothing specific that was said or done to which family members can point as evidence of another member's preferences. Indeed, their knowledge, acquired through long association and the sharing of intense life experiences, is characteristically of the sort that "transcends purely logical evidence." In addition, family members are the best candidates to act as surrogates for an incompetent patient because of their special emotional bonds to the patient. This is important because possessing deep and detailed knowledge of another can put one in an especially good position to frustrate no less than fulfill this person's desires. Family members, however, can be presumed to have a deep emotional commitment to one another, and this makes it likely that they will put their knowledge to the right use—that is, that they will decide as the patient would have wanted.

Those features of families that, in Rhoden's view, justify a legal presumption in favor of family decisionmaking for incompetent patient—intimate knowledge, caring, shared history—also provide good reasons for family involvement in the competent patients' thinking about choices. Family members would have no veto power over a patient's decision and would have to honor the choice ultimately made, no matter how foolish or idiosyncratic. But in family conferences, where the process of making a decision is shared, they could encourage the patient to evaluate different treatment options in terms of their impact on the interests of other family members, and

could attempt to persuade the patient that the best choice is one that is fair to all affected parties. In some cases, understanding what a particular treatment decision would cost other family members might give the patient a compelling reason to alter an initial choice.

For the physician, the duty to respect patient autonomy has as its corollary a duty to engage in conversation with patients and to encourage and facilitate conversation between patients and other persons to whom they are close (including family members), unless the physician has reason to think that such conversation will not in fact assist the patient in making autonomous decisions. Current medical practice does not in general reflect a commitment to foster this sort of conversation as an integral part of the physician's professional responsibility. But if, as Katz suggests, genuine respect for patient autonomy is shown not merely in accepting patients' yes or no response to a proposed intervention, but rather in facilitating patients' opportunities for serious reflection on their choices, then promoting discussion and dialogue between patient and family is an important part of the physician's duty to satisfy the patient's right of self-determination.

REFERENCES

1. John Harding, "What about the Family?" *Hastings Center Report* 10, no. 2 (1996): 5–10.
2. Hardwig's proposal to "reconstruct medical ethics in light of family interests" is novel in that it rejects the model of patient-as-primary-agent for acute care. Others have argued, along lines similar to Hardwig's, that this is not the appropriate model for home care, where family members share heavily in the burdens of care on an ongoing basis. In the view of Bart Collopy, Nancy Dubler, and Connie Zuckerman, for example, "the ethical problem for home care becomes one of gauging the interplay of agents, the relative weight to be granted to the autonomy

and interests of the family vis-à-vis those of the elderly recipient of care." While not disputing the value of the patient-centered model in acute care, these writers argue that decisionmaking in home care should be "an interactive process, invoking negotiation, compromise, and the recognition of reciprocal ties." See "The Ethics of Home Care: Autonomy and Accommodation," special supplement, *Hastings Center Report* 20, no. 2 (1990): 1–16, at 9, 10.

3. See Terrence F. Ackerman, "Why Doctors Should Intervene," *Hastings Center Report* 12. no. 4 (1982): 14–17.

4. One author who has advanced something like a communitarian position is James Lindemann Nelson. See his "Taking Families Seriously," *Hastings Center Report* 22, no. 4 (1992): 6–12.

5. Michael Sandel, *Liberalism and the Limits of Justice* (Cambridge: Cambridge University Press, 1982), pp. 170–71.

6. Badhwar, "Circumstances of Justice."

7. Jay Katz, *The Silent World of Doctor and Patient* (New York: Free Press, 1984), p. 111.

8. Nancy Rhoden, "Litigating Life and Death," *Harvard Law Review* 102, no. 2 (1988): 375–446.

POSTSCRIPT

Can Family Interests Ethically Outweigh Patient Autonomy?

A study of more than 3,000 seriously ill patients found that those who reported economic hardship as a result of their illnesses were more likely to prefer a goal of maximizing comfort than one of maximizing life expectancy. See Kenneth E. Covinsky et al., "Is Economic Hardship on the Families of the Seriously Ill Associated With Patient and Surrogate Care Preferences?" *Archives of Internal Medicine* (August 12/26, 1996). Of interest is the study's finding that economic hardship on the family does not appear to be a factor in disagreements between patients and surrogates about the goal of care. This study suggests that individual patient autonomy is often influenced by factors other than medical ones and that patients may routinely consider how the risks and benefits of a particular decision would affect others.

Bringing the Hospital Home: Ethical and Social Implications of High-Tech Home Care edited by John D. Arras (Johns Hopkins University Press, 1995) analyzes the impact on family members and patients of introducing high-technology care into a previously private and "homey" setting. The history of long-term care and practice considerations are addressed in *Long-Term Care Decisions: Ethical and Conceptual Dimensions* edited by Laurence B. McCullough and Nancy L. Wilson (Johns Hopkins University Press, 1995). See especially the chapter by Nancy S. Jecker, "What Do Husbands and Wives Owe Each Other in Old Age?" In "Adult Daughter Caregivers," *Hastings Center Report* (September–October 1994), Sarah Vaughn Brakman brings a gender-specific perspective to the care of elderly parents.

A Patient in the Family: An Ethics of Medicine and Families by Hilde Lindemann Nelson and James Lindemann Nelson (Routledge, 1995) is one of the first books to deal specifically with the question of families and medical decisions. Mark C. Kuczewski, in "Reconceiving the Family: The Process of Consent in Medical Decisionmaking," *Hastings Center Report* (March–April 1996), argues that bioethicists think about families only in terms of conflicting interests and that this is a mistake resulting from an impoverished notion of informed consent. See also James Lindemann Nelson, "Critical Interests and Sources of Familial Decision-Making Authority for Incapacitated Patients," *Journal of Law, Medicine and Ethics* (vol. 23, no. 2, 1995); Ellen H. Moskowitz, "Moral Consensus in Public Ethics: Patient Autonomy and Family Decisionmaking in the Work of One State Bioethics Commission," *The Journal of Medicine and Philosophy* (vol. 21, no. 2, 1996); and Rosalie A. Kane and Joan D. Penrod, *Family Caregiving in an Aging Society: Policy Perspectives* (Sage Publications, 1995).

ISSUE 3

Should HIV-Infected Surgeons Be Allowed to Operate?

YES: Inge B. Corless, from "Much Ado About Something: The Restriction of HIV-Infected Health-Care Providers," *AIDS and Public Policy Journal* (Summer 1992)

NO: Carson Strong, from "Should Physicians Infected With Human Immunodeficiency Virus Be Allowed to Perform Surgery?" *American Journal of Obstetrics and Gynecology* (May 1993)

ISSUE SUMMARY

YES: Nursing professor Inge B. Corless asserts that a single-minded emphasis on restricting the practice of an HIV-infected health care worker rather than insistence on universal protections to prevent infection actually puts patients at greater risk for transmission of infection.

NO: Philosopher Carson Strong argues that physicians infected with HIV should be restricted from procedures involving risks of patient exposure great enough to require informed consent or, at the least, procedures involving an open wound.

Among the more than 500,000 cases of AIDS reported in the United States to date, only six have been documented as cases of HIV transmission from a health care practitioner to a patient. And of these six—all patients of one dentist, Dr. David Acer—only one has come to symbolize public fears about this mode of transmission. That patient was Kimberly Bergalis, a 23-year-old Florida woman who died in 1991 of her disease after making impassioned pleas to legislators and public health officials to take action to prevent another case like hers. By the end of 1994 three other patients had died.

Despite extensive investigations, the Centers for Disease Control and Prevention (CDC), the federal agency responsible for monitoring disease spread and transmission in the United States, has not been able to determine definitively just what it was about Dr. Acer or the way he practiced dentistry that resulted in HIV transmission. Nevertheless, what had before been just a theoretical risk became a reality.

The CDC estimates the risk that a patient will contract HIV infection from an HIV-infected surgeon during an operation as between 1 in 42,000 and 1 in 420,000. This is less than the risk of dying because of the general anesthesia used in the operation (1 in 10,000) and about the same as the risk of contracting

HIV infection after the transfusion of blood that has been screened for the virus (1 in 60,000).

Although extensive "look-back" studies conducted among 19,000 former patients of 57 physicians who have died of AIDS (as of March 1993) have not shown any cases of transmission from doctor to patient, these studies may have missed some cases of transmission. The CDC estimates that by 1991 between 3 and 28 patients had been infected by surgeons and between 10 and 100 by dentists. Transmission from HIV-infected patients to health care practitioners is much more likely to occur. That risk is about 1 in 330.

Public opinion responded swiftly to the news about the dentist's HIV transmission and especially to the dramatic entreaties of Kimberly Bergalis. Public opinion polls showed strong support for mandatory testing of health care professionals, required disclosure of HIV infection status, and restrictions on professionals' practices.

In July 1991 the CDC recommended that "health care workers who perform exposure-prone invasive procedures should know their HIV antibody status." It rejected mandatory testing of health care professionals because the risk to patients was too low to justify this massive diversion of resources. Although some medical organizations, such as the American Medical Association, supported restrictions on HIV-infected professionals, many others rejected the CDC's recommendations. No professional group would agree to construct a list of "exposure-prone" invasive procedures because of the difficulty in defining this category in any scientific way.

The arguments for and against restricting the practice of HIV-infected professionals have several ethical dimensions: the basis of the doctor-patient relationship; the obligations of professionals to their patients to prevent harm; patients' rights of autonomy, including the right to full disclosure by the health care provider of relevant information; and the right of professionals to privacy and to be protected from discrimination based on prejudice and political pressure.

In the following selections, Inge B. Corless suggests that emphasis on a health care worker's HIV status is the wrong way to protect patients, who are much more at risk from other aspects of surgery. She stresses the importance of universal protections to prevent transmission of all infections as the most scientifically based method. Carson Strong, on the other hand, presents an ethical view that relies on the doctrine of informed consent. If the procedure is serious enough to require informed consent, an HIV-infected physician should be restricted from performing it. This would, in essence, bar HIV-infected surgeons from operating.

YES

Inge B. Corless

MUCH ADO ABOUT SOMETHING: THE RESTRICTION OF HIV-INFECTED HEALTH-CARE PROVIDERS

It is a relief to be able to say about some stressful event, "It was much ado about nothing." Such words, however, cannot be uttered in response to the putative transmission of the human immunodeficiency virus (HIV) to 5 patients by Dr. David Acer of Stuart, Florida.[1] The Acer case is indeed much ado about something; but it is the potential consequences of the way that "something" has been framed, the response to that "something," that are as dire as the events that precipitated the concern.

The facts as outlined by the Centers for Disease Control (CDC) are that 5 patients from 1 dental practice, with no other known risk factor apart from treatment by an HIV-infected dentist, became HIV-antibody positive.[2] State-of-the-art laboratory analysis by Gerald Myers of Los Alamos indicates an isomorphism in the proviral DNA sequences sampled from Dr. Acer and the 5 patients (notably in the C2-V3 region of gp 120 of the lymphocytes) —an isomorphism far greater than that observed between this group and 2 other patients from the practice with known risk factors, and 35 other HIV-antibody-positive persons residing within 90 miles.[3]

Questions have been raised about the methods employed in the CDC-Los Alamos analysis. The initial questions are about the representativeness of the local controls and the manner in which samples from these individuals were processed. Given Dr. Acer's reported penchant from privacy, should the control group also have included individuals outside the immediate area, such as individuals from Key West?[4] Time since initial infection may have been another important variable to be considered in selecting the local controls.[5] Variations in scientific method, notably the omission of the cloning step in the analysis of the samples from the local controls, introduced what may be an important source of variance.[6] Smith and Waterman also question the appropriateness of using the Wilcoxon rank-sum test, given that the date used failed to meet the assumptions of the test.[7]

The scientists at Los Alamos and CDC used several approaches to examine these complex questions and did so under the pressure of time. The difficulty is that if the method used led to a failure to uncover similarities between the dentist, the 5 patients and the controls, that failure is very serious in that it would have led to the wrong conclusions.

What does seem certain at this time is that the viral strains infecting Dr. Acer and the 5 patients were closely related. What remains a matter for dispute, in addition to some of the methodological issues, is the mode of transmission. It is known that the disinfection technique used in the practice did not meet accepted standards; that is, among other breaks in technique including re-use of gloves, instruments were reported to have been immersed in an unspecified disinfectant for variable lengths of time.[8] It is also known that the instruments used for patients were employed as well in providing dental care to Dr. Acer.[9] A review of Dr. Acer's medical records revealed that he was diagnosed with Kaposi's sarcoma following a biopsy of the palate.[10] The significance of this particular diagnosis for HIV transmission, if any, has not been considered in the CDC's discussion of the case. Moreover, at least 1 of Dr. Acer's sexual partners was also a patient in the practice. So much is known.

What is not known is how the transmission occurred.[11] Dr. Jaffe of the CDC is dubious of ever being able to determine the mode of transmission in the Acer case.[12] Meanwhile, the debate over preventive efforts has formed the basis for unprecedented political harangue and policy formulation.

The American Medical Association and the American Dental Association have asked their HIV-antibody-positive members to refrain voluntarily from engaging in invasive exposure-prone procedures.[13] The Centers for Disease Control's response to the potential for transmission of the human immunodeficiency virus in the health–care setting was to ask professional organizations to identify exposure-prone practices during which viral transmission might occur if there were injury to an HIV-infected health-care worker (HCW).[14] ...

Although prevention of inadvertent HIV transmission to patients is professionally obligatory, the means proposed are questionable. In its most recent formulation, the conditions for practice for an HIV-antibody-positive HCW will be determined by a committee composed of the health-care worker's personal physician, a specialist in infectious diseases with expertise in the epidemiology of HIV and HBV transmission, a health professional with expertise in the procedures performed by the health-care worker, and state or local public-health official(s).[15] In an earlier discussion of the management of HIV-infected workers, the CDC indicated that the infected worker's personal physician and the employer's medical advisors could make the decision as to the worker's scope of practice.[16]

Barring HIV-positive professionals from exposure-prone procedures as identified by health professionals with expertise in these procedures can be accomplished only if everyone is tested periodically or if everyone who suspects he or she is HIV-antibody positive obtains testing and, if positive or has reason to believe that he or she may be infected, voluntarily withdraws or is prohibited from engaging in invasive procedures, or both. That is, testing would be done repeatedly, and infected health-care workers would be mandated not to engage in exposure-prone invasive procedures.

There are numerous problems associated with the determination of HIV status and of conditions for practice. The American Nurses Association, the American Medical Association, and the World Health Organization have issued proclamations opposing mandatory HIV testing of nurses and physicians.[17] Another approach, self-exclusion from practice requires individual knowledge of antibody status. Moreover, even if each individual in the health-care profession who thought he or she might have been privy to even the smallest risk were to seek testing voluntarily, some HIV-infected professionals would still test antibody negative due to the window period (prior to the manifestation of HIV antibodies in the blood) or to problems with the test itself, or they would falsely test antibody positive, with a host of attendant problems.

The level of safety currently proposed for HIV-positive health-care providers who engage in invasive procedures is a standard, in some instances, that is greater than that for the screening of blood for transfusion. The CDC estimates the probability of HIV transmission as 1 in 263,158 to 1 in 2,631,579 during dental procedures in which bleeding may occur; and 1 in 41,667 to 1 in 416,667 during surgery performed by an HIV-infected surgeon.[18] Lowenfels and Wormser estimate the probability of HIV transmission from an HIV-infected surgeon to be 1 chance in 83,000 per hour of surgery with upper and lower bounds of 1 in 500,000 and 1 in 28,000.[19] When the HIV status of the surgeon is unknown, the risk is estimated to be 1 in 20 million.[20] The risk of becoming HIV "infected through blood or blood products is between 1 in 100,000 and 200,000," with

estimates as high as 1 in 60,000 per unit of transfused blood, even with prior negative screening results.[21] In either case, and with a clearer danger in the instance of the blood transfusion given the size of the potential inoculum, some persons who are HIV infected won't be detected for the previously mentioned reasons. A recent study by Conley and Holmberg found 15 persons who were infected through blood that had tested antibody negative.[22] To put these arguments regarding risks in perspective, the industry standard for manufacturing defects in condoms is 4 in 1,000![23]

The emphasis on conditions of practice, namely whether the practitioner engages in invasive exposure-prone procedures, avoids the question of fitness for practice. The occurrence of HIV-positive serostatus automatically assigns the health-care worker borderline status, wherein fitness for practice will be determined by the practice rather than the fitness. Were the emphasis given to functional capacity, the question would be similar to that for HIV testing; that is, how frequently should functional capacity be assessed? Although at first blush that may appear to be a thorny issue, an open and continuing dialogue among health-care worker, personal physician, and supervisor would allow for adjustments if and when they were appropriate.

The current emphasis on serostatus and invasive exposure-prone procedures, even without lists determined by professional organizations or the Centers for Disease Control, provides a simplistic solution that runs roughshod over the rights of health-care providers. This solution to a political problem will have multiple repercussions as organizations rush to comply with a legislative mandate that states adopt the CDC requirements or develop equivalent guidelines....

What is perplexing is that this rage to limit practice by HIV-antibody professionals is based on what is essentially one case—albeit a case involving transmission to 5 individuals. The grief of those individuals and their families and friends, however, will not be eliminated or assuaged by ill-considered actions. Douard argues that the "sloppy habits" of one health-care worker ought not to be used to develop policy for other HIV-infected health-care professionals.[24]

In other documented instances of HIV-antibody-positive health-care providers, no instances of provider-to-patient transmission have been uncovered.[25] ... As stated in a special communication by a joint committee of the Association for Practitioners in Infection Control and the Society of Hospital Epidemiologists of America, "The occurrence of a single case, or even of rare epidemiologically unrelated cases, of HCW-to-patient transmission of HIV should not be the basis upon which policy is drawn.[26] ...

Current calls for self-disclosure and withdrawal from invasive procedures will have more professional and personal consequences on health-care providers if such calls are not accompanied by opportunities for retraining. Moreover, various health-sciences disciplines may prohibit HIV-positive individuals from admission to their programs. Schools of medicine, dentistry, nursing, and perhaps even pharmacy may determine that seropositive status with regard to certain viruses constitutes ineligibility for admission. Such a determination may deprive society of highly motivated individuals interested in careers in health care.

An additional area for concern is that if HIV-positive individuals are prohibited from engaging in invasive procedures and perhaps even in health care in general, a negative message will be conveyed to all health-care professionals. Will those individuals who engage in professionally appropriate behavior by providing care to persons with HIV disease be concerned that occupationally sustained infection will be compounded by professionally imposed unemployment? Will health-care workers not seek health care, lest they discover they are, in fact, HIV seropositive? Will such delays result in more rapid downhill trajectories? Will concerns about unemployment lead to delays in obtaining health care?

The Federation of State Medical Boards considers it to be professional misconduct for those engaged in exposure-prone procedures not to know their HIV status.[27] Given that the federation represents licensing and disciplinary boards, health-care workers are threatened with a potential loss of license for failure to know their status. But how frequently will testing be necessary to avoid being out of compliance, and will the potential loss of employment pose the greater threat? If voluntary compliance is deemed desirable, then at the very least employment counseling and worker's compensation insurance must be provided for professionals in training as well as for professionally qualified practitioners who become disabled as a result of occupational practice. A similar program of counseling and retraining, minus the worker's compensation, would be helpful to all health-care providers who are HIV-antibody positive. Such counseling is provided to doctors and other health-care workers by the Medical Expertise Retention Program on a volunteer basis.[28]

But more is necessary. Science must be used as the basis for decision making in scientific issues. It is all too tempting to "play" to different audiences to achieve goals unrelated to the issue at hand. Unfortunately, a variety of agendas is being realized with this issue. Groups whose concerns are with individuals associated with various transmission groups may find an opportunity in the response to the Acer situation to enact programs of stigmatization and quarantine. HIV-infected individuals may consider these discussions to be yet one more instance of discrimination. While the discrimination may result from the political machinations associated with this situation, it is not inherent in the issue.

The issue is still what to do about something; after all, 5 people were infected with the human immunodeficiency virus in what appears to be professional negligence of some sort. As mentioned before, the emphasis needs to be on disinfection procedures and the use of universal precautions. Only such procedures will protect the public from fomite transmission, whether the source is a health-care providers or another patient. The current single-minded emphasis on the HIV-infected health-care provider actually puts patients at greater risk for transmission of infection from other patients. Adequate disinfection interrupts the chain of events that can result in patient-to-patient transmission; exclusion of seropositive health-care providers does not.

New York State's policy regarding the HIV-infected health-care worker incorporates this broader perspective by requiring training in infection control of all personnel who engage in invasive procedures as a condition for licensure, renewal of licensure, or certification.[29] The policy also contains a voluntary evaluation process that examines functional capacity and ability to comply with infection-control guidelines, among other factors.[30] This policy takes a constructive approach and appears to protect both health-care worker and patient.

The patient's right to know about conditions that could influence his or her decision making about certain health-care risks is vouchsafed by the notion of informed consent, although this concept has been applied to procedures rather than to conditions of practice. Just as the American Medical Association, as a matter of prudence (and ethics), advocates that the medical profession "err on the side of protecting patients,"[31] so too will patients as a matter of prudence err on the side of protecting themselves and their loved ones.[32] Ginzburg discusses the case of an HIV-infected surgeon whose patients, on learning of his HIV status, sought other health-care providers.[33] The effect for many health-care workers who are HIV positive and who are involved in invasive procedures, given the fear of HIV infection, will be the requirement to disclose their status to their patients or withdraw from invasive procedures (read practice) and possibly to engage in retraining.[34] A change in specialty occurs with other instances of health-care-worker impairment and is not limited to HIV disease. The argument here, however, is that HIV-antibody-positive serostatus is not necessarily equivalent to health-care-worker impairment. When health-care workers are truly impaired, it will be important to enhance employee support and retraining programs.

Focusing on a given professional's HIV status obfuscates other issues associated with illness care. The most important issues for the potential surgery patient are the numbers of persons who survive surgery, who develop iatrogenic conditions, or who survive six months after treatment by a given surgeon or physician in a given hospital. The patient clearly has the right to know about such relevant considerations for informed decision making, regardless of the practitioner's HIV status.

Daniels presents a cogent argument that the absence of practice restrictions on HIV-infected health-care workers results in fewer cases of provider-to-patient transmission than would occur if such restrictions were instituted.[35] The emphasis given by national political figures on protecting the patient from the HIV-infected health-care provider thus misdirects efforts and resources away from activities that would do the most to protect the health of the public—namely the procedures that emphasize good infection-control practice. The argument here is not intended to negate the rights of the patient nor to suggest that the health-care professional can do no wrong. Rather, this article stresses the importance of science in developing policy and abjures the mayhem and mischief of ill-considered action. Hippocrates, who is oft quoted for asserting that the doctor first and foremost do no harm, also said: "Science and opinion are two different things; science is the father of knowledge but opinion breeds ignorance."[36]

The responsibility of health-care professionals is to use science to benefit humanity. Pandering to what is politic rather than deriving policy from a foundation of science may accelerate careers, but it also betrays the trust of the public. The scientific evidence to date strongly suggests the importance of emphasizing effective disinfection practices and strict adherence to universal precautions lest we succumb to ignorance and ill-considered action.

NOTES

1. Centers for Disease Control (henceforth, CDC). "Possible Transmission of Human Immunodeficiency Virus to a Patient During an Invasive Dental Procedure," *Morbidity & Mortality Weekly Report* 39 (1990):489–93; G. Friedland, "HIV Transmission from Health Care Workers," *AIDS Clinical Care* 3, no. 4 (1991):29–30; "Changed Climate Clouds Debate," *AIDS Information Exchange* 3 (1991):5.

2. CDC, "Update: Transmission of HIV Infection During Invasive Dental Procedures—Florida," *Morbidity & Mortality Weekly Report* 40, no. 23 (1991):377–81.

3. CDC, "Update Transmission of HIV Infection"; C.Y. Ou, C.A. Ciesielski, G. Myers, *et al.*, "Molecular Epidemiology of HIV Transmission in a Dental Practice," *Science* 256 (22 May 1992): 1165–71.

4. A. Novick. Private communication with author, 3 June 1992.

5. T. F. Smith and M. S. Waterman, "The Continuing Case of the Florida Dentist," *Science* 256 (22 May 1992): 1155–56.

6. *Ibid.*, 1156; J. Palca, "CDC Closes the Case of the Florida Dentist," *Science* 256 (22 May 1992); 1130–31.

7. Smith and Waterman, "The Continuing Case."

8. D. Marianos, B. Gooch, L. Furman, *et al.*, "HIV Transmission and Infection Control in the Office of a Dentist with AIDS," in *Seventh International Conference on AIDS: Abstract Book*, vol. 1 (Florence, Italy: Seventh International Conference on AIDS, 1991), M.C. 3071; "Staff Unaware of Acer's Infection," *AIDS Alert* 6, no. 7 (July 1991):135–36.

9. "Portrait of the Infected Provider," *AIDS Alert* 6, no. 7 (July 1991):130–39.

10. C. Ciesielski, D. Marianos, and C. Y. Ou, "Transmission of Human Immunodeficiency Virus in a Dental Practice," *Annals of Internal Medicine*, 116, no. 10 (15 May 1992):798–805.

11. H. Jaffe, O. Cy, C. Ciesielski, *et al.*, "HIV Transmission to Patients During Dental Care," In *Seventh International Conference on AIDS: Abstract Book*, vol. 2, no 84 (Florence, Italy: Seventh International Conference on AIDS, 1991), TH.D. 110; D. L. Breo, "The 'Slippery Slope': Handling HIV-infected Health Workers," *Journal of the American Medical Association* 264, no. 11 (1990):1464–65.

12. H. Jaffe, "Comment During Workshop on Health Care Workers Issues II," in *Seventh International Conference on AIDS: Abstract Book*, vol. 2 (Florence, Italy: Seventh International Conference on AIDS, 1991), D. 13.

13. American Medical Association, "AMA Statement on HIV Infected Physicians," *Newsletter: American Medical Association* 8, no. 3 (1991):1–2.

14. CDC, "Process for Identifying Exposure-prone Invasive Procedures," *Morbidity & Mortality Weekly Report* 40, no. 32 (1991):565; CDC, "Recommendations for Preventing Transmission of Human Immunodeficiency Virus and Hepatitis B Virus to Patients During Exposure-Prone Invasive Procedures," *Morbidity & Mortality Weekly Report* 40, no. RR-8 (1991):1–9.

15. CDC, "Recommendations for Preventing Transmission of Human Immunodeficiency Virus and Hepatitis B Virus to Patients During Exposure-prone Invasive Procedures," 5.

16. CDC, "Guidelines for Prevention of Transmission of Human Immunodeficiency Virus and Hepatitis B. Virus to Health-care and Public Safety Workers," *Morbidity & Mortality Weekly Report* 38, no. s-6 (1989): 9.

17. B. Russell, "Testimony of the American Nurses Association on Risks of Transmission of Bloodborne Pathogens to Patients during Invasive Procedures" (Paper delivered on behalf of the American Nurses Association, 21 February 1991, at the CDC); American Medical Association, "Ethical Issues Involved in the Growing AIDS Crisis: Council on Ethical and Judicial Affairs," *Journal of the American Medical Association* 259 (1988):1360–61; World Health Organization, *Report of a Consultation on the Prevention of HBV-HIV Transmission in the Health Care Setting* (Geneva: WHO/GPA/DIR/91.5, 11–12 April 1991), 9.

18. The US Conference of Mayors, "CDC Estimates Number of Patients Infected by HCW's," *AIDS Information Exchange* 8, no. 3 (June 1991):11; M. E. Chamberland and D. M. Bell, "HIV Transmission from Health Care Worker to Patient: What Is the Risk?" *Annals of Internal Medicine* 116, no. 10 (15 May 1992):871–73.

19. A. B. Lowenfels and G. Wormser, "Risk of Transmission of HIV From Surgeon to Patient," *New England Journal of Medicine* 325, no. 12 (1991):883–89.

20. N. Daniels, "HIV-Infected Professionals, Patient Rights, and the 'Switching Dilemma'," *Journal of the American Medical Association* 267, no. 10 (1992):1368–71.

21. T. H. Murray, "The Poisoned Gift," *Milbank Quarterly* 68, Supplement 2 (1990):205–25; B. Lo and R. Steinbrook, "Health Care Workers Infected with the Human Immunodeficiency Virus," *Journal of the American Medical Association* 267, no. 8 (1992): 1101.

22. L. J. Conley and S. D. Holmberg, "Transmission of AIDS from Blood Screened Negative for Antibody to the Human Immunodeficiency Virus," *New England Journal of Medicine* 326, no. 22 (28 May 1992): 1499–1500.

23. CDC, "Condoms for Prevention of Sexually Transmitted Diseases," *Morbidity & Mortality Weekly Report* 37, no. 9 (1988):134–35.

24. J. Douard, "HIV+ Health Care Workers: Ethical Problem or Social Problem?" *AIDS and Public Policy Journal* 6, no. 4 (Winter 1991):175–80.

25. B. Mishu, W. Schaffner, J. M. Horan, *et al.*, "A Surgeon with AIDS," *Journal of the American Medical Association* 264, no. 4 (1990):467–70; J. D. Porter, J. G. Cruickshank, P. H. Gentle, *et al.*, "Management of Patients Treated by Surgeon with HIV Infection," *Lancet* 335 (1990) 113–14; J. J. Sacks, "AIDS in a Surgeon," *New England Journal of Medicine* 313, no. 16 (1985):1017–18; F. P. Armstrong, J. C. Miner, and W. H. Wolfe, "Investigation of a Health Care Worker with Symptomatic Human Immunodeficiency Virus Infection: An Epidemiologic Approach," *Military Medicine* 152, no. 8 (1987):414–18; R. W. Comer, D. R. Myers, C. D. Steadman, *et al.*, "Management Considerations for an HIV Positive Dental Student," *Journal of Dental Education* 55, no. 3 (1991):187–91; CDC, "Investigations of Patients Who Have Been Treated by HIV-Infected Health-Care Workers," *Journal of the American Medical Association* 267, no. 21 (3 June 1992):2864–65.

26. Association of Practitioners in Infection Control and the Society of Hospital Epidemiologists of America, "Position Paper: The HIV-Infected Health Care Worker," *American Journal of Infection Control* 18 (1988):373.

27. Lo and Steinbrook, "Health Care Workers Infected," 1102.

28. Medical Expertise Retention Program, Ben Schatz, Director, 273 Church St., San Francisco, CA 94114, (415) 864–0408.

29. "States Oppose Automatic Restrictions," *AIDS Alert* 7, no. 1 (January 1992): 8.

30. "Infected Workers Evaluated on Several Factors," *AIDS Alert* 7, no. 1 (January 1992): 8.

31. American Medical Association, "AMA Statement," 1–2.

32. Daniels, "HIV-Infected Professionals," 1368–71.

33. H. M. Ginzburg, "The Right of an HIV-Infected Surgeon to Practice—The Behringer Case," *Pediatric AIDS and HIV Infection: Fetus to Adolescent* 2, no. 6 (1991):366–71.

34. D. I. Schulman, "Stigma, Risk and the Florida AIDS Dental Cases," *AIDS Patient Care* 6 no. 1 (February 1992):3–4.

35. Daniels, "HIV-Infected Professionals," 1368–71.

36. J. Chadwick and W. Mann, *The Medical Works of Hippocrates* (Oxford: Blackwell Scientific Publications, 1950.)

NO

Carson Strong

SHOULD PHYSICIANS INFECTED WITH HUMAN IMMUNODEFICIENCY VIRUS BE ALLOWED TO PERFORM SURGERY?

For physicians in surgical specialties, the possible effects of becoming infected with human immunodeficiency virus (HIV) during one's practice of medicine are illustrated by the case of Dr. William Behringer. He practiced otolaryngology and facial plastic surgery at a hospital in Princeton, New Jersey, and in 1987 was diagnosed as having acquired immunodeficiency syndrome (AIDS).[1,2] The administrators of the hospital where he practiced learned about this, and meetings of the hospital board of directors were held to determine what action to take. The board decided that Dr. Behringer could continue to treat patients but that he should not perform procedures posing any risk of HIV transmission to patients. Accordingly, the board revoked his surgical privileges, against his wishes. Dr. Behringer continued in an office practice, but his surgical privileges were never reinstated. Other cases involving practice restrictions on HIV-infected physicians have arisen, including cases involving obstetrician-gynecologists in residency[3] and private practice.[4] The Centers for Disease Control and Prevention (CDC) has estimated that in the United States > 300 physicians in surgical specialties might currently be HIV positive.[5] This number could increase as the AIDS epidemic continues, and the issue of practice restrictions is likely to remain important. Such restrictions can significantly interfere with a physician's freedom to practice, as in Dr. Behringer's case. A question that should be asked is whether this intrusion is justified by the degree of risk to patients.

An important aspect of this issue is the attitudes of the public toward HIV-positive physicians. In 1988 Gerbert et al.[6] surveyed a nationwide sample of American adults, asking whether they would switch physicians if their doctor were HIV positive. Although this survey occurred before the highly publicized case of Dr. David Acer, the Florida dentist who is believed to have transmitted HIV infection to five of his patients,[7] 56% of respondents stated that they would switch.[6] After the Acer case the percentage increased, according to a similar survey conducted by *Newsweek* and The Gallup Organization.[8]

From Carson Strong, "Should Physicians Infected With Human Immunodeficiency Virus Be Allowed to Perform Surgery?" *American Journal of Obstetrics and Gynecology,* vol. 168, no. 3 (May 1993). Copyright © 1993 by Mosby-Year Book, Inc. Reprinted by permission.

The number who would switch increased to 65%, and an additional 13% stated they would continue treatment but exclude surgery or other invasive procedures. Ninety-five percent of respondents indicated that they would want to be told if their surgeon were HIV positive.[8]

Patient switching also is illustrated by the case of Dr. Behringer. This arose from a failure of the hospital at which he practiced to adequately protect this confidentiality.[1] Dr. Behringer himself had been a patient at the hospital, and his positive HIV test result was recorded in his chart. Word quickly spread among hospital staff that he was HIV positive. From there, word spread to the local community. Physician acquaintances and other friends he had not told about this condition began calling his home to express their condolences. Soon patients began calling his office to cancel appointments and request transfer of medical records. Dr. Behringer lost many patients.[1]

The attitudes of the public toward HIV-positive physicians have been described as irrational[6] and "occasionally hysterical."[9] The public is perceived to have overreacted, given the actual level of risk to patients.[10] However, even if these characterizations are true, they do not preclude the possibility that it is reasonable to restrict surgical procedures by HIV-infected physicians. This can be ascertained only after examining all sides of the issue....

ETHICAL VIEWS

Suppose an HIV-positive physician performs surgery and an accident results in patient exposure to the physician's blood. A question that arises is whether the patient should be told about this after surgery. The answer clearly is yes because the patient needs to know, to be tested and to prevent possible transmission to loved ones. Therefore consideration must be given to the patient's experiences on being told. After receiving the news, the patient will need baseline and periodic follow-up testing. All of this likely will involve considerable anxiety for the patient and the patient's family. Probably, changes in life-style will be needed, such as modifications in sexual activity. For patients of reproductive age, changes in reproductive plans might be considered. This scenario shows that the risks to patients are not limited to the risks of transmission. What often has been overlooked in discussions of this issue is the significant impact of exposure to the physician's blood on the patient's life. The likelihood that such exposure will occur can be estimated with the CDC's probability figures ... $(25/1000 \times 32/100)$, yielding a probability of 8 per 1000 surgical cases.

Although the risk of transmission might arguably be so low that it need not be revealed for informed consent, several considerations support the claim that the risk of exposure is great enough to require informed consent. Patient self-determination is supported by a legal standard of informed consent referred to as the "reasonable person" standard.[11] According to this standard, information should be provided if a reasonable person in the patient's position would find the information relevant to the decision to consent to the proposed treatment.[11] The relevance of information about risks depends on the likelihood that the risk will materialize and the seriousness of the harm that would occur.[11] A risk having a low probability can be relevant when the degree of harm is substantial. Those who have been exposed to HIV-infected blood in the health care setting have attested that the anxiety can be great.[12] Exposure has been described as an "emotional crisis" having a profound impact because of fear of AIDS and uncertainty about HIV infection.[12] A reasonably prudent patient would regard information that the surgeon is infected with HIV relevant to the decision to consent to an invasive surgical procedure because the harms associated with exposure are substantial and a probability of exposure of 8 per 1000 surgical cases, while low, is not negligible. With this information the patient has the option of avoiding this risk while obtaining the therapeutic benefit of the surgery by seeking another physician.

To push the above scenario further, suppose the patient is not told about the physician's seropositivity in advance and then learns that he or she has been exposed to the physician's blood. It seems likely that in a high percentage of such situations a lawsuit will arise. In a recent legal case, damages were awarded for emotional distress for fear of contracting AIDS after exposure to HIV-infected blood.[13] Although that case did not involve a physician, it would be a precedent for cases involving patient exposure to blood of HIV-positive physicians. Thus it is reasonable for hospitals to be concerned about liability involving HIV-positive physicians.

These considerations suggest that revealing a seropositive status is not feasible because the physician's practice likely would be disrupted, but not revealing seropositive status and performing surgery are not acceptable because the patient's right to informed consent would be violated. The only alternative is to restrict the surgical practice of HIV-positive physicians. This suggests that an ethically justifiable view is in the middle ground between the two views discussed here.

A third view, which is in the middle ground, holds that HIV-positive physicians should be restricted from performing some subset of invasive procedures involving a relatively higher risk of transmission. Several commentators have advocated this view,[2,4] and the CDC's July 12, 1991, recommendations[14] are a version of it. The shortcoming of this view is its focus on the risk of transmission rather than exposure. As discussed, it is the risk of exposure that triggers the need to reveal for purposes of informed consent. Because revealing is not feasible and operating without telling is not ethically acceptable, the risk of exposure also triggers the need for restrictions.

Therefore another middle-ground view such as the following seems indicated. HIV-infected physicians should refrain from performing procedures in which the risk of patient exposure to the physician's blood is great enough to require informed consent. If we accept the CDC exposure risk estimate as reasonable given current information, this view implies that HIV-positive physicians should refrain, at the least, from performing surgical procedures involving an open wound. Examples of procedures that the CDC study identified as involving patient exposures include abdominal and vaginal hysterectomy, ovarian cystectomy, and salpingo-oophorectomy.[15] Although cesarean sections were not observed in the CDC study, reports of hepatitis B virus transmission from infected obstetricians to patients during cesarean sections[16] suggest that there is a risk of exposure from HIV-positive physicians during such procedures. Because procedures involving small incisions such as laparoscopy were not observed in the CDC study, exposure risks associated with such procedures remain to be defined. This raises the possibility of exempting procedures involving small incisions from practice restrictions, pending availability of more data. Future empiric studies might help define more precisely those procedures in which the probability of exposure is high enough to trigger restrictions....

COMMENT

If practice restrictions are to be imposed on HIV-infected physicians in surgical specialties, it is necessary to consider what can be done to ameliorate harms to physicians whose practices are restricted. One area needing greater attention is disability insurance. Every physician at risk of acquiring HIV infection should have the opportunity to obtain disability insurance that explicitly covers HIV. Moreover, the amount of compensation should be sufficient to avoid significant loss of income. Another area needing improvement is accommodation and support by coworkers and hospitals. For physicians who are employees, reassignment to job duties not posing risks to patients should be offered by employers, rather than firing physicians because they are seropositive. Although such accommodation is required of employers by the Americans with Disabilities Act,[17] it is less clear that HIV-positive physicians in group practices have such legal protections. In one reported case an HIV-infected gynecologist was forced out of a group practice.[4] A group's desire to protect its practice provides a strong incentive for such action. Unfortunately, accommodation such as permitting an infected group member to continue in an office practice may be difficult given current public attitudes. This underscores the need for public education concerning the risks of exposure and transmission. Finally, greater attention should be given to improving surgical instruments and techniques[18] to reduce the risks of injury to patients and physicians, where possible.

REFERENCES

1. *Estate of Behringer v Medical Center at Princeton*, 592 A2d 1251 (NJ Super Ct Law Div 1991).
2. Orentlicher D. HIV-infected surgeons: Behringer v Medical Center. JAMA 1991;266:1134–7.
3. *Application of Milton S. Hershey Medical Center*, 595 A2d 1290 (Pa Super Ct 1991).
4. Gostin L. The HIV-infected health care professional: public policy, discrimination, and patient safety. Law Med Health Care 1990;18:303–10.
5. Centers for Disease Control. Estimates of the risk of endemic transmission of hepatitis B virus and human immunodeficiency virus to patients by the percutaneous route during invasive surgical and dental procedures. Atlanta: Centers for Disease Control, 1991.
6. Gerbert B, Maguire BT, Hulley SB, Coates TJ. Physicians and acquired immunodeficiency syndrome: what patients think about human immunodeficiency virus in medical practice. JAMA 1989;262:1969–72.
7. Ciesielski C, Marianos D, Ou C-Y, et al. Transmission of human immunodeficiency virus in a dental practice. Ann Intern Med 1992;116:798–805.
8. Kantrowitz B, Springer K, McCormick J, et al. Doctors and AIDS. Newsweek 1991 July 1:48–57.
9. Dickey NW. Physicians and acquired immunodeficiency syndrome: a reply to patients. JAMA 1989;262:2002.
10. Barondess JA. Working Group Convened by the New York Academy of Medicine. The risk of contracting HIV infection in the course of health care. JAMA 1991;265:1872–3.
11. *Henderson v Milobsky*, 595 F2d 654 (DC Cir 1978).
12. Henry K, Thurn J. HIV infection in healthcare workers. Postgrad Med 1991;89:30–8.
13. *Johnson v West Virginia University Hospitals, Inc.*, 413 SE2d 889 (W Va 1991).
14. Centers for Disease Control. Recommendations for preventing transmission of human immunodeficiency virus and hepatitis B virus to patients during exposure-prone invasive procedures. MMWR 1991;40:1–9.

15. Tokars JI, Bell DM, Culver DH, et al. Percutaneous injuries during surgical procedures. JAMA 1992;267:2899–904.
16. Lettau LA, Smith JD, Williams D, et al. Transmission of hepatitis B with resultant restriction of surgical practice. JAMA 1986;255:934–7.
17. Americans with Disabilities Act of 1990. Pub L No. 101–336, 104 Stat 327.
18. Burget GC, Orane AM, Teplica D. HIV-infected surgeons. JAMA 1992;267:803.

POSTSCRIPT

Should HIV-Infected Surgeons Be Allowed to Operate?

In December 1993 an Australian case was reported in which four patients were infected with HIV in a doctor's office. The doctor was not HIV-infected, but one of his patients was and he failed to sterilize his instruments. This case reemphasized the need for infection control measures to prevent patient-to-patient transmission.

In June 1992 the Centers for Disease Control and Prevention (CDC) backed away from its earlier proposals to establish a list of "exposure-prone" invasive procedures, although it did not withdraw the plan. Instead it deferred to state and local health departments in deciding on a case-by-case basis what types of care can be provided by HIV-infected health care professionals. This decision was also criticized because it left open the possibility of widely divergent policies being adopted and because it abdicated the CDC's national leadership role. Some states, such as New York, have developed policies that emphasize mandatory infection control training as a condition of licensing and relicensing and voluntary counseling and testing.

Florida has enacted legislation that allows health care professionals whose practices have been restricted because of their HIV status to be covered by disability health insurance if they have lost income. Laws in Iowa, Alabama, and Oklahoma establish review panels to determine what procedures an individual HIV-infected professional may not perform. Illinois law allows the State Health Department to notify the former patients of health care workers who have been diagnosed with AIDS.

In April 1991, in the case of Behringer v. Medical Center, a New Jersey trial court upheld a hospital's decision to restrict the surgical privileges of a doctor with AIDS. At the same time it ruled that the hospital had violated Dr. Behringer's confidentiality by failing to take reasonable precautions to prevent his AIDS diagnosis from becoming publicly known. This case is discussed in David Orentlicher, "HIV-Infected Surgeons: Behringer v. Medical Center," Journal of the American Medical Association (August 28, 1991).

One "look-back" study of the patients of an HIV-infected surgeon concluded that "the risk of HIV transmission during surgery may be so small that it will be quantified only by pooling data from multiple, methodologically similar investigations" (Audrey Smith Rogers et al., "Investigation of Potential HIV Transmission to the Patients of an HIV-Infected Surgeon," Journal of the American Medical Association, April 14, 1993). The controversy has produced a flood of articles, most of them opposing mandatory restrictions on HIV-infected health care workers. See Norman Daniels, "HIV-Infected

Professionals, Patient Rights, and the 'Switching Dilemma,'" *Journal of the American Medical Association* (March 11, 1992) for an ethical analysis concluding that all patients would be worse off if they switched to uninfected practitioners. Also see Leonard H. Glantz, Wendy K. Mariner, and George J. Annas, "Risky Business: Setting Public Health Policy for HIV-Infected Health Care Professionals," *The Milbank Quarterly* (vol. 70, no. 1, 1992); Bernard Lo and Robert Steinbrook, "Health Care Workers Infected With the Human Immunodeficiency Virus," *Journal of the American Medical Association* (February 26, 1992); and Mark Barnes et al., "The HIV-Infected Health Care Professional: Employment Policies and Public Health," *Law, Medicine and Health Care* (Winter 1990).

For arguments supporting at least some level of restriction, see Larry Gostin's "The HIV-Infected Health Care Professional: Public Policy, Discrimination, and Patient Safety," *Law, Medicine and Health Care* (Winter 1990) and "HIV-Infected Physicians and the Practice of Seriously Invasive Procedures," *Hastings Center Report* (January–February 1989), and Albert R. Jonsen, "Is Individual Responsibility a Sufficient Basis for Public Confidence?" *Archives of Internal Medicine* (April 1991). See also Gordon G. Keyes, "Health Care Professionals With AIDS: The Risk of Transmission Balanced Against the Interests of Professionals and Institutions," *Journal of College and University Law* (Spring 1990).

See also Mary E. Chamberland et al., "Health Care Workers With AIDS: National Surveillance Update," *Journal of the American Medical Association* (December 25, 1991); Richard N. Danila et al., "A Look-Back Investigation of Patients of an HIV-Infected Physician," *The New England Journal of Medicine* (November 14, 1991); and Troyen Brennan, "Transmission of the Human Immunodeficiency Virus in the Health Care Setting—Time for Action," *The New England Journal of Medicine* (May 21, 1991). For another debate on the issue, see Kenneth A. De Ville, "Nothing to Fear but Fear Itself: HIV-Infected Physicians and the Law of Informed Consent," *Journal of Law, Medicine and Ethics* (Summer 1994) and, in the same issue, Donald H. J. Hermann, "Commentary: A Call for Authoritative CDC Guidelines for HIV-Infected Health Care Workers."

In an article entitled "Human Immunodeficiency Virus-Infected Health Care Workers: The Restoration of Professional Authority," *Archives of Family Medicine* (February 1996), law professor Scott Burris argues that since judges and regulators have not been able to agree on a binding standard, the medical professional has a second chance to formulate a socially responsible, nonrestrictive policy.

An excellent source for HIV-related medical and policy information can be found at the following Web site of the *Journal of the American Medical Association:* http://www.ama-assn.org/special/hiv/hivhome.htm. This site also contains an ethics update.

PART 2

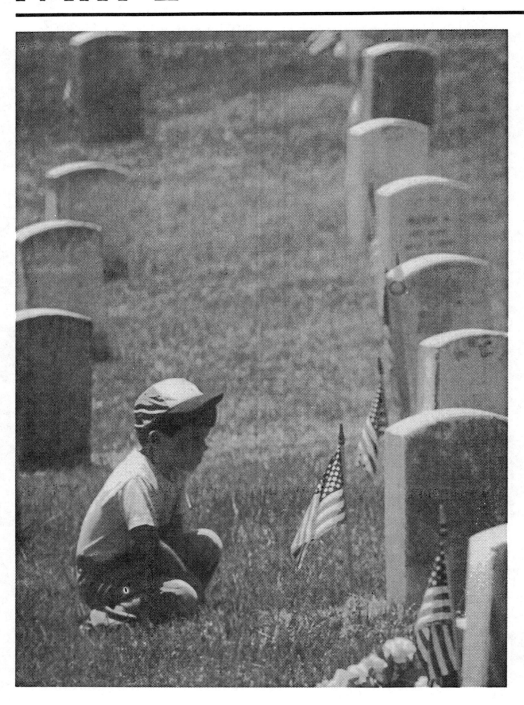

Death and Dying

What are the ethical responsibilities associated with death? Doctors are sworn "to do no harm," but this proscription is open to many different interpretations. Death is a natural event that can, in some instances, be hastened to put an end to suffering. Is it ethically necessary to prolong life at all times under all circumstances? Medical personnel as well as families often face these agonizing questions. Even the question of whether or not to tell terminally ill patients the truth about their conditions has great ethical implications. The right of an individual to decide his or her own fate may conflict with society's interest in maintaining the value of human life or in not wasting valuable resources that could be used to save other lives. This conflict is apparent in the matter of physician-assisted suicide and, in a different way, in the question of "futile" treatment. This section examines some of these anguishing questions.

- Are Some Advance Directives Too Risky for Patients?

- Should Physicians Be Allowed to Assist in Patient Suicide?

- Is It Ethical to Withhold the Truth from Dying Patients?

- Should Doctors Be Able to Refuse Demands for "Futile" Treatment?

ISSUE 4

Are Some Advance Directives Too Risky for Patients?

YES: Christopher James Ryan, from "Betting Your Life: An Argument Against Certain Advance Directives," *Journal of Medical Ethics* (vol. 22, 1996)

NO: Steven Luttrell and Ann Sommerville, from "Limiting Risks by Curtailing Rights: A Response to Dr. Ryan," *Journal of Medical Ethics* (vol. 22, 1996)

ISSUE SUMMARY

YES: Psychiatrist Christopher James Ryan argues that advance directives that refuse active treatment in situations when a patient's incompetence is potentially reversible should be abolished because healthy people are likely to underestimate their desire for treatment should they become ill.

NO: Geriatricians Steven Luttrell and Ann Sommerville assert that respect for the principle of autonomy requires that individuals be permitted to make risky choices about their own lives and that ignoring autonomous choices made by competent adults reinstates the outmoded notion of medical paternalism.

Since ancient times people have drawn up wills to determine what should be done with their property, or who should take custody of their children, after they die. In 1969 Luis Kutner, a law professor, proposed a "living will," a document that would determine the course of medical treatment should the signer become unable to express his or her wishes. A typical living will stated, "If I am permanently unconscious or there is no reasonable expectation for my recovery from a serious incapacitating or lethal illness or condition, I do not wish to be kept alive by artificial means." The proposal came at a time when the public was just beginning to be aware of the use of machines to keep people breathing and their hearts beating even though there was no possibility of regaining consciousness. In 1975 the Karen Ann Quinlan case, involving a young, permanently unconsciousness woman on a ventilator, focused ethical and legal attention on the unwanted use of medical technology.

In 1976, following the Quinlan case, California enacted the nation's first law approving the use of living wills. Nearly every state in the United States followed suit. Sometimes called "natural death acts," these laws and the wills they approved were so vaguely worded and so difficult to interpret that they were hardly ever effective in achieving their goals. It was difficult, for example, to determine what was meant by "reasonable expectation," "artificial means," or even "lethal illness."

In 1983 the President's Commission for the Study of Ethical Problems in Medicine and Biomedical and Behavioral Research recommended an alternative approach. Rather than signing a document that specified certain treatments that should be forgone, patients were encouraged to name a person who would make health care decisions in their place. This "health care proxy," it was believed, would be better able to make a judgment about what the patient would have wished, given the specific medical condition and the alternatives.

There are several types of advance directives. They can be formally written and legally authorized, or they can be informal communications with family members or health care providers. Much of the legal wrangling about withdrawal of life supports has turned on whether or not the patient expressed such desires while competent. The case of Nancy Cruzan, which eventually went to the U.S. Supreme Court, is one example. The parents of this young Missouri woman, who was permanently unconscious after an automobile accident, sued the state to have her life supports removed, claiming that this is what Nancy herself would have wanted. The state argued that there was no clear and convincing evidence that Nancy would have made the same decision. In 1990 the U.S. Supreme Court ruled that states had an interest in preserving life and could require a high standard of evidence of the patient's expressed preference for withdrawing treatment. The case then went back to the Missouri courts, which this time found the evidence convincing and agreed to allow withdrawal of life support.

To add to the weight of the Supreme Court's decision, in 1991 Congress passed the Patient Self-Determination Act (PSDA), which requires all health care providers reimbursed by Medicare to inform patients about their right to sign advance directives. By this measure Congress intended to promote the use of advance directives in hospitals and nursing homes where elderly patients are often treated.

Despite legislative and judicial approval of advance directives and widespread public opinion supporting them, such documents are still rarely signed by competent patients, and even when signed they are still rarely consulted or implemented. Studies have documented barriers such as lack of appropriate communication and physicians' disregard of the wishes expressed in the directives.

The following selections address a more basic issue: the ethical acceptability of a particular kind of advance directive. Christopher James Ryan favors the abolition of advance directives in which a healthy patient chooses withdrawal of active treatment in a future situation in which he or she is incompetent but where the incompetence is potentially reversible. Steven Luttrell and Ann Sommerville assert that advance directives are mostly made by ill patients, who do have a good idea of what they want, and that their autonomous decisions, even when risky, should be respected.

YES

Christopher James Ryan

BETTING YOUR LIFE:
AN ARGUMENT AGAINST
CERTAIN ADVANCE DIRECTIVES

A long time ago, in a country far far away, there lived a very wise old king. The king was a very ethical man and his subjects were very happy. Everyone lived together in perfect harmony and times were generally regarded as good.

One day the king introduced a new law. The law allowed his subjects to enter into a mysterious wager. Those who won the wager would receive a rich reward, but those who lost would be put to death. Entry into the wager was entirely voluntary and despite the dire consequences of losing many took up the challenge. To win, a contestant had only correctly to answer an apparently straightforward question. The question was known to all participants before they entered and all who took up the challenge were sure that they knew the answer and could not lose. Strangely, even the king's ethicists had no objection to the introduction of the law and in fact praised the king for his wisdom and progressiveness. The ethicists also believed that the answer to the question was obvious and focused only on the rich reward.

Unfortunately, however, many contestants got the answer wrong. They lost the wager and were put to an early and needless death. The question, that caused so much difficulty, was this: "Even though you are now well and healthy, imagine yourself in a situation where you have a terminal illness and are temporarily confused or unconscious. Imagine that whilst you are in this state your doctors give you a choice; either will treat you to the best of their ability and you may recover some of your health for some undefined period, or they will treat you conservatively and, though they will ensure that you are in no pain, they will not attempt to save your life. If you were in this situation what would you want the doctors to do?"

Advance directives or living wills frequently require their users to undertake the kind of task set out above; that is, to imagine themselves in a situation where they are required to make a decision about whether or not they should receive active treatment but are incompetent to do so. These have become increasingly popular over the last decade. Legislation giving statutory status

From Christopher James Ryan, "Betting Your Life: An Argument Against Certain Advance Directives," *Journal of Medical Ethics,* vol. 22 (1996), pp. 95–99. Copyright © 1996 by The British Medical Association. Reprinted by permission.

to these directives has been enacted in many parts of the Western world and planned in many others. In places where no such legislation exists living wills are thought to have increasing weight in common law.[1-3]

In this paper I oppose a common form of advance directive on ethical grounds. The basis of my argument is my contention that, like the citizens of the country above, many people who take out advance directives do so under the belief that they know the answer to the question above, when in fact they do not. In order [to] support my position I will first provide evidence which supports this contention and then demonstrate the ethical difficulties this creates for advocates of living wills.

I do not intend to provide opposition to all forms of advance directive, but will restrict my discussion to a fairly narrow but not uncommon set of criteria. I will examine only cases where an advance directive demands that the user receive only conservative or palliative care in a situation where he or she is incompetent to consent to such treatment but where that incompetence is potentially reversible.

GETTING THE ANSWER WRONG

My argument hinges on the notion that people are likely grossly to underestimate their desire to have medical intervention should they become ill; I will therefore explain why this is likely to be so on theoretical grounds and then provide some empirical evidence that suggests that this actually occurs.

Denial is a strong and largely successful mechanism for dealing with the stressors of everyday life. For the healthy person considering a terminal illness it involves the subconscious decision to re-ject the possibility that one will suffer in the way one might be expected to if one were to succumb to such an illness. There are two standard ways of going about this. The first is simply to tell yourself that terminal illnesses are things that happen to other people and that they will not happen to you. This method works reasonably well whilst one is still young and all, or most, of the people that get such illnesses are not like you at all. It starts to lose its power, however, as you grow older and terminal illnesses begin to befall your peers. Now the other people begin to look a lot like you and the only-happens-to-others strategy looks increasingly anaemic.

The second option is to use denial in a slightly more complicated manner and when confronted by the suffering of another in the midst of a terminal illness to say that this would not happen to you because, if you were in that situation, you would kill yourself before the suffering became too great. Here you have traded the real and very distressing possibility that you may develop, and suffer at the hands of, a terminal illness for the hypothetical notion of a future early death. As a hypothetical abstract your early death is unpleasant but much more bearable than the realisation that you could become so ill.

Of course once you have developed a terminal illness, this coping strategy will no longer be successful. Now the possibility of your death is no longer hypothetical and you are faced with balancing real dying with the possibility of real suffering. While there is no doubt that some individuals now decide that they would still be better off dead, I believe that the vast majority of people now decide to battle it out. Most people with terminal illnesses do not want to die and are prepared to put up with a certain amount of suffering in order to live a little longer. Now that death is no longer a hypothetical it holds little appeal and frequently denial is used again, this time to maintain hope that a cure will be found.[4]

Human beings are, I suggest, very poor at determining their attitudes to treatment for some hypothetical future terminal illness and very frequently grossly under-estimate their future desire to go on living.

Though based on psychological theorising, there is some evidence to support this contention. The first piece of evidence is admittedly anecdotal but none the less quite powerful. Healthy people frequently believe that if they were suffering a terminal illness and required various forms of medical intervention they would rather be allowed to slip away. This view is so common among healthy people that it can be regarded as perfectly normal. Among terminally ill people, however, the sustained expression of a preference not to receive treatment is very rare. Most palliative care specialists will readily recall one or two patients who persistently requested that they be allowed to die. Some will recall several. However, palliative care physicians do no report that this sustained desire is very common and certainly do not report that it is the norm. This strongly suggests that many people who, when healthy, predict they would refuse treatment in the future, will change their mind when they develop a terminal illness.

This anecdotal evidence is supported by a number of studies in the psychiatric literature. One such study by Owen *et al* found that among patients with cancer the strongest interest in euthanasia was among those patients being offered potentially curative treatment. Patients with poorer prognoses, who were only being offered palliative care, tended to reject the idea of euthanasia as a future option (p<0.05).[5] Similarly, a 1994 study by Danis *et al*, which examined the stability of future treatment preferences, found that while preferences for most remained stable over the study's two-year duration, people that had been hospitalised, had an accident or had become immobile were likely to change their health care preferences to opt for more intervention.[6] Both studies suggest that having had an episode of serious illness or a deterioration of an existing illness may make people more likely to want more intervention.

Seale and Addington-Hall asked relatives and friends of people who had died whether the dead person would have benefited from an earlier death. They found that respondents, who were not spouses, were frequently willing to say that an earlier death would have been better for the person even though the person who had died had not expressed a desire to die sooner. That is, the healthy relatives and friends were keener on euthanasia than the terminally ill patient had been. This again suggests that healthy people may view euthanasia differently from terminally ill people or at least that it is hard to empathise with the position of the terminally ill.[7]

Though it is not possible directly to equate suicide with a desire for euthanasia, one might expect that if terminally ill people increasingly wanted to die as they became sicker and sicker then suicide among patients with terminal illness would peak towards the end of their illnesses. This would be the time when pain and suffering was at its worst and when there was little to look forward to. In fact, however, completed suicide is most common in the first year after diagnosis in the terminally ill.[8] It may be that in this situation suicide more often represents an irrational reaction to the crisis of diagnosis than a reasoned decision that life has become intolerable.

Further evidence that a desire for euthanasia is uncommon in the terminally ill comes from a study by Brown and co-workers who found that among forty-four terminally ill patients, the only patients who had experienced a desire for an early death were those who were suffering from a clinical depressive illness.[9]

ARGUMENTS IN SUPPORT OF ADVANCE DIRECTIVES

Advocates of this form of advance directive argue for the documents along two lines. Firstly, they take a deontological position that the directives maximise the affected person's autonomy by allowing her some control over her medical management. They argue that since maximisation of autonomy is a legitimate aim and since living wills seem to facilitate the maximisation of autonomy, then living wills are not only ethically justified but beneficial.[10-12] Second, advocates may take a utilitarian line and argue that the directives help to facilitate the death of people who believe they would be better off dead than alive. By facilitating these deaths the directives not only end people's suffering, but spare them an undignified death. In addition the directive may ease the burden on medical staff and family of the ill individual who may find making these decisions painful. Through all these means, they argue, the directive increases the net utility of the community.[10]

Opponents of this form of advance directive usually base their opposition upon an opposition to euthanasia.[13] However, since most living will legislation throughout the world facilitates only passive euthanasia and since passive euthanasia is rarely objected to, there has been little solid opposition to this form of advance directive legislation.

My objections to these advance directives do not rely on an objection to either active or passive euthanasia. Rather my objections are based on the proposition that these living wills do not necessarily increase the user's autonomy nor society's net utility in the unproblematic way they are imagined to do, because people are much more likely to refuse treatment when faced with a future hypothetical scenario than when faced with a real here and now choice. If this contention is accepted it has a number of consequences for arguments used in support of living wills.

CONSEQUENCES FOR THE ARGUMENT FROM AUTONOMY

The principle of a right to autonomy holds that adult human beings have the right to make decisions about their lives and so direct the course of their own fate. The right to autonomy is a powerful maxim. It is the right to autonomy that underlies the notions of consent, the right to freedom and democracy itself. By grounding their support for directives in this principle proponents of living wills set up a strong case.

It is an accepted part of the principle, however, that one cannot properly exercise one's autonomy if one is not in possession of all available information that might influence one's decisions. A patient's consent to a procedure, for example, is only valid if she has been informed of all the risks and consequences. If the psychological reasoning and empirical evidence above is accepted, then a person currently using a living will does not have access to a vital piece of information that may radically alter her decision. Specifically, she does not know that it is highly likely that her decision, made now, that she would rather die if faced with a hypothetical future scenario is not what her decision would have been if she were actually faced with that scenario.

Almost everyone assumes that he knows his own mind and that he would know the choices he would make in the event of a crisis. While there is little doubt that the individual alone is in the best position to know how he would act and it is also true that some people must correctly guess how they would act, nevertheless evidence strongly suggests that many people simply get it wrong. They believe they would not opt for treatment in a hypothetical future circumstance but were they actually to face the circumstance they would opt for treatment. Most people have no experience of their reactions to a life-threatening illness, they can only guess at their reaction and they frequently guess wrong. More importantly for my argument, people do not believe in, or even know of the possibility of, an inaccurate guess. If users of advance directives do not know of the distinct possibility that their choices may be inaccurate, they lack a vital piece of information and that lack prohibits a fully informed and autonomous choice.

CONSEQUENCES FOR THE UTILITARIAN ARGUMENT

The possibility that a large number of people are dying when they would not have wanted to because of the introduction of advance directives, directly threatens the utilitarian argument offered in support of these directives.

The utilitarian argument draws its strength from the hope that the existence of advance directives will end the suffering of people with terminal illnesses who have decided that they would be better off dead. It is assumed that they have come to this opinion by weighing up the benefits of their continued existence with the pain and suffering of their terminal illness. There is an additional hidden assumption that the affected individuals can accurately estimate this balance from the safety of health and happiness prior to their illness. If this additional assumption is unjustified then the utilitarian argument is undermined.

CONCLUSIONS REGARDING LIVING WILLS

With the argument from autonomy and the utilitarian argument both undermined, ethical support for living wills of this sort is seriously diminished. The effect this diminution will have upon one's attitudes to living wills will depend on both the seriousness with which one takes the evidence for the inaccuracy of people's choices and one's beliefs about how well this inaccuracy can be addressed through changes to legislation and education.

At a minimum one should require significant changes in legislation to address users' ignorance of their likelihood of wrong decisions. The principle of autonomy demands that the individual making the choice be given all available relevant information, therefore those making living wills must be informed of the apparent likelihood that their decision to refuse treatment now may not accurately reflect the decision they would make in the future, were they competent at the time. To my knowledge, no piece of living will legislation currently refers to this likelihood. Though there are numerous published advance directive forms and more publications to assist in filling them in, none of them inform the potential user of the likely inaccuracy of their current decision.[10, 11, 14, 15]

While such a change may satisfy strong advocates of advance directives that autonomy is now again maximised, I would remain dubious that this were the case. The logistics of giving such warnings to all people filling in living wills will necessarily mean that the warnings will be scant and superficial. The belief that one knows one's own mind now and in the future is understandably held with some vehemence by most of the community. The psychological needs met by the belief that one would rather be dead in a future tragic situation are strong and deeply ingrained. An insignificant warning is unlikely to have any impact upon this belief and many people will continue falsely to believe they definitely know what they would want in the hypothetical scenario.

This kind of reasoning leads me to believe that it will be practically impossible to allow people to make an autonomous choice about this kind of advance directive and therefore on the grounds that such directives will neither increase autonomy nor increase the community's level of utility I believe that this type of living will should be abolished.

It is important to note that this line of argument will not demand the abandonment of all varieties of advance directive. It will not, for example, apply to advance directives where the ability to consent to treatment is irreversibly lost. In this situation there will be no possibility of the person recovering to give carers a more accurate report of her current desire for treatment. Carers would then be justified in taking their best guess as to the affected individual's preferences, no matter how inaccurate it is likely to be. Moreover, this best guess will be substantially improved if the person has taken out a living will. Neither will it affect advance directives made by people who are already critically ill and who are, for example, giving instruction that they should not be resuscitated in the event of cardiac arrest. These people are already critically ill and therefore are able correctly to determine their preferences for what is essentially their current situation.

The argument applies only to advance directives made by essentially healthy individuals who opt for withdrawal of active care in a situation where their inability to consent is potentially reversible. In these situations, patients should be resuscitated and their opinions regarding future treatment sought again now that they are in the scenario that they had previously only imagined. For some no doubt this will lead to considerable hardship, as they must again state their preference that they would rather be allowed to die, but for others, perhaps the majority, it will provide a safety net and a chance to reconsider their decision with all available information.

Those who would have wished to see the King's wager abolished because of the needless deaths it seemed to cause must be similarly troubled by this form of living will.

REFERENCES

1. Mendelson D. The Medical Treatment (Enduring Power of Attorney) Act and assisted suicide: the legal position in Victoria. *Bioethics News* 1993; **12:** 34–42.
2. Stern K. Living wills in English law. *Palliative Medicine* 1993; **7:** 283–8.
3. Greco PJ, Schulman KA, Lavizzo-Mourey R, Hansen-Flaschen J. The Patient Self-Determination Act and the future of advance directives. *Annals of Internal Medicine* 1991; **115:** 639–43.
4. Kübler-Ross E. *On death and dying.* New York: Macmillan, 1969.
5. Owen C, Tennant C, Levis J. Jones M. Suicide and euthanasia: patient attitudes in the context of cancer. *Psycho-Oncology* 1992; **1:** 79–88.
6. Danis M, Garrett J, Harris R, Patrick DL. Stability of choices about life-sustaining treatments. *Annals of Internal Medicine* 1994; **120:** 567–73.
7. Dillner L. Relatives keener on euthanasia than patients. *British Medical Journal* 1994; *309:* 1107.
8. Allebeck P, Bolund C, Ringback G. Increased suicide rate in cancer patients. *Journal of Clinical Epidemiology* 1989; **42:** 611–6.
9. Brown JH, Henteleff P, Barakat S, Rowe CJ. Is it normal for terminally ill patients to desire death? *American Journal of Psychiatry* 1986; **143:** 208–11.
10. Molloy W, Mepham V, Clarnette R. *Let me decide.* Melbourne: Penguin, 1993.
11. Quill TE. *Death and dignity. Making choices and taking charge.* New York: WW Norton, 1993.
12. Charlesworth M. A good death. In: Kuhse H, ed. *Willing to listen—waiting to die.* Melbourne: Penguin, 1994: 203–16.
13. Marker R. *Deadly compassion. The death of Ann Humphry and the case against euthanisia.* London: Harper Collins, 1994.
14. Humphry D. *Dying with dignity: understanding euthanasia.* New York: Birch Lane Press, 1992.
15. Kennedy L. *Euthanasia.* London: Chatto & Windus, 1990.

NO
Steven Luttrell and Ann Sommerville

LIMITING RISKS BY CURTAILING RIGHTS: A RESPONSE TO DR. RYAN

Decisions about life-sustaining medical treatment should really be left to doctors. That is the core message of "betting your life" by Dr C J Ryan.[1] Although he focuses on only one type of decision—when the patient's mental incompetence is potentially reversible—the implication is that healthy people cannot validly appreciate the dimensions of the risk involved when they seek to limit in advance the scope of their own medical treatment. The danger of such miscalculation is said to be so profound that their right to take the risk must be curtailed for their own good. The general argument is not new. As the House of Lords Select Committee on Medical Ethics noted: "Disabled individuals are commonly more satisfied with their life than able-bodied people expect to be with the disability. The healthy do not choose in the same way as the sick".[2] But does this mean healthy people are to be deprived of the opportunity to make the attempt?

Some of the existing criticism of advance decision-making has been preoccupied with personal identity and the continuity of mind and mental state as the important criteria. According to such arguments, the rupture caused by loss of competence is so great that it makes nonsense of the concept of personal continuity. A competent individual is not making advance decisions for herself but for the future relict of who she once was. Dr Ryan's argument is a variation on this theme and seeks to prove that in advance of disability, people are in such a totally different mind-set that they are "likely to grossly under-estimate their desire for medical intervention should they become ill".[1]

We do not agree with Dr Ryan's view that advance directives dealing with situations where the deterioration in mental capacity is potentially reversible should be abolished and take issue with him on the following points:

(1) His argument hinges on the notion that people are likely to under-estimate substantially their desire to have medical intervention should they become ill. The evidence for this is not convincing. Emanuel *et al* following a prospective study of 495 HIV-positive or oncology out-patients and 102 members of the public concluded that most people made moderately sta-

From Steven Luttrell and Ann Sommerville, "Limiting Risks by Curtailing Rights: A Response to Dr. Ryan," *Journal of Medical Ethics*, vol. 22 (1996), pp. 100–104. Copyright © 1996 by The British Medical Association. Reprinted by permission.

ble treatment choices and that recent hospitalisation did not decrease that stability.[3]

Even if it is the case that in general the sick do not make the same choices as the healthy, there is evidence that this does not apply to people who have completed an advance directive. Although Danis *et al* found that patients who were hospitalised one or more times between baseline and follow-up interviews were more likely to change their choices and desire more treatment, patients who had a living will were more likely to maintain stable preferences. Indeed, patients who had living wills and chose the least amount of care at their initial interview had extremely stable preferences (96 per cent unchanged).[4]

There appears to be little evidence that healthy people consider making treatment decisions in advance. Even in the United States, where living wills have been in existence much longer than in Britain, there is a wide disparity between the large percentage of people who indicate a desire to die without heroic measures and the small percentage who have made advance directives.[5] The scant UK evidence[6] supports American findings that interest in living wills is primarily shown by people who are educated, articulate and already have a diagnosis. (In the USA, the obligation for hospitals to raise the subject of advance decision-making arose only with patients who were checking in for treatment and therefore, by definition, were not a healthy population.) Part of the increased interest in this mechanism in the UK has been as a result of a small but well-informed population of HIV-positive patients witnessing the terminal treatment of friends and partners. Indeed, one of the limitations of advance statements is their lack of ready accessibility to people with differing levels of education, experience and literacy.

(ii) Dr Ryan states that it is an accepted principle that one cannot properly exercise one's autonomy if one is not in possession of all available information that might influence one's decisions and that a patient's consent to a procedure is only valid if she has been informed of all the risks and consequences. We take issue with this view. It implicitly denies the option of consciously deciding from a knowingly incomplete knowledge base and the option to decide validly to allow another person to decide on one's behalf. It is not necessarily obligatory for an individual to know each and every one of the risks implicit in a course of action. Indeed, if this were the case, no person could ever make a valid decision. As human beings, our motivation is often intuitive or emotional as well as cognitive and we sometimes exercise autonomy by choosing not to know or at least not to recognise the full import of our actions. It is arguably not necessary to examine all the implications in order for a person to be clear that she does not want to go on living indefinitely with a restricted range of competency or mobility, even if some small improvement is possible. If applied to other spheres of medicine, Dr Ryan's principle would mean that people cannot make valid decisions about childbearing without taking account of potentially available genetic information or pre-natal testing.

Arguably, therefore, it cannot be assumed that in real life, people who make advance refusals want to know everything or, if having chosen not to be fully informed of every detail, are incapable of understanding the implications of their decision. Nevertheless, the *Code of Practice on Advance Statements*, published by the British Medical Association, sees health professionals as obliged to make all appropriate efforts to raise patients' awareness at the drafting stage about the risks and disadvantages, as well as the benefits, of advance statements.[7] As a matter of law in the UK, a patient's consent to a procedure is valid if he understands in general terms the nature of the intervention. There is no legal obligation to explain *all* the risks and benefits.[8]

(iii) Even if people do make unwise choices, we believe that this should not be used as a reason to curtail their autonomy. Society generally recognises that individuals sometimes make bad or risky choices in the way they shape their lives. In our society, the libertarian legacy of Mill, however, assumes that individual choices should be permitted, unless they impinge on the rights of others. Mill's famous dictum was that "the sole end for which mankind are warranted, individually or collectively, in interfering with the liberty of action of any of their number is self-protection" and that an individual "cannot rightfully be compelled to do or forbear because it will be better for him to do so, because it will make him happier, because in the opinions of others to do so would be wise or even right".[9] So, does it damage the fabric of society or the rights of other people to allow Jehovah's Witnesses, for example, the right to refuse in advance the administration of blood products in all circumstances, even when their condition is curable? Or should they, as Dr Ryan suggests, be forcibly treated and only then "their opinions regarding future treatment be sought again now that they are in the scenario that they had previously only imagined"?[1]

COMMON SENSE

It is trite to observe that people's views change with their circumstances. The philosopher, Parfit, for example, discussing different stages of individual development, talks about "my most recent self", "one of my earlier selves" and "one of my distant selves"; each of these showing a different degree of psychological connectedness with the present self.[10] From a practical perspective, would this mean that greater weight must automatically be attached to an advance directive made comparatively recently by an individual who is still more or less the same self? Common sense would seem to support such a view even if the individual was completely healthy when making the directive and now is in an altered psychological state. Simply acknowledging varying degrees of psychological continuity or disparity with regard to former and future selves does not answer the question of whether it is morally correct for subsequent selves to be treated in contravention of an advance directive reflecting their former interests.

(iv) We believe that a retreat to medical paternalism is not a practical option in societies increasingly aware of patient charters and consumer rights. Many forms of advance directives offer the drafter a choice of specifying personal instructions and/or nominating a proxy to decide. American surveys show that the option most commonly chosen is for people to select decision-making by a family member or other proxy despite the evidence of a variable correlation between the judgments of nominated proxy decision-makers and the patients' own prior wishes.[11] One study indicated that of 104 patients with life-threatening illness who were offered advance directives, 69 took up the offer and most asked for non-aggressive treatment if "the burdens of treatment outweigh the expected benefits". None, however, gave any other personal instructions,[12] although evidence suggests that proxies are more likely than patients themselves to opt for life-prolonging treatment, ie, to support more conservative choices than the individual would have made if competent and in that situation.[13]

Dr Ryan contests one specific type of advance directive on grounds of utility and autonomy. He argues that it is contrary to utility to permit people to die when their lives could be prolonged and their condition improved. This might be true if utility were a matter of simply prolonging life rather than also a question of maximising happiness and choice and reducing misery, including the misery of families who may see their relative being resuscitated contrary to an informed and competent advance refusal.

TWO AUTONOMIES

Nor is autonomy a simple matter. When an individual is conscious but mentally incapacitated, in Dworkin's view, "two autonomies are in play: the autonomy of the demented patient and the autonomy of the person who became demented. These two autonomies can conflict, and the resulting problems are complex and difficult".[14] Of course, some philosophers solve this by attributing no autonomy to the demented person and recognising the "residual interests" of the previously competent individual as paramount. A range of psychological and philosophical questions arise here about our ability to decide now life and death matters for the people we will be in the future when some part of what makes us the individ-

uals we are—our awareness of ourselves, our past and continuity—has been lost. Dworkin seems to support Dr Ryan's approach in seeing the competent person who makes the anticipatory decision as fundamentally different from and other to the incapacitated individual who lives out (or not) the consequences of the decision. It is widely accepted that individuals can only make advance directives for "themselves". A person who becomes severely mentally disordered, however, is in some sense no longer "herself". Nevertheless, despite the lack of continuity, the former, competent "self" should arguably still retain moral rights about how the later, incompetent self is treated.[15] Even if acknowledged as being not quite the same person, the claim of the competent to decide on behalf of the later incompetent self still appears stronger than the claims of other players, especially bearing in mind the above-mentioned tendency for proxy decision-makers to choose options inconsistent with the individual's own values.

There is a danger that health professionals and nominated proxies will not take full account of the complex mixture of reasoning which leads some people to choose to forego treatment even in situations where medicine can offer them an extension of life. Although doctors' decisions about lifesaving treatment correlate with their own estimate of subsequent quality of life, they significantly underestimate their elderly patients' quality of life compared with the views of the patients themselves.[16] For some people, medical views of quality of life or possibility of improvement may not be a central issue. Just as Dr Ryan points out that it is difficult for healthy people convincingly to imagine themselves with disability, so it is often hard for the young or middle-aged to envisage that there may be a stage when we have simply lived long enough and the burdens of further treatment no longer outweigh the benefits. We may then wish to opt out even at the risk of potentially missing out on a slightly prolonged lifespan.

(v) We do not agree that advance directives for conditions of temporary mental incapacity should be less valid than advance directives for conditions of permanent mental incapacity. We question the logic of such a distinction. Dr Ryan concedes that his argument does not apply where loss of mental capacity is permanent. He distinguishes this situation as there "will be no possibility of the person recovering to give carers a more accurate report of her current desire for treatment"[1] and therefore they should be guided by an existing living will. He recognises that an accurate report of individual wishes is of value and therefore should be respected. If, however, a Jehovah's Witness, for example, repeatedly states that under no circumstances does he want a transfusion with blood products, Dr Ryan would urge us to ignore this directive if mental incapacity is temporarily impaired. There is no logical reason why the situation where mental incapacity is temporary should be treated in a different way from the situation where the incapacity is permanent. We feel that in both cases an appropriately worded advance directive should be equally applicable.

INFORMATION-SHARING

(vi) Even if Dr Ryan's arguments are accepted, we do not agree that "there is the possibility of large numbers of people dying when they would not have wanted to" although it may be that some will die when doctors would prefer to keep them alive. Doctors hostile to the concept of advance decision-making can limit or otherwise influence patients' choices. The acceptance or refusal of treatment is highly dependent on the amount and manner of information-sharing about the treatment options.[17] Discussion with elderly outpatients about limiting treatment rarely occurs[18] and in Emanuel's survey of patient and public opinion, the lack of physician initiative was the most frequently mentioned perceived barrier to the making of advance directives. In this survey of 405 out-patients and 102 members of the public, 93 per cent of the former and 89 per cent of the latter claimed to desire advance directives but considered their doctors to be reluctant.[19] Yet it is to be strongly advised that advance directives are only made in conjunction with advice and information from health professionals.[20]

Dr Ryan's arguments only apply to advance directives which withhold consent to treatment where there has been a temporary loss of mental capacity. We agree that the greatest value of advance directives is their use in situations where the loss of mental capacity is not reversible, such as in cases of dementia, chronic stroke or chronic brain injury due to trauma.

Nevertheless, we refute his thesis that large numbers of people will die unnecessarily since we believe it unlikely that many people will draft advance directives specifically indicating that they would not want treatment if they were to suffer temporary mental incapacity. Examples of common clinical situations where a reduction in mental capacity is potentially reversible include the acute confusional state in an older person, the early phase of recovery from an acute stroke, and the early stage of recovery from head trauma and psychiatric illness. We agree that the advance directive is of more limited application in these situations as it may be very difficult to envisage what degree of recovery will occur. Certainly, with respect to mental illness, if a patient is detained under a section of the Mental Health Act 1983, treatment under the Act will override any refusal of treatment of mental disorder set out in an advance directive.

If one examines the standard forms for advance directives in the UK, many emphasise that for the decision to be implementable the deterioration in mental capacity must be considered permanent or where life is nearing its end due to a terminal physical illness. People may draft their decisions in any form but many use standard documents which direct attention to irreversible conditions. One of the most common living wills, the Terrence Higgins Trust model, is not unique in allowing drafters the option of choosing to have all available treatment as well as refusing interventions in three situations:

- When there is a life-threatening illness *from which there is no likelihood of recovery* and it is so serious that life is nearing its end;
- When *mental functions become permanently impaired with no likelihood of improvement* and the impairment is so severe that the drafter does not understand what is happening and medical treatment is needed to keep him alive;
- When the drafter is *permanently unconscious* with no likelihood of regaining consciousness.[21]

Dr Ryan's argument is based on the fact that the sick do not make the same choices as the healthy. He does not point out, however, that in many instances advance directives are made by people who are already sick. Indeed, the mechanism is probably most useful for those people who have already been diagnosed as having a chronic illness for which there is no adequate curative treatment and where there is likely to be a predictable pattern of deterioration, for example, patients with AIDS or dementia. Moreover, even if an advance directive is made while the drafter is healthy, he or she will often have the opportunity of revoking or changing it when illness occurs as long as mental capacity is retained.

CONCLUSION

For the reasons outlined in this paper, we maintain that advance directives refusing treatment during periods of temporary incapacity should be respected. We acknowledge, however, that there are difficulties for healthy people trying to make decisions for future events. It is important that patients are made aware of these difficulties and not discouraged by medical reluctance to discuss the matter so that they draft directives in isolation. Emanuel found that those patients who had discussion with their physicians made the most stable decisions.[3] We would therefore urge any person making an advance directive about medical therapy to discuss the directive with a medical practitioner.

REFERENCES

1. Ryan J. Betting your life: an argument against certain advance directives. *Journal of Medical Ethics* 1996; **22**: 95–9.
2. House of Lords Select Committee on Medical Ethics. *Report from the Select Committee on Medical Ethics.* London: HMSO, 1994: **1**: 41.

3. Emanuel L, Emanuel E, Stoeckle, *et al*. Advance directives, stability of patient's treatment choices. *Archives of Internal Medicine* 1994; **154:** 209–17.
4. Danis M, Garret J, Harris R, *et al*. Stability of choices about life sustaining treatments. *Annals of Internal Medicine* 1994; **120:** 567–73.
5. Menikoff JA, Sachs GA, Seigler M. Beyond advance directives: health care surrogate laws. *New England Journal of Medicine* 1992; **327:** 1165–9.
6. Meadows P. Use of living wills in HIV infection and AIDS. *Lancet* 1994; **334:** 1509. Calvert GM. The completion of living wills: an examination of the demographics, completion and issues raised by the living will. London: Terrence Higgins Trust, 1994. Schlyter C. *Advance directives and AIDS: an empirical study of the interest in living wills and proxy decision making in the context of HIV/AIDs care.* London: Centre of Medical Law and Ethics, Kings College, 1992.
7. Sommerville A. *Advance statements about medical treatment.* London: BMJ Publishing Group, 1995: 23.
8. Sidaway v Board of Governors of the Bethlem Royal Hospital and the Maudsley Hospital [1985] AC 871.
9. Mill JS. *On liberty.* London: Parker and Son, 1859: 68.
10. Parfit D. Personal identity. In: Honderich T. Burnyeat M, eds. *Philosophy as it is.* Harmondsworth: Pelican, 1979: 186–211.
11. For example see Seckler AB, Meier DE, Mulvihill M, Cammer Paris BE: Substituted judgement: how accurate are proxy predictions? *Annuals of Internal Medicine* 1991: **115:** 92–8. Ouslander JG, Tymchuk AJ, Rhabar B. Health care decisions among elderly long care residents and their potential proxies. *Archives of Internal Medicine*

1989; **149:** 1367–72. Emanuel BJ, Emanuel LL. Proxy decision making for incompetent patients: an ethical and empirical analysis. *Journal of the American Medical Association* 1992; **267:** 2067–71.
12. Schneiderman L, *et al*. Effects of offering advance directives on medical treatments and costs. *Annals of Internal Medicine* 1992; **117:** 599–606.
13. See reference 11: Seckler AB, *et al*.
14. Dworkin R. *Life's dominion.* London: Harper Collins, 1993.
15. Sommerville A. Are advance directives the answer? In: Maclean S, ed. *Death, dying and the law.* Aldershot: Dartmouth Press, 1996.
16. Uhlmann RF, Pearlman RA. Perceived quality of life and preferences for life sustaining treatment in older adults. *Archives of Internal Medicine* 1991; **151:** 495–7.
17. Ainslie A, Beisecker A. Changes in treatment decisions by elderly persons based on treatment descriptions. *Archives of Internal Medicine* 1994; **154:** 2225–33. Malloy TR, Wigton RS, Meeske J, Tape TG. The influence of treatment descriptions on advance directive decisions. *Journal of the American Geriatric Society* 1992; **40:** 1255–60.
18. Goold SD, Arnold RM, Siminoff LA. Discussion about limiting treatment in a geriatric clinic. *Journal of the American Geriatric Society* 1993; **41:** 277–81.
19. Emanuel LL, Barry MJ, Stoeckle JD, *et al*. Advance directives for medical care—a case for greater use. *New England Journal of Medicine* 1991; **324:** 889–95.
20. Mower WR, Baraff LJ. Advance directives, effect of type of directive on physicians' therapeutic decisions. *Archives of Internal Medicine* 1993; **153:** 375–81.
21. Living will drawn up by Terrence Higgins Trust and King's College Centre for Medical Ethics and Law.

POSTSCRIPT

Are Some Advance Directives Too Risky for Patients?

In November 1995 a major two-year study indicated that there are substantial shortcomings in the care of seriously ill hospitalized patients, despite an intervention that tried to improve communication between physicians and patients and their families about preferences regarding end-of-life treatment. The Study to Understand Prognoses and Preferences for Outcomes and Risks of Treatment, or SUPPORT study, concluded that the intervention failed to improve care or patient outcomes and that more forceful measures may be needed to change established practices. See "A Controlled Trial to Improve Care for Seriously Ill Hospitalized Patients," *Journal of the American Medical Association* (November 22/29, 1995).

A study of the impact of ethnicity on knowledge about and completion of advance directives found that advance directives seem to fit best with the prevailing beliefs of European Americans. By contrast, African Americans tended to have a positive view of advance directives but less knowledge about them. Mexican Americans tended to have negative attitudes, and Korean Americans were almost completely unaware of advance directives and reported negative reactions to the concept. See Sheila T. Murphy et al., "Ethnicity and Advance Care Directives," *Journal of Law, Medicine and Ethics* (Summer 1996).

Linda Emanuel, in "Structured Advance Planning: Is It Finally Time for Physician Action and Reimbursement?" *Journal of the American Medical Association* (August 9, 1995), suggests that an immediate agenda to bring advance directives into more widespread use would include encouraging physicians to co-sign the documents, providing worksheets that are easy to use in hospitals and doctors' offices, educating physicians in discussing advance directives, and reimbursing physicians for time spent discussing advance directives.

Nancy M. P. King argues in favor of advance directives in *Making Sense of Advance Directives*, rev. ed. (Georgetown University Press, 1996). Among her major points are that advance directives are just one piece of a larger picture of common law and statutory principles and that advance directives are only one procedural mechanism for implementing an individual's constitutional right to make decisions concerning his or her own body. Ultimately, King believes, physicians have a strong moral obligation to honor patients' deeply held values and preferences. Another book is *Planning for Uncertainty: A Guide to Living Wills and Other Advance Directives for Health Care* by D. J. Doukas and W. Reichel (Johns Hopkins University Press, 1993). In collaboration with the American Medical Association and the American Bar Association, the American Association of Retired Persons has prepared a booklet called *A Matter of Choice: Planning Ahead for Health Care Decisions* (AARP, 1919 K Street, Washington, D.C. 20049). Many hospitals and bioethics groups also have educational materials concerning advance directives that conform to their state laws.

For more information on advance directives and living wills, see the following Web sites: `http://mel.lib.mi.us/social/SOC-wills.html` and `http://www.aarp.org/programs/advdir/adirhow.html`.

ISSUE 5

Should Physicians Be Allowed to Assist in Patient Suicide?

YES: Timothy E. Quill, from "Death and Dignity: A Case of Individualized Decision Making," *The New England Journal of Medicine* (March 7, 1991)

NO: Herbert Hendin, from "Selling Death and Dignity," *Hastings Center Report* (May–June 1995)

ISSUE SUMMARY

YES: Physician Timothy E. Quill discusses the case of his patient "Diane" in arguing that in some cases, physicians' indirect assistance in suicide honors patients' choices and prevents severe suffering.

NO: Psychiatrist Herbert Hendin asserts that individual cases presented to justify legalizing physician-assisted suicide fail to deal with the underlying medical failures to control pain, create an illusion of control over death, and do not acknowledge the likelihood that the practice will kill thousands of patients inappropriately.

Since the early 1980s physicians, lawyers, philosophers, and judges have examined questions about withholding life-sustaining treatment. Their deliberations have resulted in a broad consensus that competent adults have the right to make decisions about their medical care, even if those decisions seem unjustifiable to others and even if they result in death. Furthermore, the right of individuals to name others to carry out their prior wishes or to make decisions if they should become incompetent is now well established. Thirty-eight states now have legislation allowing advance directives (commonly known as "living wills").

The debate in specific cases continues (for example, on withholding food and water), but on the whole, patients' rights to self-determination have been bolstered by 80 or more legal cases, dozens of reports, and statements made by medical societies and other organizations.

As often occurs in bioethical debate, the resolution of one issue only highlights the lack of resolution about another. There is clearly no consensus about either euthanasia or physician-assisted suicide.

Like truth telling, euthanasia is an old problem given new dimensions by the ability of modern medical technology to prolong life. The word itself is Greek (literally, *happy death*), and the Greeks wrestled with the question of whether, in some cases, people would be better off dead. But the Hippocratic

Oath in this instance was clear: "I will neither give a deadly drug to anybody if asked for it, nor will I make a suggestion to that effect." On the other hand, if the goal of medicine is not simply to prolong life but to reduce suffering, at some point the question of what measures should be taken or withdrawn will inevitably arise. The problem is, when death is inevitable, how far should one go in hastening it?

The majority of cases in which euthanasia is raised as a possibility are among the most difficult ethical issues to resolve, for they involve the conflict between a physician's duty to preserve life and the burden on the patient and the family that is created by fulfilling that duty. One common distinction is between *active* euthanasia (that is, some positive act such as administering a lethal injection) and *passive* euthanasia (that is, an inaction such as deciding not to administer antibiotics when the patient has a severe infection). Another common distinction is between *voluntary* euthanasia (that is, the patient wishes to die and consents to the action that will make it happen) and *involuntary*—or better, *nonvoluntary*—euthanasia (that is, the patient is unable to consent, perhaps because he or she is in a coma).

The two selections that follow take up one aspect of this large issue: the question of whether or not physicians may ethically assist in a hopelessly ill patient's suicide. Physician Timothy E. Quill describes himself as a "longtime advocate of active, informed patient choice of treatment or nontreatment, and of a patient's right to die with as much control and dignity as possible." In the case of "Diane," a patient with leukemia, this advocacy included prescribing drugs in dosages that he knew she would use to kill herself. Although he acknowledges that this decision could have subjected him to criminal prosecution, he believes that it was justified to empower her and to prevent severe suffering. Psychiatrist Herbert Hendin argues that euthanasia and assisted suicide are being promoted through "marketing techniques," including the use of case histories designed to present the practice as justifiable and compassionate. Even in these cases, he says, the patient's wishes are often manipulated. He believes that the fundamental problems involve a cultural resistance to facing death, inadequate pain control, and the failure to provide meaningful care at the end of life.

YES
Timothy E. Quill

DEATH AND DIGNITY: A CASE OF INDIVIDUALIZED DECISION MAKING

Diane was feeling tired and had a rash. A common scenario, though there was something subliminally worrisome that prompted me to check her blood count. Her hematocrit was 22, and the white-cell count was 4.3 with some metamyelocytes and unusual white cells. I wanted it to be viral, trying to deny what was staring me in the face. Perhaps in a repeated count it would disappear. I called Diane and told her it might be more serious than I had initially thought—that the test needed to be repeated and that if she felt worse, we might have to move quickly. When she pressed for the possibilities, I reluctantly opened the door to leukemia. Hearing the word seemed to make it exist. "Oh, shit!" she said. "Don't tell me that." Oh, shit! I thought, I wish I didn't have to.

Diane was no ordinary person (although no one I have ever come to know has been really ordinary). She was raised in an alcoholic family and had felt alone for much of her life. She had vaginal cancer as a young woman. Through much of her adult life, she had struggled with depression and her own alcoholism. I had come to know, respect, and admire her over the previous eight years as she confronted these problems and gradually overcame them. She was an incredibly clear, at times brutally honest, thinker and communicator. As she took control of her life, she developed a strong sense of independence and confidence. In the previous 3 1/2 years, her hard work had paid off. She was completely abstinent from alcohol, she had established much deeper connections with her husband, college-age son, and several friends, and her business and her artistic work were blossoming. She felt she was really living fully for the first time.

Not surprisingly, the repeated blood count was abnormal, and detailed examination of the peripheral-blood smear showed myelocytes. I advised her to come into the hospital, explaining that we needed to do a bone marrow biopsy and make some decisions relatively rapidly. She came to the hospital knowing what we would find. She was terrified, angry, and sad. Although we knew the odds, we both clung to the thread of possibility that it might be something else.

From Timothy E. Quill, "Death and Dignity: A Case of Individualized Decision Making," *The New England Journal of Medicine*, vol. 324, no. 10 (March 7, 1991), pp. 691–694. Copyright © 1991 by The Massachusetts Medical Society. Reprinted by permission.

The bone marrow confirmed the worst: acute myelomonocytic leukemia. In the face of this tragedy, we looked for signs of hope. This is an area of medicine in which technological intervention has been successful, with cures 25 percent of the time —long-term cures. As I probed the costs of these cures, I heard about induction chemotherapy (three weeks in the hospital, prolonged neutropenia, probable infectious complications, and hair loss; 75 percent of patients respond, 25 percent do not). For the survivors, this is followed by consolidation chemotherapy (with similar side effects; another 25 percent die, for a net survival of 50 percent). Those still alive, to have a reasonable chance of long-term survival, then need bone marrow transplantation (hospitalization for two months and whole-body irradiation, with complete killing of the bone marrow, infectious complications, and the possibility for graft-versus-host disease—with a survival of approximately 50 percent, or 25 percent of the original group). Though hematologists may argue over the exact percentages, they don't argue about the outcome of no treatment—certain death in days, weeks, or at most a few months.

Believing that delay was dangerous, our oncologist broke the news to Diane and began making plans to insert a Hickman catheter and begin induction chemotherapy that afternoon. When I saw her shortly thereafter, she was enraged at his presumption that she would want treatment, and devastated by the finality of the diagnosis. All she wanted to do was go home and be with her family. She had no further questions about treatment and in fact had decided that she wanted none. Together we lamented her tragedy and the unfairness of life. Before she left, I felt the need to be sure that she and her husband understood that there was some risk in delay, that the problem was not going to go away, and that we needed to keep considering the options over the next several days. We agreed to meet in two days.

She returned in two days with her husband and son. They had talked extensively about the problem and the options. She remained very clear about her wish not to undergo chemotherapy and to live whatever time she had left outside the hospital. As we explored her thinking further, it became clear that she was convinced she would die during the period of treatment and would suffer unspeakably in the process (from hospitalization, from lack of control over her body, from the side effects of chemotherapy, and from pain and anguish). Although I could offer support and my best effort to minimize her suffering if she chose treatment, there was no way I could say any of this would not occur. In fact, the last four patients with acute leukemia at our hospital had died very painful deaths in the hospital during various stages of treatment (a fact I did not share with her). Her family wished she would choose treatment but sadly accepted her decision. She articulated very clearly that it was she who would be experiencing all the side effects of treatment and that odds of 25 percent were not good enough for her to undergo so toxic a course of therapy, given her expectations of chemotherapy and hospitalization and the absence of a closely matched bone marrow donor. I had her repeat her understanding of the treatment, the odds, and what to expect if there were no treatment. I clarified a few misunderstandings, but she had a remarkable grasp of the options and implications.

I have been a longtime advocate of active, informed patient choice of treatment or nontreatment, and of a patient's right to die with as much control and dignity as possible. Yet there was something about her giving up a 25 percent chance of long-term survival in favor of almost certain death that disturbed me. I had seen Diane fight and use her considerable inner resources to overcome alcoholism and depression, and I half expected her to change her mind over the next week. Since the window of time in which effective treatment can be initiated is rather narrow, we met several times that week. We obtained a second hematology consultation and talked at length about the meaning and implications of treatment and nontreatment. She talked to a psychologist she had seen in the past. I gradually understood the decision from her perspective and became convinced that it was the right decision for her. We arranged for home hospice care (although at that time Diane felt reasonably well, was active, and looked healthy), left the door open for her to change her mind, and tried to anticipate how to keep her comfortable in the time she had left.

Just as I was adjusting to her decision, she opened up another area that would stretch me profoundly. It was extraordinarily important to Diane to maintain control of herself and her own dignity during the time remaining to her. When this was no longer possible, she clearly wanted to die. As a former director of a hospice program, I know how to use pain medicines to keep patients comfortable and lessen suffering. I explained the philosophy of comfort care, which I strongly believe in. Although Diane understood and appreciated this, she had known of people lingering in what was called relative comfort, and she wanted no part

of it. When the time came, she wanted to take her life in the least painful way possible. Knowing of her desire for independence and her decision to stay in control, I thought this request made perfect sense. I acknowledged and explored this wish but also thought that it was out of the realm of currently accepted medical practice and that it was more than I could offer or promise. In our discussion, it became clear that preoccupation with her fear of a lingering death would interfere with Diane's getting the most out of the time she had left until she found a safe way to ensure her death. I feared the effects of a violent death on her family, the consequences of an ineffective suicide that would leave her lingering in precisely the state she dreaded so much, and the possibility that a family member would be forced to assist her, with all the legal and personal repercussions that would follow. She discussed this at length with her family. They believed that they should respect her choice. With this in mind, I told Diane that information was available from the Hemlock Society that might be helpful to her.

A week later she phoned me with a request for barbiturates for sleep. Since I knew that this was an essential ingredient in a Hemlock Society suicide, I asked her to come to the office to talk things over. She was more than willing to protect me by participating in a superficial conversation about her insomnia, but it was important to me to know how she planned to use the drugs and to be sure that she was not in despair or overwhelmed in a way that might color her judgment. In our discussion, it was apparent that she was having trouble sleeping, but it was also evident that the security of having enough barbiturates available to commit suicide when and if the time came would leave her secure enough to live fully and concentrate on the present. It was clear that she was not despondent and that in fact she was making deep, personal connections with her family and close friends. I made sure that she knew how to use the barbiturates for sleep, and also that she knew the amount needed to commit suicide. We agreed to meet regularly, and she promised to meet with me before taking her life, to ensure that all other avenues had been exhausted. I wrote the prescription with an uneasy feeling about the boundaries I was exploring—spiritual, legal, professional, and personal. Yet I also felt strongly that I was setting her free to get the most out of the time she had left, and to maintain dignity and control on her own terms until her death.

The next several months were very intense and important for Diane. Her son stayed home from college, and they were able to be with one another and say much that had not been said earlier. Her husband did his work at home so that he and Diane could spend more time together. She spent time with her closest friends. I had her come into the hospital for a conference with our residents, at which she illustrated in a most profound and personal way the importance of informed decision making, the right to refuse treatment, and the extraordinarily personal effects of illness and interaction with the medical system. There were emotional and physical hardships as well. She had periods of intense sadness and anger. Several times she became very weak, but she received transfusions as an outpatient and responded with marked improvement of symptoms. She had two serious infections that responded surprisingly well to empirical courses of oral antibiotics. After three tumultuous months, there were two weeks of relative calm and well-being, and fantasies of a miracle began to surface.

Unfortunately, we had no miracle. Bone pain, weakness, fatigue, and fevers began to dominate her life. Although the hospice workers, family members, and I tried our best to minimize the suffering and promote comfort, it was clear that the end was approaching. Diane's immediate future held what she feared the most—increasing discomfort, dependence, and hard choices between pain and sedation. She called up her closest friends and asked them to come over to say goodbye, telling them that she would be leaving soon. As we had agreed, she let me know as well. When we met, it was clear that she knew what she was doing, that she was sad and frightened to be leaving, but that she would be even more terrified to stay and suffer. In our tearful goodbye, she promised a reunion in the future at her favorite spot on the edge of Lake Geneva, with dragons swimming in the sunset.

Two days later her husband called to say that Diane had died. She had said her final goodbyes to her husband and son that morning, and asked them to leave her alone for an hour. After an hour, which must have seemed an eternity, they found her on the couch, lying very still and covered by her favorite shawl. There was no sign of struggle. She seemed to be at peace. They called me for advice about how to proceed. When I arrived at their house, Diane indeed seemed peaceful. Her husband and son were quiet. We talked about what a remarkable person she had been. They seemed to have no doubts about the course she had chosen or about their cooperation, although the unfairness of her illness and the finality of her death were overwhelming to us all.

I called the medical examiner to inform him that a hospice patient had died. When asked about the cause of death, I said, "acute leukemia." He said that was fine and that we should call a funeral director. Although acute leukemia was the truth, it was not the whole story. Yet any mention of suicide would have given rise to a police investigation and probably brought the arrival of an ambulance crew for resuscitation. Diane would have become a "coroner's case," and the decision to perform an autopsy would have been made at the discretion of the medical examiner. The family or I could have been subject to criminal prosecution, and I to professional review, for our roles in support of Diane's choices. Although I truly believe that the family and I gave her the best care possible, allowing her to define her limits and directions as much as possible, I am not sure the law, society, or the medical profession would agree. So I said "acute leukemia" to protect all of us, to protect Diane from an invasion into her past and her body, and to continue to shield society from the knowledge of the degree of suffering that people often undergo in the process of dying. Suffering can be lessened to some extent, but in no way eliminated or made benign, by the careful intervention of a competent, caring physician, given current social constraints.

Diane taught me about the range of help I can provide if I know people well and if I allow them to say what they really want. She taught me about life, death, and honesty and about taking charge and facing tragedy squarely when it strikes. She taught me that I can take small risks for people that I really know and care about. Although I did not assist in her suicide directly, I helped indirectly to make it possible, successful, and relatively painless. Although I know we have measures to help control pain and lessen suffering, to think that people do not suffer in the process of dying is an illusion. Prolonged dying can occasionally be peaceful, but more often the role of the physician and family is limited to lessening but not eliminating severe suffering.

I wonder how many families and physicians secretly help patients over the edge into death in the face of such severe suffering. I wonder how many severely ill or dying patients secretly take their lives, dying alone in despair. I wonder whether the image of Diane's final aloneness will persist in the minds of her family, or if they will remember more the intense, meaningful months they had together before she died. I wonder whether Diane struggled in that last hour, and whether the Hemlock Society's way of death by suicide is the most benign. I wonder why Diane, who gave so much to so many of us, had to be alone for the last hour of her life. I wonder whether I will see Diane again, on the shore of Lake Geneva at sunset, with dragons swimming on the horizon.

NO

Herbert Hendin

SELLING DEATH AND DIGNITY

Dying is hard to market. Voters, many repelled by the image of doctors giving their patients lethal injections, rejected euthanasia initiatives in Washington and California. Learning from these defeats, Oregon sponsors of a similar measure limited it to assisted suicide, while still casting the patient in the role familiar from euthanasia advertising: the noble individualist fighting to exercise the right to die.

Although both assisted suicide and euthanasia have been presented as empowering patients by giving them control over their death, assisted suicide has been seen as protecting against potential medical abuse since the final act is in the patient's hands. Yet opponents see little protection in assisted suicide: people who are helpless or seriously ill are vulnerable to influence or coercion by physicians or relatives who can achieve the same ends with or without direct action.[1] How could advocates counteract not only images of lethal physicians but images of grasping relatives, eager to be rid of a burden or to gain an inheritance by coercing death?

Supporters of assisted suicide and euthanasia have found the ultimate marketing technique to promote the normalization of assisted suicide and euthanasia: the presentation of a case history designed to show how necessary assisted suicide or euthanasia was in that particular instance. Such cases may rely either on nightmarish images of unnecessarily prolonged dying or on predictions of severe disability. The instance in which it is felt that most would agree it was desirable to end life is represented as typical. Those who participate in the death (the relatives, the euthanasia advocates, the physician) are celebrated as enhancing the dignity of the patient, who is usually presented as a heroic, fully independent figure.

How much truth is there in this advertising? Does this accurately describe what happens? Even in cases advocates believe best illustrate the desirability of legalizing assisted suicide or euthanasia, there is ample room to question whether the death administered in fact realizes the patient's wishes and meets his or her needs. Advocates' desire to dramatize these model cases, moreover, requires that they be presented in some detail—and this creates

From Herbert Hendin, "Selling Death and Dignity," *Hastings Center Report,* vol. 25, no. 3 (May–June 1995). Copyright © 1995 by The Hastings Center. Reprinted by permission.

the opportunity to see the discrepancy between theory and practice with regard to assisted suicide and euthanasia.

DEATH ON REQUEST

The ultimate attempt to normalize euthanasia in the Netherlands and make it seem an ordinary part of everyday life was the showing in the fall of 1994 on Dutch television of *Death on Request*,[2] a film of a patient being put to death by euthanasia. Maarten Nederhurst, who created the film, found an agreeable patient and doctor by contacting the Dutch Voluntary Euthanasia Society.

The patient, Cees van Wendel, had been diagnosed as having amyotrophic lateral sclerosis in June 1993; he expressed his wish for euthanasia a month later. Severe muscular weakness confined him to a wheel chair; his speech was barely audible.

Almost 700,000 people saw the first showing of the film in the Netherlands. Subsequently, the right to show the film has been acquired by countries throughout the world. *Prime Time Live* excerpted and showed a representative segment to American viewers with a voiceover in English. Sam Donaldson introduced the program saying that it took no sides on the issue but added, "It is a story of courage and love."[3] Only for the most gullible viewer.

In point of fact, the doctor, Wilfred van Oijen, is the film's most significant person. He is the manager who can make "everything"—even death—happen. He is presented as someone who has accepted the burden of all phases of experience. The patient is nearly invisible.

The film opens with a chilly scene in winter—trees are bare of leaves, it is cold, wet, inhospitable—not a bad time to die. In an undershirt in his bathroom, the doctor combs his hair getting ready for just another day. His encounters will include treating a child of about ten months, a pregnant woman and a baby, and bringing death to Cees. The purpose of the film is to include euthanasia both as part of his daily burden as a doctor and as the natural course of events.

In the two house calls van Oijen makes to Cees, of most interest is the tension between the film's professed message—that all want release from illness, the patient most of all—and the message conveyed by what is actually filmed. The relationship depicted is between van Oijen and Antoinette, the patient's wife, who has called the doctor and clearly wants her husband to die.

The wife appears repulsed by her husband's illness, never touching him during their conversation and never permitting Cees to answer any question the doctor asks directly. She "translates" for him, although Cees is at this point in his illness intelligible, able to communicate verbally, but slowly, and able to type out messages on his computer. The doctor asks him if he wants euthanasia, but his wife replies. When Cees begins to cry, the doctor moves sympathetically toward him to touch his arm, but his wife tells the doctor to move away and says it is better to let him cry alone. During his weeping she continues to talk to the doctor. The doctor at no time asks to speak to Cees alone; neither does he ask if anything would make it easier for him to communicate or if additional help in his care would make him want to live.

Virtually the entire film is set up to avoid confronting any of the patient's feelings or how the relationship with his wife affects his agreeing to die. Cees is never seen alone. Van Oijen is obliged to obtain a second opinion from a consultant. The consultant, who appears well known to the doctor, also makes no attempt to communicate with Cees alone, and he too permits the wife to answer all the questions put to Cees. When the consultant asks the pro forma question if Cees is sure he wants to go ahead, Antoinette answers for him. The consultant seems uncomfortable, asks a few more questions, and leaves. The consultation takes practically no time at all. The pharmacist who supplies the lethal medication—one shot to put Cees to sleep and another to help him die—seems only another player in this carefully orchestrated event.

Antoinette visits the doctor to ask where "we stand." She wants the euthanasia over with. Cees has set several dates, but keeps moving them back. Now he has settled on his birthday, and they arrange for van Oijen to do it at eight o'clock after Cees celebrates by drinking a glass of port. Cees makes a joke that sleeping is a little death but this time his sleep will be a lot of death. Van Oijen tries to laugh warmly. Antoinette keeps her distance from the two and remarks that the day has gone slowly and it seemed eight o'clock would never come.

Antoinette helps Cees into bed in preparation for van Oijen to administer the first shot. Van Oijen smiles, gives the injection, and explains the medication will take a while to put Cees into a deep sleep. No one says goodbye. Only after the shot has put Cees to sleep does Antoinette murmur something to her husband. She then moves into the other room with the doctor to permit Cees to sink into a deeper sleep. After a few minutes, they return. When the doctor wants to place Cees in a more comfortable position, she withdraws again. After the second shot is administered, Antoinette and van Oijen sit next to the bed, both holding the arm that has received the injections. Antoinette asks if this was good, presumably wanting to know if it was "good" to kill Cees. Van Oijen reassures her. They leave Cees alone very quickly. On the way into the next room, Antoinette takes a note Cees wrote to her about their relationship and what it meant to him and reads it to the doctor. She seems to want to convey to him that they in fact once had a relationship.

From the beginning, the loneliness and isolation of the husband haunts the film. Only because he is treated from the start as an object does his death seem inevitable. One leaves the film feeling that death with dignity requires more than effective management; it requires being accorded personhood even though one's speech is slurred or one needs to point to letters on a board or communicate through writing on one's computer. Throughout the film, Cee's wife denies him such personhood, as does the doctor, who never questions her control over all of the patient's communication and even the doctor's communication with Cees. The doctor and wife took away Cees's personhood before ALS had claimed it.

A GOOD DEATH FOR LOUISE

An article featured on the cover of the *New York Times Magazine* in the fall of 1993 also used a case description to try to prove the value of assisted suicide to an American audience.[4] The article described the assisted suicide of Louise, a Seattle woman whose death was arranged by her doctor and the Reverend Ralph Mero, head of Compassion in Dying, a group that champions legalizing assisted suicide. Members of the group counsel the terminally ill, offer advice on lethal doses, convince cautious doctors to become involved, and are present during the death. Mero and his followers do not provide the means for suicide (the patients obtain such help from their doctors) and claim not to encourage the patients to seek suicide.

Mero arranged for a *Times* reporter to interview Louise in the last weeks of her life, offering Louise's death as an illustration of the beneficial effects of the organization's work. Yet the account serves equally to illustrate how assisted suicide made both life and death miserable for Louise.

Louise, who was referred to Mero by her doctor, had been ill with an unnamed, degenerative neurological disease. The reporter tells us that "Louise had mentioned suicide periodically during her six years of illness, but the subject came into sudden focus in May during a somber visit to her doctor's office." As Louise recounted it, "I really wasn't having any different symptoms, I just knew something had changed. I looked the doctor right in the eye and said, 'I'm starting to die.' And she said, 'I've had the same impression for a couple of days.' " An MRI scan confirmed that the frontal lobes of Louise's brain had begun to deteriorate, a sign that led her doctor to warn Louise that her life would most likely be measured in months, perhaps weeks. Louise said her doctor explained that "she didn't want to scare me... she just wanted to be honest. She told me that once the disease becomes active, it progresses very fast, that I would become mentally incapacitated and wouldn't be myself, couldn't care for myself anymore. She would have to look into hospice care, or the hospital, or some other facility where I would stay until I died."

We are told that Louise did not hesitate with her answer. "I can't do that...I don't want that." The reporter continues, "Her doctor, Louise thought, looked both sad and relieved. 'I know, I know,' the doctor said. 'But it has to come from you.' " Louise makes sure that they are both talking about suicide and says, "That's what I'd like to do, go for as long as I can and then end it."

What has happened between Louise and her doctor? The doctor's quick affirmation that Louise is starting to die, even before the MRI scan confirms her decline, is disturbing. She prefaces a grim description of Louise's prognosis with assurance that she does not want to scare her. The doctor's relief when Louise indicates that she is choosing suicide gives us some feeling about her attitudes toward patients in Louise's condition.

As the account continues, the doctor indicates that she would be willing to help, had recently helped another patient whom Louise knew, and said she would prescribe enough barbiturates to kill Louise. To avoid legal trouble, she would not be there when Louise committed suicide. They exchanged several hugs and Louise went home. The doctor called Compassion in Dying for advice. The reporter quotes the doctor as saying about contacting Mero, "I was ecstatic to find someone who's doing what he's doing... I loved the fact that there were guidelines."

On the phone, Mero advises the doctor on the medication to prescribe and then visits Louise, suggesting that he is prepared to help Louise die before knowing or even meeting her or in any way determining whether she meets any guidelines. When he does meet Louise, she asks him at once if he will help her with her suicide and be there when she does it and she is almost tearfully grateful when he says yes. He repeats many times that it has to be her choice. Louise affirms that it is, saying that all she wants "these next few weeks is to live as peacefully as possible." Louise seems concerned with being close to others during her final time and with spending what is left of her life in an environment of love leave-taking.

The doctor is concerned that Louise's judgment might soon become impaired: "The question is, at what point is her will going to be affected, and, if suicide is what she wants, does she have the right to do it when she still has the will?" The doctor, like Mero, says she does not want to influence the patient, but worries that Louise might not act in time. "If she loses her mind and doesn't do this, she's going into the hospital. But the last thing I want to do is pressure her to do this."

Yet the closeness before dying that Louise seemed to want is lost in the flurry of activity and planning for her death as each of those involved with her dying pursues his or her own requirements. At a subsequent meeting of Mero and Louise, with Louise's mother and her doctor also present, Mero gives Louise a checklist in which he reviews steps to be taken during the suicide, from the food to be eaten to how the doctor would call the medical examiner.

The doctor indicates she will be out of town for the next week, but that she has told her partner of Louise's plans. "You don't have to wait for me to get back," she tells Louise, hinting, the reporter tells us, that it might be a good idea not to wait. The doctor was more direct when alone with Louise's mother, telling her that she was afraid Louise might not be coherent enough to act if she waited past the coming weekend.

The doctor and Mero discuss how pointed they can be with Louise, wanting her to make an informed decision without frightening her into acting sooner than she was ready. They hoped "she would read between the lines." Mero assures the reporter that he always wants to err on the side of caution. Nonetheless, a few days after the meeting, Mero called the reporter in New York, asking her to come to Seattle as soon as possible. He knew she was planning to come the following week, but he warned her not to wait that long.

The reporter leaves immediately for Seattle and finds Louise in a debilitated condition. She is in pain, getting weaker, and speaks of wanting to end her life while she can still be in control. She says she is almost ready, but not quite. She needs about a week, mainly to relax and be with her mother.

The reporter blurted out, "Your doctor feels that if you don't act by this weekend you may not be able to." Her words are met with a "wrenching silence" and Louise, looking sharply at her mother, indicates that she hadn't been told that. Her mother says gently that is what the doctor had told her. Louise looks terrified and her mother tells her it's OK to be afraid. "I'm not afraid. I just feel as if everyone is ganging up on me, pressuring me," Louise said, "I just want some time."

Louise's mother was growing less certain that Louise would actually take her own life. When she tried to ask her directly, Louise replied, "I feel like it's all we ever talk about." A friend who had agreed to be with Louise during the suicide is also uncomfortable with Louise's ambivalence but is inclined to attribute her irritability and uncertainty to her mental decline. When Louise indicates that she would wait for Mero to return from a trip and ask his opinion on her holding on for a few days, the friend indicates that this was a bad idea since the change in her mood might be missed by someone like Mero who did not know her well.

Like many people in extreme situations, Louise has expressed two conflicting wishes—to live and to die—and found support only for the latter. The anxiety of her doctor, Mero, her mother, and her friend that Louise might change her mind or lose her "will" may originate in their desire to honor Louise's wishes, or even in their own view of what kind of life is worth living, but eventually overrides the emotions Louise is clearly feeling and comes to affect what happens more than Louise's will. Although those around her act in the name of supporting Louise's autonomy, Louise begins to lose her own death.

Despite predictions, Louise makes it through the weekend. Over the next days she speaks with Mero by phone, but he tells the reporter he kept the conversations short because he was uncomfortable with her growing dependence on his opinion. Nevertheless, after a few such conversations, the contents of which are not revealed, Louise indicated she was ready; that evening Mero came and the assisted suicide was performed. A detailed description of the death scene provides the beginning, the end, and the drama of the published story. Louise did not die immediately but lingered for seven hours. Had she not died from the pills, Mero subsequently implied to the reporter, he would have used a plastic bag to suffocate her, although this violates the Compassion in Dying guidelines.

Everyone—Mero, the friend, the mother, the doctor, and the reporter—all became part of a network pressuring Louise to stick to her decision and to do so in a timely manner. The death was virtually clocked by their anxiety that she might want to live. Mero and the doctor influence the feelings of the mother and the friend so that the issue is not their warm leave-taking and the affection they have had for Louise, but whether they can get her to die according to the time requirements of Mero, the doctor (who probably cannot stay away indefinitely), the reporter (who has her own deadlines), and the disease, which turns out to be on a more flexible schedule than previously thought. Louise is explicit that the doctor, mother, friend, and reporter have become instruments of pressure in moving her along. Mero appears to act more subtly and indirectly through his effect on the others involved with Louise.

Without a death there is, of course, no story, and Mero and the reporter have a stake in the story, although Mero has criticized Jack Kevorkian to the reporter for wanting publicity. The doctor develops a time frame for Louise; her own past troubling experience with a patient who was a friend seems to color the doctor's need to have things over with quickly and in her absence if possible. Louise is clearly frustrated by not having someone to talk to who has no stake in persuading her.

Individually and collectively those involved engender a terror in Louise with which she must struggle alone, while they reassure each other that they are gratifying her last wishes. The end of her life does not seem like death with dignity; nor is there much compassion conveyed in the way Louise was helped to die. Compassion is not an easy emotion to express in the context of an imminent loss. It requires that we look beyond our own pain to convey the power and meaning of all that has gone before in our life with another. Although the mother, friend, and physician may have acted out of good intentions in assisting the suicide, none appears to have honored Louise's need for a "peaceful" parting. None seems to have been able to accept the difficult emotions involved in loving someone who is dying and knowing there is little one can do but convey love and respect for the life that has been lived. The effort to deal with the discomfort of Louise's situation seems to drive the others to "do something" to eliminate the situation.

Watching someone die can be intolerably painful for those who care for the patient. Their wish to have it over with quickly is understandable. Their feeling can become a form of pressure on the patient and must be separated from what the patient actually wants. The patient who wants to live until the end but sense his family cannot tolerate watching him die is familiar to those who care for the terminally ill. Once those close to the patient decide to assist in the suicide, their desire to have it over with can make the pressure put on the patient many times greater. The mood of those assisting is reflected in Macbeth's famous line, "If it were done when 'tis done, then 'twere well it were done quickly."

Certainly assisted *suicide*—the fact that she took the lethal medication herself—offered no protection to Louise. Short of actually murdering her, it is hard to see how her doctor, Mero, her mother, her friend, and the reporter could have done more to rush her toward death. Case vignetttes limited to one or two paragraphs describing the patient's medical symptoms, and leaving out the social context in which euthanasia is being considered, obscure such complex—and often subtle —pressures on patients' "autonomous" decisions to seek death.

EMPOWERMENT FOR WHOM?

Our culture supports the feeling that we should not tolerate situations we cannot control. "Death," Arnold Toynbee has said, "is un-American." The physician who feels a sense of failure and helplessness in the face of incurable disease, or the relative who cannot bear the emotions of loss and separation, finds in assisted suicide and euthanasia an illusion of mastery over the disease and the accompanying feelings of helplessness. Determining when death will occur becomes a way of dealing with frustration.

In the selling of assisted suicide and euthanasia words like "empowerment" and "dignity" are associated only with the choice for dying. But who is being empowered? The more one knows about individual cases, the more apparent it becomes that needs other than those of the patient often prevail. "Empowerment" flows toward the relatives, the doctor who offers a speedy way out if he cannot offer a cure, or the activists who have found in death a cause that gives meaning to their lives. The patient, who may have said she wants to die in the hope of receiving emotional reassurance that all around her want her to live, may find that like Louise she has set in motion a process whose momentum she cannot control. If death with dignity is to be a fact and not a selling slogan, surely what is required is a loving parting that acknowledges the value of the life lived and affirms its continuing meaning.

Euthanasia advocates try to use the individual case to demonstrate that there are some cases of rational or justifiable assisted suicide or euthanasia. If they can demonstrate that there are *some* such cases, they believe that would justify legalizing euthanasia.

Their argument recalls Abraham's approach in persuading God not to go ahead with his intention to destroy everyone in Sodom. Abraham asks if it would be right for God to destroy Sodom if there were fifty who were righteous within the city. When God agrees to spare Sodom if there were fifty who were righteous, Abraham asks what about forty-five, gradually reduces the number to ten, and gets God to spare the city for the time being for the sake of the ten.

Abraham, however, is arguing in favor of saving life; we want him to succeed and are relieved that he does. Euthanasia advocates are arguing that if there are ten cases where euthanasia might be appropriate, we should legalize a practice that is likely to kill thousands inappropriately.

The appeal of assisted suicide and euthanasia are a symptom of our failure to develop a better response to death and the fear of intolerable pain or artificial prolongation of life. The United States needs a national commission to explore and develop a consensus on the care and treatment of the seriously or terminally ill—a scientific commission similar to the President's Commission that in 1983 gave us guidelines about forgoing life-sustaining treatment with dying patients. Work of a wider scope needs to be done now. There is a great deal of evidence that doctors are not sufficiently trained in relieving pain and other symptoms in the terminally ill. Hospice care is in its infancy. We have not yet educated the public as to the choices they have in refusing or terminating treatment nor has the medical profession learned how best to avoid setting in motion the technology that only prolongs a painful process of dying. And we have not devoted enough time in our medical schools or hospitals to educating future physicians about coming to terms with the painful truth that there will be patients they will not be able to save but whose needs they must address.

How we deal with illness, age, and decline says a great deal about who and what we are, both as individuals and as a society. We should not buy into the view of those who are engulfed by fear of death or by suicidal despair that death is the preferred solution to the problems of illness, age, and depression. We would be encouraging the worst tendencies of depressed patients, most of whom can be helped to overcome their condition. By rushing to "normalize" euthanasia as a medical option along with accepting or refusing treatment, we are inevitably laying the groundwork for a culture that will not only turn euthanasia into a "cure" for depression but may prove to exert a coercion to die on patients when they are most vulnerable. Death ought to be hard to sell.

REFERENCES

1. Yale Kamisar, "Physician-Assisted Suicide: The Last Bridge to Active Voluntary Euthanasia," in *Examining Euthanasia*, ed. John Keown (Cambridge: Cambridge University Press, in press); Yale Kamisar, "Are Laws against Assisted Suicide Unconstitutional?" *Hastings Center Report* 23, no. 3 (1993): 33–41; Herbert Hendin, "Seduced by Death: Doctors, Patients and the Dutch Cure," *Issues in Law and Medicine* 10, no. 2 (1994): 123–68; Carlos Gomez, *Regulating Death: Euthanasia and the Case of the Netherlands* (New York: Free Press, 1991).
2. "Death on Request," Ikon Television Network, 1994.
3. "Death on Request," *Prime Time Live*, 8 December 1994.
4. Lisa Belken, "There's No Simple Suicide," *New York Times Magazine*, 14 November 1993.

POSTSCRIPT

Should Physicians Be Allowed to Assist in Patient Suicide?

Two recent federal court decisions have furthered the likelihood that physician-assisted suicide will be legalized in some form. In March 1996 the U.S. Court of Appeals for the Ninth Circuit, which has jurisdiction over nine western states, overturned a Washington state law that made assisted suicide a felony. The court cited the "powerful precedent" of the U.S. Supreme Court's abortion rulings, noting that the decision by a mentally competent, terminally ill person of how and when to die is similar to a woman's right to choose abortion. In April 1996 the U.S. Court of Appeals for the Second Circuit, which covers New York, Vermont, and Connecticut, ruled that New York's law banning physician-assisted suicide was also unconstitutional (Quill was one of the people who brought the case against the state). Two judges said that under the "equal protection" clause of the Constitution it would not be illegal for a physician to respond to a request for assistance in committing suicide as long as the state allows people to hasten death by refusing medical treatment. Another judge agreed with the ruling but wrote that the legislature could bar the practice of physician-assisted suicide constitutionally with legislation that used modern medical, legal, and ethical standards. In October 1996 the U.S. Supreme Court agreed to review both decisions.

For more analysis on the ethics of physician-assisted suicide, see John Keown, ed., *Euthanasia Examined: Ethical, Clinical and Legal Perspectives*, (Cambridge University Press, 1995). Also see the collection of essays in the May–June 1995 *Hastings Center Report* and in the special section entitled "Physician-Aided Death: The Escalating Debate" in *Cambridge Quarterly of Healthcare Ethics* (vol. 5, no. 1, 1996). In addition to the concerns raised about vulnerable groups such as people who are mentally incompetent or severely disabled, Susan M. Wolf introduces the issue of gender as a risk factor in "Gender, Feminism, and Death: Physician-Assisted Suicide," in Susan M. Wolf, ed., *Feminism and Bioethics: Beyond Reproduction* (Oxford University Press, 1996). The impact of patient prognosis and other factors on end-of-life decisions are explored by Peter A. Singer et al. in "Public Opinion Regarding End-of-Life Decisions: Influence of Prognosis, Practice and Process," *Social Science and Medicine* (vol. 41, no. 11, 1995). A recent survey of Michigan physicians found that most prefer either legalization or no law at all and that fewer than 20 percent want physician-assisted suicide completely banned. See "Attitudes of Michigan Physicians and the Public Toward Legalizing Physician-Assisted Suicide and Voluntary Euthanasia," *The New England Journal of Medicine* (February 1, 1996).

ISSUE 6

Is It Ethical to Withhold the Truth from Dying Patients?

YES: Bernard C. Meyer, from "Truth and the Physician," in E. Fuller Torrey, ed., *Ethical Issues in Medicine* (Little, Brown, 1968)

NO: Sissela Bok, from *Lying: Moral Choice in Public and Private Life* (Pantheon Books, 1978)

ISSUE SUMMARY

YES: Physician Bernard C. Meyer argues that physicians must use discretion in communicating bad news to patients. Adherence to a rigid formula of truth telling fails to appreciate the differences in patients' readiness to hear and understand the information.

NO: Philosopher Sissela Bok challenges the traditional physician's view by arguing that the harm resulting from disclosure is less than they think and is outweighed by the benefits, including the important one of giving the patient the right to choose among treatments.

In his powerful short story "The Death of Ivan Ilych," Leo Tolstoy graphically portrays the physical agony and the social isolation of a dying man. However, "What tormented Ivan Ilych most was the deception, the lie, which for some reason they all accepted, that he was not dying but was simply ill, and that he only need keep quiet and undergo a treatment and then something very good would result." Instrumental in setting up the deception is Ivan's doctor, who reassures him to the very end that all will be well. Hearing the banal news from his doctor once again, "Ivan Ilych looks at him as much as to say: 'Are you really never ashamed of lying?' But the doctor does not wish to understand this question."

Unlike many of the ethical issues discussed in this volume, which have arisen as a result of modern scientific knowledge and technology, the question of whether or not to tell dying patients the truth is an old and persistent one. But this debate has been given a new urgency because medical practices today are so complex that it is often difficult to know just what the "truth" really is. A dying patient's life can often be prolonged, although at great financial and personal cost, and many people differ over the definition of a terminal illness.

What must be balanced in this decision are two significant principles of ethical conduct: the obligation to tell the truth and the obligation not to harm others. Moral philosophers, beginning with Aristotle, have regarded truth as either an absolute value or one that, at the very least, is preferable to deception. The great nineteenth-century German philosopher Immanuel Kant argued that there is no justification for lying (although some later commentators feel that his absolutist position has been overstated). Other philosophers have argued that deception is sometimes justified. For example, Henry Sidgwick, an early-twentieth-century British philosopher, believed that it was entirely acceptable to lie to invalids and children to protect them from the shock of the truth. Although the question has been debated for centuries, no clear-cut answer has been reached. In fact, the case of a benevolent lie to a dying patient is often given as the prime example of an excusable deception.

If moral philosophers cannot agree, what guidance is there for the physician torn between the desire for truth and the desire to protect the patient from harm (and the admittedly paternalistic conviction that the doctor knows best what will harm the patient)? None of the early medical codes and oaths offered any advice to physicians on what to tell patients, although they were quite explicit about the physician's obligation to keep confidential whatever a patient revealed. The American Medical Association's (AMA) 1847 "Code of Ethics" did endorse some forms of deception by noting that the physician has a sacred duty "to avoid all things which have a tendency to discourage the patient and to depress his spirits." The most recent (1980) AMA "Principles of Medical Ethics" say only that "a physician shall deal honestly with patients and colleagues." However, the American Hospital Association's "Patient's Bill of Rights," adopted in 1972, is more specific: "The patient has the right to obtain from his physician complete current information concerning his diagnosis, treatment, and prognosis in terms the patient can reasonably be expected to understand. When it is not medically advisable to give such information to the patient, the information should be made available to an appropriate person in his behalf."

In the following selections, Bernard C. Meyer argues for an ethic that transcends the virtue of uttering truth for truth's sake. He believes that the physician's prime responsibility is contained in the Hippocratic Oath—"So far as possible, do no harm." Sissela Bok counters with evidence that physicians often misread patients' wishes and that withholding the truth can often harm them more than disclosure.

YES

Bernard C. Meyer

TRUTH AND THE PHYSICIAN

Truth does not do so much good in this world as the semblance of it does harm.

—La Rochefoucauld

Among the reminiscences of his Alsatian boyhood, my father related the story of the local functionary who was berated for the crude and blunt manner in which he went from house to house announcing to wives and mothers news of battle casualties befalling men from the village. On the next occasion, mindful of the injunctions to be more tactful and to soften the impact of his doleful message, he rapped gently on the door and, when it opened, inquired, "Is the widow Schmidt at home?"

Insofar as this essay is concerned with the subject of truth it is only proper to add that when I told this story to a colleague, he already knew it and claimed that it concerned a woman named Braun who lived in a small town in Austria. By this time it would not surprise me to learn that the episode is a well-known vignette in the folklore of Tennessee where it is attributed to a woman named Smith or Brown whose husband was killed at the battle of Shiloh. Ultimately, we may find that all three versions are plagiarized accounts of an occurrence during the Trojan War.

COMMUNICATION BETWEEN PHYSICIAN AND PATIENT

Apocryphal or not, the story illustrates a few of the vexing aspects of the problem of conveying unpalatable news, notably the difficulty of doing so in a manner that causes a minimum amount of pain, and also the realization that not everyone is capable of learning how to do it. Both aspects find their application in the field of medicine where the imparting of the grim facts of diagnosis and prognosis is a constant and recurring issue. Nor does it seem likely that for all our learning we doctors are particularly endowed with superior talents and techniques for coping with these problems. On the contrary, for reasons to be given later, there is cause to believe that in not a few instances, elements in his own psychological makeup may cause the physician to be singularly ill-equipped to be the bearer of bad tidings. It should be observed, moreover, that until comparatively recent times, the subject of communication between physician and patient received little attention in medical curriculum and medical literature.

Within the past decade or so, coincident with an expanded recognition of the significance of emotional factors in all medical practice, an impressive number of books and articles by physicians, paramedical personnel, and others have been published, attesting to both the growing awareness of the importance of the subject and an apparent willingness to face it. An especially noteworthy example of this trend was provided by a three-day meeting in February, 1967, sponsored by the New York Academy of Sciences, on the subject of *The Care of Patients with Fatal Illness*. The problem of communicating with such patients and their families was a recurring theme in most of the papers presented.

Both at this conference and in the literature, particular emphasis has been focused on the patient with cancer, which is hardly surprising in light of its frequency and of the extraordinary emotional reactions that it unleashes not only in the patient and in his kinsmen but in the physician himself. At the same time, it should be noted that the accent on the cancer patient or the dying patient may foster the impression that in less grave conditions this dialogue between patient and physician hardly warrants much concern or discussion. Such a view is unfounded, however, and could only be espoused by someone who has had the good fortune to escape the experience of being ill and hospitalized. Those less fortunate will recall the emotional stresses induced by hospitalization, even when the condition requiring it is relatively banal.

A striking example of such stress may sometimes be seen when the patient who is hospitalized, say, for repair of an inguinal hernia, happens to be a physician. All the usual anxieties confronting a prospective surgical subject tend to become greatly amplified and garnished with a generous sprinkling of hypochondriasis in the physician-turned-patient. Wavering unsteadily between these two roles, he conjures up visions of all the complications of anesthesia, of wound dehiscence or infection, of embolization, cardiac arrest, and whatnot that he has ever heard or read about. To him, lying between hospital sheets, clad in impersonal hospital clothes, divested of his watch and the keys to his car, the hospital suddenly takes on a different appearance from the place he may have known in a professional capacity. Even his colleagues—the anesthetist who will put him to sleep or cause a temporary motor and sensory paralysis of the lower half of his body, and the surgeon who will incise it—appear different. He would like to have a little talk with them, a very professional talk to be sure, although in his heart he may know that the talk will also be different. And if they are in tune with the situation, they too know that it will be different, that beneath the restrained tones of sober and factual conversation is the thumping anxiety of a man who seeks words of reassurance. With some embarrassment he may introduce his anxieties with the phrase, "I suppose this is going to seem a little silly, but...""; and from this point on he may sound like any other individual confronted by the ordeal of surgical experience.[1] Indeed, it would appear that under these circumstances, to say nothing of more ominous ones, most people, regardless of their experience, knowledge, maturity or sophistication, are assailed by more or less similar psychological pressures, from which they seek relief not through pharmacological sedation, but through the more calming influence of the spoken word.

Seen in this light the question of what to tell the patient about his illness is but one facet of the practice of medicine as an art, a particular example of that spoken and mute dialogue between patient and physician which has always been and will always be an indispensable ingredient in the therapeutic process. How to carry on this dialogue, what to say and when to say it, and what not to say, are questions not unlike those posed by an awkward suitor; like him, those not naturally versed in this art may find themselves discomfited and needful of the promptings of some Cyrano who will whisper those words and phrases that ultimately will wing their way to soothe an anguished heart.

EMOTIONAL REACTIONS OF PHYSICIAN

The difficulties besetting the physician under these circumstances, however, cannot be ascribed simply to his mere lack of experience or innate eloquence. For like the stammering suitor, the doctor seeking to communicate with his patient may have an emotional stake in his message. When that message contains an ominous significance, he may find himself too troubled to use words wisely, too ridden with anxiety to be kind, and too depressed to convey hope. An understanding of such reactions touches upon a recognition of some of the several psychological motivations that have led some individuals to choose a medical career. There is evidence that at times that choice has been dictated by what might be viewed as counterphobic forces. Having in childhood experienced recurring brushes with illness and having encountered a deep and abiding fear of death and dying, such persons may embrace a medical career as if it will confer upon them a magical immunity from a repetition of those dreaded eventualities; for them the letters M.D. constitute a talisman bestowing upon the wearer a sense of invulnerability and a pass of safe conduct through the perilous frontiers of life. There are others for whom the choice of a career dedicated to helping and healing appears to have arisen as a reaction formation against earlier impulses to wound and to destroy.[2] For still others among us, the practice of medicine serves as the professional enactment of a long-standing rescue fantasy.

It is readily apparent in these examples (which by no means exhaust the catalogue of motives leading to the choice of a medical career) that confrontation by the failure of one's efforts and by the need to announce it may unloose a variety of inner psychological disturbances: faced by the gravely ill or dying patient the "counterphobic" doctor may feel personally vulnerable again; the "reaction-formation" doctor, evil and guilty; and the "rescuer," worthless and impotent. For such as these, words cannot come readily in their discourse with the seriously or perilously ill. Indeed, they may curtail their communications; and, what is no less meaningful to their patients, withdraw their physical presence. Thus the patient with inoperable cancer and his family may discover that the physician, who at a more hopeful moment in the course of the illness had been both articulate and supportive, has become remote both in his speech and in his behavior. Nor is the patient uncomprehending of the significance of the change in his doctor's attitude. Observers have recorded the verbal expressions of patients who sensed the feelings of futility and depression in their physicians. Seeking to account for their own reluctance to ask questions (a reluctance based partly upon their own disinclination to face a grim reality), one such patient said, "He looked so tired." Another stated, "I don't want to upset him because he has tried so hard to help me"; and another, "I know he feels so badly already and is doing his best" (Abrams, 1966). To paraphrase a celebrated utterance, one might suppose that these remarks were dictated by the maxim: "Ask not what your doctor can do for you; ask what you can do for your doctor."[3]

ADHERENCE TO A FORMULA

In the dilemma created both by a natural disinclination to be a bearer of bad news and by those other considerations already cited, many a physician is tempted to abandon personal judgment and authorship in his discourse with his patients, and to rely instead upon a set formula which he employs with dogged and indiscriminate consistency. Thus, in determining what to say to patients with cancer, there are exponents of standard policies that are applied routinely in seeming disregard of the overall clinical picture and of the personality or psychological makeup of the patient. In general, two such schools of thought prevail; i.e., those that always tell and those that never do. Each of these is amply supplied with statistical anecdotal evidence proving the correctness of the policy. Yet even if the figures were accurate —and not infrequently they are obtained via a questionnaire, itself a rather opaque window to the human mind—all they demonstrate is that more rather than less of a given proportion of the cancer population profited by the policy employed. This would provide small comfort, one might suppose, to the patients and their families that constitute the minority of the sample.

TRUTH AS ABSTRACT PRINCIPLE

At times adherence to such a rigid formula is dressed up in the vestments of slick and facile morality. Thus a theologian has insisted that the physician has a moral obligation to tell the truth and that his withholding it constitutes a deprivation of the patient's right; therefore it is "theft, therefore unjust, therefore immoral" (Fletcher, 1954). "Can it be," he asks, "that doctors who practice professional deception would, if the roles were reversed, want to be coddled or deceived?" To which, as many physicians can assert, the answer is distinctly yes. Indeed so adamant is this writer upon the right of the patient to know the facts of his illness that in the event he refuses to hear what the doctor is trying to say, the latter should "ask leave to withdraw from the case, urging that another physician be called in his place."[4] (Once there were three boy scouts who were sent away from a campfire and told not to return until each had done his good turn for the day. In 20 minutes all three had returned, and curiously each one reported that he had helped a little old lady to cross a street. The scoutmaster's surprise was even greater when he learned that in each case it was the same little old lady, prompting him to inquire why it took the three of them to perform this one simple good deed. "Well, sir," replied one of the boys, "you see she really didn't want to cross the street at all.")

In this casuistry wherein so much attention is focused upon abstract principle and so little upon humanity, one is reminded of the no less specious arguments of those who assert that the thwarting of suicide and the involuntary hospitalization of the mentally deranged constitute violations of personal freedom and human right.[5] It is surely irregular for a fire engine to travel in the wrong direction on a one-way street, but if one is not averse to putting out fires and saving lives, the traffic violation looms as a conspicuous irrelevancy. No less irrelevant is the obsessional concern with meticulous definitions of truth in an enterprise where kindness, charity, and the relief of human suffering are the ethical verities. "The letter killeth," say the Scriptures, "but the spirit giveth life."

Problem of Definition

Nor should it be forgotten that in the healing arts, the matter of truth is not always susceptible to easy definition. Consider for a moment the question of the hopeless diagnosis. It was not so long ago that such a designation was appropriate for subacute bacterial endocarditis, pneumococcal meningitis, pernicious anemia, and a number of other conditions which today are no longer incurable, while those diseases which today are deemed hopeless may cease to be so by tomorrow. Experience has proved, too, the unreliability of obdurate opinions concerning prognosis even in those conditions where all the clinical evidence and the known behavior of a given disease should leave no room for doubt. To paraphrase Clemenceau, to

insist that a patient is hopelessly ill may at times be worse than a crime; it may be a mistake.

Problem of Determining Patient's Desires

There are other pitfalls, moreover, that complicate the problem of telling patients the truth about their illness. There is the naive notion, for example, that when the patient asserts that what he is seeking is the plain truth he means just that. But as more than one observer has noted, this is sometimes the last thing the patient really wants. Such assertions may be voiced with particular emphasis by patients who happen to be physicians and who strive to display a professional and scientifically objective attitude toward their own condition. Yet to accept such assertions at their face value may sometimes lead to tragic consequences, as in the following incident.

A distinguished urological surgeon was hospitalized for a hypernephroma, which diagnosis had been withheld from him. One day he summoned the intern into his room, and after appealing to the latter on the basis of we're-both-doctors-and-grown-up-men, succeeded in getting the unwary younger man to divulge the facts. Not long afterward, while the nurse was momentarily absent from the room, the patient opened a window and leaped to his death.

Role of Secrecy in Creating Anxiety

Another common error is the assumption that until someone has been formally told the truth he doesn't know it. Such self-deception is often present when parents feel moved to supply their pubertal children with the sexual facts of life. With much embarrassment and a good deal of backing and filling on the subjects of eggs, bees, and babies, sexual information is imparted to a child who often not only already knows it but is uncomfortable in hearing it from that particular source. There is indeed a general tendency to underestimate the perceptiveness of children not only about such matters but where graver issues, notably illness and death, are concerned. As a consequence, attitudes of secrecy and overprotection designed to shield children from painful realities may result paradoxically in creating an atmosphere that is saturated with suspicion, distrust, perplexity, and intolerable anxiety. Caught between trust in their own intuitive perceptions and the deceptions practiced by the adults about them, such children may suffer greatly from a lack of opportunity of coming to terms emotionally with some of the vicissitudes of existence that in the end are inescapable. A refreshing contrast to this approach has been presented in a paper entitled "Who's Afraid of Death on a Leukemia Ward?" (Vernick and Karon, 1965). Recognizing that most of the children afflicted with this disease had some knowledge of its seriousness, and that all were worried about it, the hospital staff abandoned the traditional custom of protection and secrecy, providing instead an atmosphere in which the children could feel free to express their fears and their concerns and could openly acknowledge the fact of death when one of the group passed away. The result of this measure was immensely salutary.

Similar miscalculations of the accuracy of inner perceptions may be noted in dealing with adults. Thus, in a study entitled "Mongolism: When Should Parents Be Told?" (Drillien and Wilkinson, 1964), it was found that in nearly half the cases the mothers declared they had realized before being told that something was seriously wrong with the child's development, a figure which obviously excludes the mothers who refused consciously to acknowledge their suspicions. On the basis of their findings the authors concluded that a full explanation given in the early months, coupled with regular support thereafter, appeared to facilitate the mother's acceptance of and adjustment to her child's handicap.

A pointless and sometimes deleterious withholding of truth is a common practice in dealing with elderly people. "Don't tell Mother" often seems to be an almost reflex maxim among some adults in the face of any misfortune, large or small. Here, too, elaborate efforts at camouflage may backfire, for, sensing that he is being shielded from some ostensibly intolerable secret, not only is the elderly one deprived of the opportunity of reacting appropriately to it, but he is being tacitly encouraged to conjure up something in his imagination that may be infinitely worse.

Discussion of Known Truth

Still another misconception is the belief that if it is certain that the truth is known it is all right to discuss it. How mistaken such an assumption may be was illustrated by the violent rage which a recent widow continued to harbor toward a friend for having alluded to cancer in the presence of her late husband. Hearing her outburst one would have concluded that until the ominous word had been uttered, her husband had been ignorant of the nature of his condition. The facts, however, were different, as the unhappy woman knew, for it had been her husband who originally had told the friend what the diagnosis was.

DENIAL AND REPRESSION

The psychological devices that make such seeming inconsistencies of thought and knowledge possible are the mechanisms of repression and denial. It is indeed the remarkable capacity to bury or conceal more or less transparent truth that makes the problem of telling it so sticky and difficult a matter, and one that is so unsusceptible to simple rule-of-thumb formulas. For while in some instances the maintenance of denial may lead to severe emotional distress, in others it may serve as a merciful shield. For example,

A physician with a reputation for considerable diagnostic acumen developed a painless jaundice. When, not surprisingly, a laparotomy revealed a carcinoma of the head of the pancreas, the surgeon relocated the biliary outflow so that postoperatively the jaundice subsided. This seeming improvement was consistent with the surgeon's explanation to the patient that the operation had revealed a hepatitis. Immensely relieved, the patient chided himself for not having anticipated the "correct" diagnosis. "What a fool I was!" he declared, obviously alluding to an earlier, albeit unspoken, fear of cancer.

Among less sophisticated persons the play of denial may assume a more primitive expression. Thus a woman who had ignored the growth of a breast cancer to a point where it had produced spinal metastases and paraplegia, attributed the latter to "arthritis" and asked whether the breast would grow back again. The same mental mechanism allowed another woman to ignore dangerous rectal bleeding by ascribing it to menstruation, although she was well beyond the menopause.

In contrast to these examples is a case reported by Winkelstein and Blacher of a man who, awaiting the report of a cervical node biopsy, asserted that if it showed cancer he wouldn't want to live, and that if it didn't he wouldn't believe it (Winkelstein and Blacher, 1967). Yet despite this seemingly unambiguous willingness to deal with raw reality, when the chips were down, as will be described later, this man too was able to protect himself through the use of denial.

From the foregoing it should be self-evident that what is imparted to a patient about his illness should be planned with the same care and executed with the same skill that are demanded by any potentially therapeutic measure. Like the transfusion of blood, the dispensing of certain information must be distinctly indicated, the amount given consonant with the needs of the recipient, and the type chosen with the view of avoiding untoward reactions. This means that only in selected instances is there any justification for telling a patient the precise figures of his blood pressure, and that the question of revealing interesting but asymptomatic congenital anomalies should be considered in light of the possibility of evoking either hypochondriacal ruminations or narcissistic gratification.

Under graver circumstances the choices of confronting the physician rest upon more crucial psychological issues. In principle, we should strive to make the patient sufficiently aware of the facts of his condition to facilitate his participation in the treatment without at the same time giving him cause to believe that such participation is futile. "The indispensable ingredient of this therapeutic approach," write Stehlin and Beach, "is free communication between [physician] and patient, in which the latter is sustained by hope within a framework of reality" (Stehlin and Beach, 1966). What this may mean in many instances is neither outright truth nor outright falsehood but a carefully modulated formulation that neither overtaxes human credulity nor invites despair. Thus a sophisticated woman might be expected to reject with complete disbelief the notion that she has had to undergo mastectomy for a benign cyst, but she may at the same time accept postoperative radiation as a prophylactic measure rather than as evidence of metastasis.

A doctor's wife was found to have ovarian carcinoma with widespread metastases. Although the surgeon was convinced she would not survive for more than three or four months, he wished to try the effects of radiotherapy and chemotherapy. After some discussion of the problem with a psychiatrist, he addressed himself to the patient as follows: to his surprise, when examined under the microscope the tumor in her abdomen proved to be cancerous; he fully believed he had removed it entirely; to feel perfectly safe, however, he intended to give her radiation and chemical therapies over an indeterminate period of time. The patient was highly gratified by his frankness and proceeded to live for nearly three more *years*, during which time she enjoyed an active and a productive life.

A rather similar approach was utilized in the case of Winkelstein and Blacher previously mentioned (Winkelstein and Blacher, 1967). In the presence of his wife the patient was told by the resident surgeon, upon the advice of the psychiatrist, that the biopsy of the cervical node showed cancer; that he had a cancerous growth in the abdomen; that it was the type of cancer that responds well to chemotherapy; that if the latter produced any discomfort he would receive medi-

cation for its relief; and finally that the doctors were very hopeful for a successful outcome. The patient, who, it will be recalled, had declared he wouldn't want to live if the doctors found cancer, was obviously gratified. Immediately he telephoned members of his family to tell them the news, gratuitously adding that the tumor was of low-grade malignancy. That night he slept well for the first time since entering the hospital and he continued to do so during the balance of his stay. Just before leaving he confessed that he had known all along about the existence of the abdominal mass but that he had concealed his knowledge to see what the doctors would tell him. Upon arriving home he wrote a warm letter of thanks and admiration to the resident surgeon.

It should be emphasized that although in both of these instances the advice of a psychiatrist was instrumental in formulating the discussion of the facts of the illness, it was the surgeon, not the psychiatrist, who did the talking. The importance of this point cannot be exaggerated, for since it is the surgeon who plays the central and crucial role in such cases, it is to him, and not to some substitute mouthpiece, that the patient looks for enlightenment and for hope. As noted earlier, it is not every surgeon who can bring himself to speak in this fashion to his patient; and for some there may be a strong temptation to take refuge in a sterotyped formula, or to pass the buck altogether. The surgical resident, in the last case cited, for example, was both appalled and distressed when he was advised what to do. Yet he steeled himself, looked the patient straight in the eye and spoke with conviction. When he saw the result, he was both relieved and gratified. Indeed, he emerged from the experience a far wiser man and a better physician.

THE DYING PATIENT

The general point of view expressed in the foregoing pages has been espoused by others in considering the problem of communicating with the dying patient. Aldrich stresses the importance of providing such persons with an appropriately timed opportunity of selecting acceptance or denial of the truth in their efforts to cope with their plight (Aldrich, 1963). Weisman and Hackett believe that for the majority of patients it is likely that there is neither complete acceptance nor total repudiation of the imminence of death (Weismann and Hackett, 1961). "To deny this 'middle knowledge' of approaching death," they assert,

> ... is to deny the responsiveness of the mind to both internal perceptions and external information. There is always a psychological sampling of the physiological stream; fever, weakness, anorexia, weight loss and pain are subjective counterparts of homeostatic alteration.... If to this are added changes in those close to the patient, the knowledge of approaching death is confirmed.

Other observers agree that a patient who is sick enough to die often knows it without being told, and that what he seeks from his physician are no longer statements concerning diagnosis and prognosis, but earnest manifestations of his unwavering concern and devotion. As noted earlier, it is at such times that for reason of their own psychological makeup some physicians become deeply troubled and are most prone to drift away, thereby adding, to the dying patient's physical suffering, the suffering that is caused by a sense of abandonment, isolation, and emotional deprivation.

In contrast, it should be stressed that no less potent than morphine nor less effective than an array of tranquilizers is the steadfast and serious concern of the physician for those often numerous and relatively minor complaints of the dying patient. To this beneficent manifestation of psychological denial, which may at times attain hypochondriacal proportions, the physician ideally should respond in kind, shifting his gaze from the lethal process he is now helpless to arrest to the living being whose discomfort and distress he is still able to assuage. In these, the final measures of the dance of life, it may then appear as if both partners had reached a tacit and a mutual understanding, an unspoken pledge to ignore the dark shadow of impending death and to resume those turns and rhythms that were familiar figures in a more felicitious past. If in this he is possessed of enough grace and elegance to play his part the doctor may well succeed in fulfilling the assertion of Oliver Wendell Holmes that if one of the functions of the physician is to assist at the coming in, another is to assist at the going out.

If what has been set down here should prove uncongenial to some strict moralists, one can only observe that there is a hierarchy of morality, and that ours is a profession which traditionally has been guided by a precept that transends the virtue of uttering truth for truth's sake; that is, "So far as possible, do no harm." Where it concerns the communication between the physician and his patient, the attainment of this goal demands an ear that is sensitive to both what is said and what is not said, a mind that is capable of understanding what has been heard, and a heart that can respond to what has been understood. Here, as in many difficult human enterprises, it may prove easier to learn the words than to sing the tune.

We did not dare to breathe a prayer
Or give our anguish scope!
Something was dead in each of us,
And what was dead was Hope!

—Oscar Wilde,
The Ballad of Reading Gaol

NOTES

1. It should be observed, however, that while the emotional conflicts of the sick doctor may contribute to the ambiguity of his position, that ambiguity may be abetted by the treating physician, who in turn may experience difficulty in assigning to his ailing colleague the unequivocal status of patient. Indeed the latter may be more or less tacitly invited to share the responsibility in the diagnosis and care of his own illness to a degree that in some instances he is virtually a consultant on his own case.

A similar lack of a clear-cut definition of role is not uncommon when members of a doctor's family are ill. Here a further muddying of the waters may be caused by the time-honored practice of extending so-called courtesy—i.e., free care—to physicians and their families, a custom which, however well intentioned, may place its presumed beneficiaries in a moral straitjacket that discourages them from making rather ordinary demands on the treating physician, to say nothing of discharging him. It is not surprising that the care of physicians and their families occasionally evokes an atmosphere of bitterness and rancor.

2. The notion that at heart some doctors are killers is a common theme in literature. It is claimed that when in a fit of despondency Napoleon Bonaparte declared he should have been a physician, Talleyrand commented: "*Toujours assassin.*"

3. This aspect of the patient-doctor relationship has not received the attention it deserves. Moreover, aside from being a therapeutic success, there are other ways in which his patients may support the doctor's psychological needs. His self-esteem, no less than his economic well-being, may be nourished by an ever-growing roster of devoted patients, particularly when the latter include celebrities and other persons of prominence. How important this can be may be judged by the not too uncommon indiscretions perpetrated by some physicians (and sometimes by their wives) in leaking confidential matters pertaining to their practice, notably the identity of their patients.

4. The same writer relaxes his position when it concerns psychiatric patients. Here he would sanction the withholding of knowledge "precisely because he may prevent the patient's recovery by revealing it." But in this, too, the writer is in error, in double error, it would seem, for, first, it is artificial and inexact to make a sharp distinction between psychiatric and nonpsychiatric patterns—the seriously sick and the dying are not infrequently conspicuously emotionally disturbed: and second, because it may at times be therapeutically advisable to acquaint the psychiatric patient with the facts of his illness.

5. Proponents of these views have seemingly overlooked the unconscious elements in human behavior and thought. Paradoxical though it may seem, the would-be suicide may wish to live: what he seeks to destroy may be restricted to that part of the self that has become burdensome or hateful. By the same token, despite his manifest combativeness, a psychotic individual is often inwardly grateful for the restraints imposed upon his dangerous aggression. There can be no logical objection to designating such persons as "prisoners," as Szasz would have it, provided we apply the same term to breathless individuals who are "incarcerated" in oxygen tents.

REFERENCES

Abrams, R.D. The patient with cancer—His changing pattern of communication. *New Eng. J. Med.* 274:317, 1966.

Aldrich, C.K. The dying patient's grief. *J.A.M.A.* 184:329, 1963.

Drillien, C.M., and Wilkinson, E.M. Mongolism: When should parents be told? *Brit. Med. J.* 2:1306, 1964.

Fletcher, J. *Morals and Medicine.* Princeton: Princeton University Press, 1954.

Stehlin, J.S., and Beach, K.A. Psychological aspects of cancer therapy. *J.A.M.A.* 197:100, 1966.

Vernick, J., and Karon, M. Who's afraid of death on a leukemia ward? *Amer. J. Dis. Child*, 109:393, 1965.

Weisman, A.D., and Hackett, T. Predilection to death: Death and dying as a psychiatric problem. *Psychosom. Med.* 23:232, 1961.

Winkelstein, C., and Blacher, R. Personal communication, 1967.

NO

Sissela Bok

LIES TO THE SICK AND DYING

DECEPTION AS THERAPY

A forty-six-year-old man, coming to a clinic for a routine physical check-up needed for insurance purposes, is diagnosed as having a form of cancer likely to cause him to die within six months. No known cure exists for it. Chemotherapy may prolong life by a few extra months, but will have side effects the physician does not think warranted in this case. In addition, he believes that such therapy should be reserved for patients with a chance for recovery or remission. The patient has no symptoms giving him any reason to believe that he is not perfectly healthy. He expects to take a short vacation in a week.

For the physician, there are now several choices involving truthfulness. Ought he to tell the patient what he has learned, or conceal it? If asked, should he deny it? If he decides to reveal the diagnosis, should he delay doing so until after the patient returns from his vacation? Finally, even if he does reveal the serious nature of the diagnosis, should he mention the possibility of chemotherapy and his reasons for not recommending it in this case? Or should he encourage every last effort to postpone death?

In this particular case, the physician chose to inform the patient of his diagnosis right away. He did not, however, mention the possibility of chemotherapy. A medical student working under him disagreed; several nurses also thought that the patient should have been informed of this possibility. They tried, unsuccessfully, to persuade the physician that this was the patient's right. When persuasion had failed, the student elected to disobey the doctor by informing the patient of the alternative of chemotherapy. After consultation with family members, the patient chose to ask for the treatment.

Doctors confront such choices often and urgently. What they reveal, hold back, or distort will matter profoundly to their patients. Doctors stress with corresponding vehemence their reasons for the distortion or concealment: not to confuse the sick person needlessly, or cause what may well be unnecessary pain or discomfort, as in the case of the cancer patient; not to leave a patient without hope, as in those many cases where the dying are not told the truth about their condition; or to improve the chances of cure, as where unwarranted optimism is expressed about some form of therapy. Doctors use information as part of the therapeutic regimen; it is given out in amounts, in admixtures, and according to timing believed best for patients. Accuracy, by comparison, matters far less.

Lying to patients has, therefore, seemed an especially excusable act. Some would argue that doctors, and *only* doctors, should be granted the right to manipulate the truth in ways so undesirable for politicians, lawyers, and others. Doctors are trained to help patients; their relationship to patients carries special obligations, and they know much more than laymen about what helps and hinders recovery and survival.

Even the most conscientious doctors, then, who hold themselves at a distance from the quacks and the purveyors of false remedies, hesitate to forswear all lying. Lying is usually wrong, they argue, but less so than allowing the truth to harm patients. B. C. Meyer echoes this very common view:

[O]urs is a profession which traditionally has been guided by a precept that transcends the virtue of uttering truth for truth's sake, and that is, "so far as possible, do no harm."

Truth, for Meyer, may be important, but not when it endangers the health and well-being of patients. This has seemed self-evident to many physicians in the past—so much so that we find very few mentions of veracity in the codes and oaths and writings by physicians through the centuries. This absence is all the more striking as other principles of ethics have been consistently and movingly expressed in the same documents....

Given such freedom, a physician can decide to tell as much or as little as he wants the patient to know, so long as he breaks no law. In the case of the man mentioned at the beginning of this chapter, some physicians might feel justified in lying for the good of the patient, others might be truthful. Some may conceal alternatives to the treatment they recommend; others not. In each case, they could appeal to the A.M.A. Principles of Ethics. A great many would choose to be able to lie. They would claim that not only can a lie avoid harm for the patient, but that it is also hard to know whether they have been right in the first place in making their pessimistic diagnosis; a "truthful" statement could therefore turn out to hurt patients unnecessarily. The concern for curing and for supporting those who cannot be cured then runs counter to the desire to be completely open. This concern is especially strong where the prognosis is bleak; even more so when patients are so affected by their illness or their medication that they are more dependent than usual, perhaps more easily depressed or irrational.

Physicians know only too well how uncertain a diagnosis or prognosis can be. They know how hard it is to give meaningful and correct answers regarding health and illness. They also know that disclosing their own uncertainty or fears can reduce those benefits that depend upon faith in recovery. They fear, too, that revealing grave risks, no matter how unlikely it is that these will come about, may exercise the pull of the "self-fulfilling prophecy." They dislike being the bearers of uncertain or bad news as much as anyone else. And last, but not least, sitting down to discuss an illness truthfully and sensitively may take much-needed time away from other patients.

These reasons help explain why nurses and physicians and relatives of the sick and dying prefer not to be bound by rules that might limit their ability to suppress, delay, or distort information. This is not to say that they necessarily plan to lie much of the time. They merely want to have the freedom to do so when they believe it wise. And the reluctance to see lying prohibited explains, in turn, the failure of the codes and oaths to come to grips with the problems of truth-telling and lying.

But sharp conflicts are now arising. Doctors no longer work alone with patients. They have to consult with others much more than before; if they choose to lie, the choice may not be met with approval by all who take part in the care of the patient. A nurse expresses the difficulty which results as follows:

> From personal experience I would say that the patients who aren't told about their terminal illness have so many verbal and mental questions unanswered that many will begin to realize that their illness is more serious than they're being told....

The doctor's choice to lie increasingly involves coworkers in acting a part they find neither humane nor wise. The fact that these problems have not been carefully thought through within the medical profession, nor seriously addressed in medical education, merely serves to intensify the conflicts. Different doctors then respond very differently to patients in exactly similar predicaments. The friction is increased by the fact that relatives often disagree even where those giving medical care to a patient are in accord on how to approach the patient. Here again, because physicians have not worked out to common satisfaction the question of whether relatives have the right to make such requests, the problems are allowed to be haphazardly resolved by each physician as he sees fit.

THE PATIENT'S PERSPECTIVE

The turmoil in the medical profession regarding truth-telling is further augmented by the pressures that patients themselves now bring to bear and by empirical data coming to light. Challenges are growing to the three major arguments for lying to patients: that truthfulness is impossible; that patients do not want bad news; and that truthful information harms them.

The first of these arguments... confuses "truth" and "truthfulness" so as to clear the way for occasional lying on grounds supported by the second and third arguments. At this point, we can see more clearly that it is a strategic move intended to discourage the question of truthfulness from carrying much weight in the first place, and thus to leave the choice of what to say and how to say it up to the physician. To claim that "since telling the truth is impossible, there can be no sharp distinction between what is true and what is false" is to try to defeat objections to lying before even discussing them. One need only imagine how such an argument would be received, were it made by a car salesman or a real estate dealer, to see how fallacious it is.

In medicine, however, the argument is supported by a subsidiary point: even if people might ordinarily understand what is spoken to them, patients are often not in a position to do so. This is where paternalism enters in. When we buy cars or houses, the paternalist will argue, we need to have all our wits about us; but when we are ill, we cannot always do so. We need help in making choices, even if help can be given only by keeping us in the dark. And the physician is trained and willing to provide such help.

It is certainly true that some patients cannot make the best choices for themselves when weakened by illness or drugs. But most still can. And even those who are incompetent have a right to have someone—their guardian or spouse perhaps—receive the correct information.

The paternalistic assumption of superiority to patients also carries great dangers for physicians themselves—it risks turning to contempt. The following view was recently expressed in a letter to a medical journal:

> As a radiologist who has been sued, I have reflected earnestly on advice to obtain Informed Consent but have decided to "take the risks without informing the patient" and trust to "God, judge, and jury" rather than evade responsibility through a legal gimmick....
>
> [I]n a general radiologic practice many of our patients are uninformable and we would never get through the day if we had to obtain their consent to every potentially harmful study....

The argument which rejects informing patients because adequate truthful information is impossible in itself or because patients are lacking in understanding, must itself be rejected when looked at from the point of view of patients. They know that liberties granted to the most conscientious and altruistic doctors will be exercised also in the "Medicaid Mills"; that the choices thus kept from patients will be exercised by not only competent but incompetent physicians; and that even the best doctors can make choices patients would want to make differently for themselves.

The second argument for deceiving patients refers specifically to giving them news of a frightening or depressing kind. It holds that patients do not, in fact, generally want such information, that they prefer not to have to face up to serious illness and death. On the basis of such a belief, most doctors in a number of surveys stated that they do not, as a rule, inform patients that they have an illness such as cancer.

When studies are made of what patients desire to know, on the other hand, a large majority say that they *would* like to be told of such a diagnosis. All these studies need updating and should be done with larger numbers of patients and non-patients. But they do show that there is generally a dramatic divergence between physicians and patients on the factual question of whether patients want to know what ails them in cases of serious illness such as cancer. In most of the studies, over 80 percent of the persons asked indicated that they would want to be told.

Sometimes this discrepancy is set aside by doctors who want to retain the view that patients do not want unhappy news. In reality, they claim, the fact that patients say they want it has to be discounted. The more someone asks to know, the more he suffers from fear which will lead to the denial of the information even if it is given. Informing patients is, therefore, useless; they resist and deny having been told what they cannot assimilate. According to this view, empirical studies of what patients say they want are worthless since they do not probe deeply enough to uncover this universal resistance to the contemplation of one's own death.

This view is only partially correct. For some patients, denial is indeed well established in medical experience. A number of patients (estimated at between 15 percent and 25 percent) will give evidence of denial of having been told about their illness, even when they repeatedly ask and are repeatedly informed. And nearly everyone experiences a period of denial at some point in the course of approaching death. Elisabeth Kübler-Ross sees denial as resulting often from premature and abrupt information by a stranger who goes through the process quickly to "get it over with." She holds that denial functions as a buffer after unexpected shocking news, permitting individuals to collect themselves and to mobilize other defenses. She describes prolonged denial in one patient as follows:

> She was convinced that the X-rays were "mixed up"; she asked for reassurance that her pathology report could not possibly be back so soon and that another patient's report must have been marked with her name. When none of this could be confirmed, she quickly asked to leave the hospital, looking for another physician in the vain hope "to get a better explanation for my troubles." This patient went "shopping around" for many doctors, some of whom gave her reassuring answers, other of whom confirmed the previous suspicion. Whether confirmed or not, she reacted in the same manner; she asked for examination and reexamination. . . .

But to say that denial is universal flies in the face of all evidence. And to take any claim to the contrary as "symptomatic" of deeper denial leaves no room for reasoned discourse. There is no way that such universal denial can be proved true or false. To believe in it is a metaphysical belief about

man's condition, not a statement about what patients do and do not want. It is true that we can never completely understand the possibility of our own death, any more than being alive in the first place. But people certainly differ in the degree to which they can approach such knowledge, take it into account in their plans, and make their peace with it.

Montaigne claimed that in order to learn both to live and to die, men have to think about death and be prepared to accept it. To stick one's head in the sand, or to be prevented by lies from trying to discern what is to come, hampers freedom—freedom to consider one's life as a whole, with a beginning, a duration, an end. Some may request to be deceived rather than to see their lives as thus finite; others reject the information which would require them to do so; but most say that they want to know. Their concern for knowing about their condition goes far beyond mere curiosity or the wish to make isolated personal choices in the short time left to them; their stance toward the entire life they have lived, and their ability to give it meaning and completion, are at stake. In lying or withholding the facts which permit such discernment, doctors may reflect their own fears (which, according to one study, are much stronger than those of laymen) of facing questions about the meaning of one's life and the inevitability of death.

Beyond the fundamental deprivation that can result from deception, we are also becoming increasingly aware of all that can befall patients in the course of their illness when information is denied or distorted. Lies place them in a position where they no longer participate in choices concerning their own health, including the choice of whether to be a "patient" in the first place. A terminally ill person who is not informed that his illness is incurable and that he is near death cannot make decisions about the end of his life: about whether or not to enter a hospital, or to have surgery; where and with whom to spend his last days; how to put his affairs in order—these most personal choices cannot be made if he is kept in the dark, or given contradictory hints and clues.

It has always been especially easy to keep knowledge from terminally ill patients. They are most vulnerable, least able to take action to learn what they need to know, or to protect their autonomy. The very fact of being so ill greatly increases the likelihood of control by others. And the fear of being helpless in the face of such control is growing. At the same time, the period of dependency and slow deterioration of health and strength that people undergo has lengthened. There has been a dramatic shift toward institutionalization of the aged and those near death. (Over 80 percent of Americans now die in a hospital or other institution.)

Patients who are severely ill often suffer a further distancing and loss of control over their most basic functions. Electrical wiring, machines, intravenous administration of liquids, all create new dependency and at the same time new distance between the patient and all who come near. Curable patients are often willing to undergo such procedures; but when no cure is possible, these procedures merely intensify the sense of distance and uncertainty and can even become a substitute for comforting human acts. Yet those who suffer in this way often fear to seem troublesome by complaining. Lying to them, perhaps for the most charitable of purposes, can then cause them to slip unwittingly into

subjection to new procedures, perhaps new surgery, where death is held at bay through transfusions, respirators, even resuscitation far beyond what most would wish.

Seeing relatives in such predicaments has caused a great upsurge of worrying about death and dying. At the root of this fear is not a growing terror of the *moment* of death, or even the instants before it. Nor is there greater fear of *being* dead. In contrast to the centuries of lives lived in dread of the punishments to be inflicted after death, many would now accept the view expressed by Epicurus, who died in 270 B.C.:

> Death, therefore, the most awful of evils, is nothing to us, seeing that, when we are, death is not come, and, when death is come, we are not.

The growing fear, if it is not of the moment of dying nor of being dead, is of all that which now precedes dying for so many: the possibility of prolonged pain, the increasing weakness, the uncertainty, the loss of powers and chance of senility, the sense of being a burden. This fear is further nourished by the loss of trust in health professionals. In part, the loss of trust results from the abuses which have been exposed—the Medicaid scandals, the old-age home profiteering, the commercial exploitation of those who seek remedies for their ailments; in part also because of the deceptive practices patients suspect, having seen how friends and relatives were kept in the dark; in part, finally, because of the sheer numbers of persons, often strangers, participating in the care of any one patient. Trust which might have gone to a doctor long known to the patient goes less easily to a team of strangers, no matter how expert or well-meaning.

It is with the working out of all that *informed consent*[1] implies and the information it presupposes that truth-telling is coming to be discussed in a serious way for the first time in the health professions. Informed consent is a farce if the information provided is distorted or withheld. And even complete information regarding surgical procedures or medication is obviously useless unless the patient also knows what the condition is that these are supposed to correct.

Bills of rights for patients, similarly stressing the right to be informed, are now gaining acceptance. This right is not new, but the effort to implement it is. Nevertheless, even where patients are handed the most elegantly phrased Bill of Rights, their right to a truthful diagnosis and prognosis is by no means always respected.

The reason why even doctors who recognize a patient's right to have information might still not provide it brings us to the third argument against telling all patients the truth. It holds that the information given might hurt the patient and that the concern for the right to such information is therefore a threat to proper health care. A patient, these doctors argue, may wish to commit suicide after being given discouraging news, or suffer a cardiac arrest, or simply cease to struggle, and thus not grasp the small remaining chance for recovery. And even where the outlook for a patient is very good, the disclosure of a minute risk can shock some patients or cause them to reject needed protection such as a vaccination or antibiotics.

The factual basis for this argument has been challenged from two points of view. The damages associated with the disclosure of sad news or risks are rarer than physicians believe; and the *benefits* which result from being informed are more substantial, even measurably so. Pain is tolerated more easily, recovery from surgery is quicker, and cooperation with therapy is greatly improved. The attitude that "what you don't know won't hurt you" is proving unrealistic; it is what patients do not know but vaguely suspect that causes them corrosive worry.

It is certain that no answers to this question of harm from information are the same for all patients. If we look, first, at the fear expressed by physicians that informing patients of even remote or unlikely risks connected with a drug prescription or operation might shock some and make others refuse the treatment that would have been best for them, it appears to be unfounded for the great majority of patients. Studies show that very few patients respond to being told of such risks by withdrawing their consent to the procedure and that those who do withdraw are the very ones who might well have been upset enough to sue the physician had they not been asked to consent before hand. It is possible that on even rarer occasions especially susceptible persons might manifest physical deterioration from shock; some physicians have even asked whether patients who die after giving informed consent to an operation, but before it actually takes place, somehow expire because of the information given to them. While such questions are unanswerable in any one case, they certainly argue in favor of caution, a real concern for the person to whom one is recounting the risks he or she will face, and sensitivity to all signs of distress.

The situation is quite different when persons who are already ill, perhaps already quite weak and discouraged, are told of a very serious prognosis. Physicians fear that such knowledge may cause the patients to commit suicide, or to be frightened or depressed to the point that their illness takes a downward turn. The fear that great numbers of patients will commit suicide appears to be unfounded. And if some do, is that a response so unreasonable, so much against the patient's best interest that physicians ought to make it a reason for concealment or lies? Many societies have allowed suicide in the past; our own has decriminalized it; and some are coming to make distinctions among the many suicides which ought to be prevented if at all possible, and those which ought to be respected.

Another possible response to very bleak news is the triggering of physiological mechanisms which allow death to come more quickly—a form of giving up or of preparing for the inevitable, depending on one's outlook. Lewis Thomas, studying responses in humans and animals, holds it not unlikely that:

> ... there is a pivotal movement at some stage in the body's reaction to injury or disease, maybe in aging as well, when the organism concedes that it is finished and the time for dying is at hand, and at this moment the events that lead to death are launched, as a coordinated mechanism. Functions are then shut off, in sequence, irreversibly, and, while this is going on, a neural mechanism, held ready for this occasion, is switched on. ...

Such a response may be appropriate, in which case it makes the moments of dying as peaceful as those who have died and been resuscitated so often testify. But it may also be brought on inappropriately, when the organism could have lived on, perhaps even induced malevolently, by external acts intended to kill. Thomas speculates that some of the deaths resulting from "hexing" are due to such responses. Levi-Strauss describes deaths from exorcism and the casting of spells in ways which suggest that the same process may then be brought on by the community.

It is not inconceivable that unhappy news abruptly conveyed, or a great shock given to someone unable to tolerate it, could also bring on such a "dying response," quite unintended by the speaker. There is every reason to be cautious and to try to know ahead of time how susceptible a patient might be to the accidental triggering—however rare—of such a response. One has to assume, however, that most of those who have survived long enough to be in a situation where their informed consent is asked have a very robust resistance to such accidental triggering of processes leading to death.

When, on the other hand, one considers those who are already near death, the "dying response" may be much less inappropriate, much less accidental, much less unreasonable. In most societies, long before the advent of modern medicine, human beings have made themselves ready for death once they felt its approach. Philippe Aries describes how many in the Middle Ages prepared themselves for death when they "felt the end approach." They awaited death lying down, surrounded by friends and relatives. They recollected all they had lived through and done, pardoning all who stood near their deathbed, calling on God to bless them, and finally praying. "After the final prayer all that remained was to wait for death, and there was no reason for death to tarry."

Modern medicine, in its valiant efforts to defeat disease and to save lives, may be dislocating the conscious as well as the purely organic responses allowing death to come when it is inevitable, thus denying those who are dying the benefits of the traditional approach to death. In lying to them, and in pressing medical efforts to cure them long past the point of possible recovery, physicians may thus rob individuals of an autonomy few would choose to give up.

Sometimes, then, the "dying response" is a natural organic reaction at the time when the body has no further defense. Sometimes it is inappropriately brought on by news too shocking or given in too abrupt a manner. We need to learn a great deal more about this last category, no matter how small. But there is no evidence that patients in general will be debilitated by truthful information about their condition.

Apart from the possible harm from information, we are coming to learn much more about the benefits it can bring patients. People follow instructions more carefully if they know what their disease is and why they are asked to take medication; any benefits from those procedures are therefore much more likely to come about.[2] Similarly, people recover faster from surgery and tolerate pain with less medication if they understand what ails them and what can be done for them.[3]

RESPECT AND TRUTHFULNESS

Taken all together, the three arguments defending lies to patients stand on much shakier ground as a counterweight to the right to be informed than is often thought. The common view that many patients cannot understand, do not want, and may be harmed by, knowledge of their condition, and that lying to them is either morally neutral or even to be recommended, must be set aside. Instead, we have to make a more complex comparison. Over against the right of patients to knowledge concerning themselves, the medical and psychological benefits to them from this knowledge, the unnecessary and sometimes harmful treatment to which they can be subjected if ignorant, and the harm to physicians, their profession, and other patients from deceptive practices, we have to set a severely restricted and narrowed paternalistic view—that *some* patients cannot understand, *some* do not want, and *some* may be harmed by, knowledge of their condition, and that they ought not to have to be treated like everyone else if this is not in their best interest.

Such a view is persuasive. A few patients openly request not to be given bad news. Others give clear signals to that effect, or are demonstrably vulnerable to the shock or anguish such news might call forth. Can one not in such cases infer implied consent to being deceived?

Concealment, evasion, withholding of information may at times be necessary. But if someone contemplates lying to a patient or concealing the truth, the burden of proof must shift. It must rest, here, as with all deception, on those who advocate it in any one instance. They must show why they fear a patient may be harmed or how they know that another cannot cope with the truthful knowledge. A decision to deceive must be seen as a very unusual step, to be talked over with colleagues and others who participate in the care of the patient. Reasons must be set forth and debated, alternatives weighed carefully. At all times, the correct information must go to *someone* closely related to the patient.

NOTES

1. The law requires that inroads made upon a person's body take place only with the informed voluntary consent of that person. The term "informed consent" came into common use only after 1960, when it was used by the Kansas Supreme Court in Nathanson vs. Kline, 186 Kan. 393, 350, p. 2d, 1093 (1960). The patient is now entitled to full disclosure of risks, benefits, and alternative treatments to any proposed procedure, both in therapy and in medical experimentation, except in emergencies or when the patient is incompetent, in which case proxy consent is required.

2. Barbara S. Hulka, J. C. Cassel, et al. "Communication, Compliance, and Concordance between Physicians and Patients with Prescribed Medications," *American Journal of Public Health*, Sept. 1976, pp. 847–53. The study shows that of the nearly half of all patients who do not follow the prescriptions of the doctors (thus foregoing the intended effect of these prescriptions), many will follow them if adequately informed about the nature of their illness and what the proposed medication will do.

3. See Lawrence D. Egbert, George E. Batitt, et al., "Reduction of Postoperative Pain by Encouragement and Instruction of Patients," *New England Journal of Medicine*, 270, pp. 825–27, 1964.

See also: Howard Waitzskin and John D. Stoeckle, "The Communication of Information about Illness," *Advances in Psychosomatic Medicine*, Vol. 8, 1972, pp. 185–215.

POSTSCRIPT

Is It Ethical to Withhold the Truth from Dying Patients?

In its 1983 report *Making Health Care Decisions*, the President's Commission for the Study of Ethical Problems in Medicine and Biomedical and Behavioral Research cited evidence from a survey it conducted indicating that 94 percent of the public would "want to know everything" about a diagnosis and prognosis, and 96 percent would want to know specifically about a diagnosis of cancer. To the question "If you had a type of cancer that usually leads to death in less than a year, would you want your doctor to give you a realistic estimate of how long you had to live, or would you prefer that he not tell you?" 85 percent said that they would want the realistic estimate. However, when physicians were asked a similar question about what they would disclose to a patient, only 13 percent would give a "straight, statistical prognosis," and a third said that they would not give a definite time period but would stress that it would not be a long one. Physicians, it appears, are more reluctant to tell the truth than the public (at least when faced with a hypothetical choice) is to hear it. Dennis H. Novack et al., in "Physicians' Attitudes Toward Using Deception to Resolve Difficult Ethical Problems," *Journal of the American Medical Association* (May 26, 1989), report on a survey conducted by a group from the Brown University Program in Medicine. Researchers found that 87 percent of 109 physicians "indicated that deception is acceptable on rare occasions."

An important, recent legal case concerning truth telling and informed consent is *Arcato v. Avedon*. Mr. Arcato, a California electrical contractor, was operated on in 1980 to remove a kidney that was not functioning. The surgeons also removed a tumor from his pancreas, but neither they nor the oncologist to whom they referred Arcato told him that approximately 95 percent of people with pancreatic cancer die within a year. Arcato died one year after the cancer had been diagnosed. His wife and children sued the doctors, claiming that California's informed-consent doctrine required the disclosure of the withheld information. If he had been told the truth, his family argued, he might not have undergone the difficult and unsuccessful experimental treatment his oncologist offered. The case ultimately went to the California Supreme Court, which in 1993 upheld the trial court's ruling in favor of the physicians. For more on the case, see George Annas, "Informed Consent, Cancer, and Truth in Prognosis," *The New England Journal of Medicine* (January 20, 1994), in which the author argues that the real issue was not the statistics on life expectancy but the impact of the proposed treatment in terms of prospects for long-term survival and quality of life.

For a strong defense of the patient's right to know the truth, see chapter 6 of Robert M. Veatch, *Death, Dying, and the Biological Revolution* (Yale University Press, 1976). A philosophical argument with a different view is Donald Van DeVeer's article "The Contractual Argument for Withholding Information," *Philosophy and Public Affairs* (Winter 1980). See also Mark Sheldon, "Truth Telling in Medicine," *Journal of the American Medical Association* (February 5, 1982) and Thurstan B. Brewin, "Truth, Trust, and Paternalism," *The Lancet* (August 31, 1985).

Two books that stress the importance of communication in the doctor-patient relationship are Jay Katz, *The Silent World of Doctor and Patient* (Free Press, 1984) and Eric J. Cassell, *Talking With Patients*, 2 vols. (MIT Press, 1985). Susan J. Barnes edited a symposium called "Perspectives on J. Katz, *The Silent World of Doctor and Patient*," which appeared in the *Western New England Law Review* (vol. 9, no. 1, 1987).

Most of the literature on withholding the truth from patients concerns cancer. Drs. Margaret A. Drickamer and Mark S. Lachs address a different disease in their essay "Should Patients With Alzheimer's Disease Be Told Their Diagnosis?" *The New England Journal of Medicine* (April 2, 1992). Although they favor truth telling, they present the case for not telling, including such factors as the difficulty of conclusive diagnosis, the impaired decision-making capacity and competence of patients with Alzheimer's, and the limited therapeutic options. A cultural difference can be seen in Antonella Surbone's "Truth Telling to the Patient," *Journal of the American Medical Association* (October 7, 1992), in which she describes the practice of withholding information from seriously ill patients in Italy. The same issue contains an accompanying editorial by Edmund D. Pellegrino.

Cultural differences are a strong determinant in people's attitudes about what to tell or not to tell dying patients. Leslie Blackhall et al. found that Korean Americans and Mexican Americans were much less likely to believe that a patient should be told of a terminal prognosis than European Americans or African Americans (see "Ethnicity and Attitudes Toward Patient Autonomy," *Journal of the American Medical Association*, September 13, 1995). Nevertheless, not all families in each ethnic category held the same beliefs, and the authors caution against hasty generalizations.

ISSUE 7

Should Doctors Be Able to Refuse Demands for "Futile" Treatment?

YES: Steven H. Miles, from "Informed Demand for 'Non-Beneficial' Medical Treatment," *The New England Journal of Medicine* (August 15, 1991)

NO: Felicia Ackerman, from "The Significance of a Wish," *Hastings Center Report* (July/August 1991)

ISSUE SUMMARY

YES: Physician Steven H. Miles maintains that physicians' duty to follow patients' wishes ends when the requests are inconsistent with what medical care can reasonably be expected to achieve, when they violate community standards of care, and when they consume an unfair share of collective resources.

NO: Philosopher Felicia Ackerman contends that it is ethically inappropriate for physicians to decide what kind of life is worth prolonging and that decisions involving personal values should be made by the patient or family.

In the typical controversy involving life-prolonging treatment, it is the patient or patient's family who wants to stop treatment and the doctor or hospital administrator who wants to continue it. That line of cases began, most prominently, with the *Quinlan* case (1976) and was most recently decided in the *Cruzan* case (1990). Another scenario, however, is emerging. What happens when the patient or family demands that treatment be continued past the point that doctors or hospital administrators feel it is warranted? Families may hope for a miracle and want "everything possible" done to preserve life. In the case of "Baby L," described by John Paris, Robert K. Crone, and Frank Reardon in *The New England Journal of Medicine* (April 5, 1990), pediatricians refused a mother's request to start ventilator treatment for a severely compromised, blind, deaf, and neurologically impaired child who had spent all 28 months of her life in intensive care.

In other cases, patients or families may act out of religious convictions that life is a God-given gift that must be preserved at all costs. In her book *Ethics on Call* (Crown Publishers, 1992), Nancy Dubler describes the case of "Joseph," a devoutly religious man who interpreted Jewish law to mean that life can be taken only by God, and that he must take whatever measures are available to sustain his life, no matter what suffering was entailed. There may even be cases in which a criminal prosecution may hinge on whether a patient dies or not, or there may be financial motivations to preserving life.

These cases stretch the limits of patient autonomy and come to a full stop when they reach the boundaries of professional responsibility. Just as patients are moral agents, so too are physicians. Their professional ethic begins with the Hippocratic injunction "First, do no harm." Beyond avoiding harm, they are guided by the obligation to do good—to provide benefit to patients within the limits of their expertise. Since ancient times physicians have felt it is their prerogative to determine whether or not treatment is justified. The writings of Hippocrates and Plato warn physicians to acknowledge when their art is doomed to fail.

In modern times the Vatican's 1980 *Declaration on Euthanasia* places a strong emphasis on physician judgment, pointing out that "[doctors] may . . . judge that the investment in instruments and personnel is disproportionate to the results foreseen; they may also judge that the techniques applied impose on the patient strain or suffering out of proportion with the benefits." The U.S. President's Commission for the Study of Bioethical Problems in Medicine concluded in 1983 that "health care professionals or institutions may decline to provide a particular option because that choice may violate their conscience or professional judgement, though, in doing so they may not abandon a patient." Even more recently (December 1990), the Society of Critical Care Medicine declared that "treatments that offer no benefit and serve to prolong the dying process should not be employed."

As frequently happens in bioethics, one case—not necessarily the first to arise—serves to focus the arguments. In the area of demands for "nonbeneficial" treatment, that case involved the treatment of Helga Wanglie, an elderly Minnesota woman who suffered a series of medical problems, culminating in a year and a half spent unconscious on a respirator in a persistent vegetative state. Her physicians asked her husband to consent to withdrawing treatment; his refusal set off a chain of events described in the following selections.

Steven H. Miles, a gerontologist and ethics consultant to Mrs. Wanglie's physicians, argues that Mrs. Wanglie was "overmastered" by her disease and that continued intensive care was inappropriate and inconsistent with reasonable medical expectations of benefit. Felicia Ackerman maintains that decisions about what lives are worth living properly fall to those who share the values of the patient—in this case, the family.

YES

Steven H. Miles

INFORMED DEMAND FOR "NON-BENEFICIAL" MEDICAL TREATMENT

An 85-year-old woman was taken from a nursing home to Hennepin County Medical Center on January 1, 1990, for emergency treatment of dyspnea [shortness of breath] from chronic bronchiectasis [widening of the air passages]. The patient, Mrs. Helga Wanglie, required emergency intubation [insertion of a tube] and was placed on a respirator. She occasionally acknowledged discomfort and recognized her family but could not communicate clearly. In May, after attempts to wean her from the respirator failed, she was discharged to a chronic care hospital. One week later, her heart stopped during a weaning attempt; she was resuscitated and taken to another hospital for intensive care. She remained unconscious, and a physician suggested that it would be appropriate to consider withdrawing life support. In response, the family transferred her back to the medical center on May 31. Two weeks later, physicians concluded that she was in a persistent vegetative state.... She was maintained on a respirator, with repeated courses of antibiotics, frequent airway suctioning, tube feedings, an air flotation bed, and biochemical monitoring.

In June and July of 1990, physicians suggested that life-sustaining treatment be withdrawn since it was not benefiting the patient. Her husband, daughter, and son insisted on continued treatment. They stated their view that physicians should not play God, that the patient would not be better off dead, that removing life support showed moral decay in our civilization, and that a miracle could occur. Her husband told a physician that his wife had never stated her preferences concerning life-sustaining treatment. He believed that the cardiac arrest would not have occurred if she had not been transferred from Hennepin County Medical Center in May. The family reluctantly accepted a do-not-resuscitate order based on the improbability of Mrs. Wanglie's surviving a cardiac arrest. In June, an ethics committee consultant recommended continued counseling for the family. The family declined counseling, including the counsel of their own pastor, and in late July asked

From Steven H. Miles, "Informed Demand for 'Non-Beneficial' Medical Treatment," *The New England Journal of Medicine*, vol. 325, no. 7 (August 15, 1991), pp. 512–515. Copyright © 1991 by The Massachusetts Medical Society. Reprinted by permission.

that the respirator not be discussed again. In August, nurses expressed their consensus that continued life support did not seem appropriate, and I, as the newly appointed ethics consultant, counseled them.

In October 1990, a new attending physician consulted with specialists and confirmed the permanence of the patient's cerebral and pulmonary conditions. He concluded that she was at the end of her life and that the respirator was "non-beneficial," in that it could not heal her lungs, palliate her suffering, or enable this unconscious and permanently respirator-dependent woman to experience the benefit of the life afforded by respirator support. Because the respirator could prolong life, it was not characterized as "futile."[1] In November, the physician, with my concurrence, told the family that he was not willing to continue to prescribe the respirator. The husband, an attorney, rejected proposals to transfer the patient to another facility or to seek a court order mandating this unusual treatment. The hospital told the family that it would ask a court to decide whether members of its staff were obliged to continue treatment. A second conference two weeks later, after the family had hired an attorney, confirmed these positions, and the husband asserted that the patient had consistently said she wanted respirator support for such a condition.

In December, the medical director and hospital administrator asked the Hennepin County Board of Commissioners (the medical center's board of directors) to allow the hospital to go to court to resolve the dispute. In January, the county board gave permission by a 4-to-3 vote. Neither the hospital nor the county had a financial interest in terminating treatment. Medicare largely financed the $200,000 for the first hospitalization at Hennepin County; a private insurer would pay the $500,000 bill for the second. From February through May of 1991, the family and its attorney unsuccessfully searched for another health care facility that would admit Mrs. Wanglie. Facilities with empty beds cited her poor potential for rehabilitation.

The hospital chose a two-step legal procedure, first asking for the appointment of an independent conservator to decide whether the respirator was beneficial to the patient and second, if the conservator found it was not, for a second hearing on whether it was obliged to provide the respirator. The husband cross-filed, requesting to be appointed conservator. After a hearing in late May, the trial court on July 1, 1991, appointed the husband, as best able to represent the patient's interests. It noted that no request to stop treatment had been made and declined to speculate on the legality of such an order.[2] The hospital said that it would continue to provide the respirator in the light of continuing uncertainty about its legal obligation to provide it....

DISCUSSION

This sad story illustrates the problem of what to do when a family demands medical treatment that the attending physician concludes cannot benefit the patient. Only 600 elderly people are treated with respirators for more than six months in the United States each year.[3] Presumably, most of these people are actually or potentially conscious. It is common practice to discontinue the use of a respirator before death when it can no longer benefit a patient.[4,5]

We do not know Mrs. Wanglie's treatment preferences. A large majority of elderly people prefer not to receive prolonged respirator support for irreversible unconsciousness.[6] Studies show that an older person's designated family proxy overestimates that person's preference for life-sustaining treatment in a hypothetical coma.[7-9] The implications of this research for clinical decision making have not been cogently analyzed.

A patient's request for a treatment does not necessarily oblige a provider or the health care system. Patients may not demand that physicians injure them (for example, by mutilation), or provide plausible but inappropriate therapies (for example, amphetamines for weight reduction), or therapies that have no value (such as laetrile for cancer). Physicians are not obliged to violate their personal moral views on medical care so long as patients' rights are served. Minnesota's Living Will law says that physicians are "legally bound to act consistently within my wishes within limits of reasonable medical practice" in acting on requests and refusals of treatment.[10] Minnesota's Bill of Patients' Rights says that patients "have the right to appropriate medical... care based on individual needs... [which is] limited where the service is not reimbursable."[11] Mrs. Wanglie also had aortic insufficiency. Had this condition worsened, a surgeon's refusal to perform a life-prolonging valve replacement as medically inappropriate would hardly occasion public controversy. As the Minneapolis *Star Tribune* said in an editorial on the eve of the trial,

> The hospital's plea is born of realism, not hubris.... It advances the claim that physicians should not be slaves to technology—any more than patients should be its prisoners. They should be free to deliver, and act on, an honest and

time-honored message: "Sorry, there's nothing more we can do."[12]

Disputes between physicians and patients about treatment plans are often handled by transferring patients to the care of other providers. In this case, every provider contacted by the hospital or the family refused to treat this patient with a respirator. These refusals occurred before and after this case became a matter of public controversy and despite the availability of third-party reimbursement. We believe they represent a medical consensus that respirator support is inappropriate in such a case.

The handling of this case is compatible with current practices regarding informed consent, respect for patients' autonomy, and the right to health care. Doctors should inform patients of all medically reasonable treatments, even those available from other providers. Patients can refuse any prescribed treatment or choose among any medical alternatives that physicians are willing to prescribe. Respect for autonomy does not empower patients to oblige physicians to prescribe treatments in ways that are fruitless or inappropriate. Previous "right to die" cases address the different situations of a patient's right to choose to be free of a prescribed therapy. This case is more about the nature of the patient's choice in using that entitlement.

The proposal that this family's preference for this unusual and costly treatment, which is commonly regarded as inappropriate, establishes a right to such treatment is ironic, given that preference does not create a right to other needed, efficacious, and widely desired treatments in the United States. We could not afford a universal health care system based on patients' demands. Such a system would irrationally allocate health care to socially powerful people with strong preferences for immediate treatment to the disadvantage of those with less power or less immediate needs.

After the conclusion was reached that the respirator was not benefiting the patient, the decision to seek a review of the duty to provide it was based on an ethic of "stewardship." Even though the insurer played no part in this case, physicians' discretion to prescribe requires responsible handling of requests for inappropriate treatment. Physicians exercise this stewardship by counseling against or denying such treatment or by submitting such requests to external review. This stewardship is not aimed at protecting the assets of insurance companies but rests on fairness to people who have pooled their resources to insure their collective access to appropriate health care. Several citizens complained to Hennepin County Medical Center that Mrs. Wanglie was receiving expensive treatment paid for by people who had not consented to underwrite a level of medical care whose appropriateness was defined by family demands.

Procedures for addressing this kind of dispute are at an early stage of development. Though the American Medical Association[13] and the Society of Critical Care Medicine[14] also support some decisions to withhold requested treatment, the medical center's reasoning most closely follows the guidelines of the American Thoracic Society.[15] The statements of these professional organizations do not clarify when or how a physician may legally withdraw or withhold demanded life-sustaining treatments. The request for a conservator to review the medical conclusion before considering the medical obligation was often misconstrued as implying that the husband was incompetent or ill motivated. The medical center intended to emphasize the desirability of an independent review of its medical conclusion before its obligation to provide the respirator was reviewed by the court. I believe that the grieving husband was simply mistaken about whether the respirator was benefiting his wife. A direct request to remove the respirator seems to center procedural oversight on the soundness of the medical decision making rather than on the nature of the patient's need. Clearly, the gravity of these decisions merits openness, due process, and meticulous accountability. The relative merits of various procedures need further study.

Ultimately, procedures for addressing requests for futile, marginally effective, or inappropriate therapies require a statutory framework, case law, professional standards, a social consensus, and the exercise of professional responsibility. Appropriate ends for medicine are defined by public and professional consensus. Laws can, and do, say that patients may choose only among medically appropriate options, but legislatures are ill suited to define medical appropriateness. Similarly, health-facility policies on this issue will be difficult to design and will focus on due process rather than on specific clinical situations. Public or private payers will ration according to cost and overall efficacy, a rationing that will become more onerous as therapies are misapplied in individual cases. I believe there is a social consensus that intensive care for a person as "overmastered" by disease as this woman was is inappropriate.

Each case must be evaluated individually. In this case, the husband's request seemed entirely inconsistent with what medical care could do for his wife, the standards of the community, and his fair share of resources that many people pooled for their collective medical care. This case is about limits to what can be achieved at the end of life.

REFERENCES

1. Tomlinson T. Brody H. Futility and the ethics of resuscitation. JAMA 1990; 264:1276–80.
2. In re Helga Wanglie, Fourth Judicial District (Dist. Ct., Probate Ct. Div.) PX-91-283. Minnesota, Hennepin County.
3. Office of Technology Assessment Task Force. Life-sustaining technologies and the elderly. Washington, D.C.: Government Printing Office, 1987.
4. Smedira NG, Evans BH, Grais LS, et al. Withholding and withdrawal of life support from the critically ill. N Engl J Med 1990; 322: 309–15.
5. Lantos JD, Singer PA, Walker RM, et al. The illusion of futility in clinical practice. Am J Med 1989; 87:81–4.
6. Emanuel LL, Barry MJ, Stoeckle JD, Ettelson LM, Emanuel EJ. Advance directives for medical care —a case for greater use. N Engl J Med 1991; 324:889–95.
7. Zweibel NR, Cassel CK. Treatment choices at the end of life: a comparison of decisions by older patients and their physician-selected proxies. Gerontologist 1989; 29:615–21.
8. Tomlinson T, Howe K, Notman M, Rossmiller D. An empirical study of proxy consent for elderly persons. Gerontologist 1990; 30:54–64.
9. Danis M, Southerland LI, Garrett JM, et al. A prospective study of advance directives for life-sustaining care. N Engl J Med 1991; 324:882–8.
10. Minnesota Statutes. Adult Health Care Decisions Act. 145b.04.
11. Minnesota Statutes. Patients and residents of health care facilities: Bill of rights. 144.651: Subd. 6.
12. Helga Wanglie's life. Minneapolis Star Tribune. May 26, 1991:18A.
13. Council on Ethical and Judicial Affairs. American Medical Association. Guidelines for the appropriate use of do-not-resuscitate orders JAMA 1991; 265:1868–71.
14. Task Force on Ethics of the Society of Critical Care Medicine. Consensus report on the ethics of foregoing life-sustaining treatments in the critically ill. Crit Care Med 1990; 18:1435–9.
15. American Thoracic Society. Withholding and withdrawing life-sustaining therapy. Am Rev Respir Dis (in press).

NO

Felicia Ackerman

THE SIGNIFICANCE OF A WISH

The case of Helga Wanglie should be seen in the general context of conflicts that can arise over whether a patient should be maintained on life-support systems. Well-publicized conflicts of this sort usually involve an institution seeking to prolong the life of a patient diagnosed as terminally ill and/or permanently comatose, versus a family that claims, with varying degrees of substantiation, that the patient would not have wanted to be kept alive under these circumstances. But other sorts of conflicts about prolonging life also occur. Patients who have indicated a desire to stay alive may face opposition from family or medical staff who think these patients' lives are not worth prolonging. Such cases can go badly for patients, who may have difficulty getting their preferences even believed, let alone respected.[1]

Helga Wanglie's case is not as clear cut. But in view of the fact that keeping her on a respirator will prolong her life, that there is more reason to believe she would have wanted this than to believe she would not have wanted it, that medical diagnoses of irreversible unconsciousness are not infallible, and that her private health insurance plan has not objected to paying for her respirator support and in fact has publicly taken the position that cost should not be a factor in treatment decisions, I believe HCMC [Hennepin County Medical Center] should continue to maintain Mrs. Wanglie on a respirator. This respirator support is medically and economically feasible, and it serves a recognized medical goal—that of prolonging life and allowing a chance at a possible, albeit highly unlikely, return to consciousness.

THE SIGNIFICANCE OF MEDICAL EXPERTISE

Dr. Steven Miles, ethics consultant at HCMC, has argued that continued respirator support is "medically inappropriate" for Mrs. Wanglie. The argument is based on a criterion of medical appropriateness that allows doctors to prescribe respirators for any of three purposes: to allow healing, to alleviate suffering, and to enable otherwise disabled persons to continue to enjoy life. Since keeping Mrs. Wanglie on a respirator serves none of these ends, it is argued, such treatment is medically inappropriate.

From Felicia Ackerman, "The Significance of a Wish," *Hastings Center Report*, vol. 21, no. 4 (July/August 1991). Copyright © 1991 by The Hastings Center. Reprinted by permission.

But just what does "medically inappropriate" mean here? A clear case of medical inappropriateness would be an attempt to cure cancer with laetrile, since medicine has presumably shown that laetrile cannot cure cancer. Moreover, since laetrile's clinical ineffectiveness is a technical medical fact about which doctors are supposed to have professional expertise, it is professionally appropriate for doctors to refuse to grant a patient's request to have laetrile prescribed for cancer. But HCMC's disagreement with Mrs. Wanglie's family is not a technical dispute about a matter where doctors can be presumed to have greater expertise than laymen. The parties to the dispute do not disagree about whether maintaining Mrs. Wanglie on a respirator is likely to prolong her life; they disagree about whether her life is worth prolonging. This is not a medical question, but a question of values. Hence the term "medically inappropriate," with its implication of the relevance of technical medical expertise, is itself inappropriate in this context. It is as presumptuous and *ethically* inappropriate for doctors to suppose that their professional expertise qualifies them to know what kind of life is worth prolonging as it would be for meteorologists to suppose their professional expertise qualifies them to know what kind of destination is worth a long drive in the rain.

It has also been argued that continued respirator support does not serve Mrs. Wanglie's interests since a permanently unconscious person cannot "enjoy any realization of the quality of life."[2] Yet were this approach to be applied consistently, it would undermine the idea frequently advanced in other life-support cases that it is in the interests of the irreversibly comatose to be "allowed" to die "with dignity." Such people are not suffering or even conscious, so how can death benefit them or serve their interests? The obvious reply in both cases is that there is a sense in which it is in a permanently comatose person's interests to have his or her previous wishes and values respected. And there is some evidence that Mrs. Wanglie would want to be kept alive.

But why suppose doctors are any more obliged to serve this want than they would be to help gratify some nonmedical desire such as a desire to be remembered in a certain way? An obvious answer is that prolonging life is a medical function, as is allowing a possible return to consciousness. Medical diagnoses of irreversible coma are not infallible, as the recent case of Carrie Coons clearly demonstrates. The court order to remove her feeding tube, requested by her family, was rescinded after Mrs. Coons regained consciousness following five and a half months in what was diagnosed as an irreversible vegetative state.[3] Such cases cast additional light on the claim that respirator support is medically inappropriate and not in Mrs. Wanglie's interests. When the alternative is death, the question of whether going for a long-shot chance of recovering consciousness is worth it is quite obviously a question of values, rather than a technical medical question doctors are especially professionally qualified to decide.

THE SIGNIFICANCE OF QUALITY OF LIFE

Medical ethicists who take into account the possibility that seemingly irreversibly comatose patients might regain consciousness have offered further general arguments against maintaining such patients on life-support systems. One such argument relies on the fact that "the few patients who have recovered consciousness after a prolonged period of unconsciousness were severely disabled,"[4] with disabilities including blindness, inability to speak, permanent distortion of limbs, and paralysis. Since many blind, mute, and/or paralyzed people seem to find their lives well worth living, however, the assumption that disability is a fate worse than death seems highly questionable. Moreover, when the patient's views on the matter are unknown, maintaining him on a respirator to give him a chance to regain consciousness and then decide whether to continue his disabled existence seems preferable to denying him even the possibility of a choice by deciding in advance that he would be better off dead. Keeping alive someone who would want to die and "allowing" to die someone who would want a chance of regained consciousness are not parallel wrongs. While both obviously go against the patient's values, only the latter has the additional flaw of doing this in a way that could actually affect his conscious experience.

The other argument asserts that since long-term treatment imposes emotional and often financial burdens on the comatose patient's family and most patients, before losing consciousness, place a high value on their families' welfare, presumably these patients would rather die than be a burden to their loved ones.[5] Though very popular nowadays, this latter sort of argument is cruel because it attributes extreme self-abnegation to those unable to speak for themselves. It is also biased because it assumes great sacrificial love on the part of the patient, but not the family. Why not argue instead that a loving family will not want to deny a beloved member a last chance at regained consciousness and hence that it is *not* in the interest of the patient's loved ones to withdraw life supports? Mrs. Wanglie's family clearly wants her kept alive.[6]

THE SIGNIFICANCE OF A GESTURE

Mrs. Wanglie's family claims that she would want to be kept alive. Yet Dr. Cranford suggests that her family at first denied having previously discussed the matter with her, and that it was only after the HCMC committed itself to going to court that the family claimed Mrs. Wanglie had said she would want to be kept alive. Dr. Miles mentions that during the months when she was on a respirator before becoming unconscious, Mrs. Wanglie at times pulled at her respirator tubing.

I agree that Mrs. Wanglie's views are less than certain. Yet for reasons given above and also because death is irrevocable, there should be a presumption in favor of life when a patient's views are unclear or unknown. Pulling at a respirator tube is obviously insufficient evidence of even a fleeting desire to die; it may simply be a semi-automatic attempt to relieve discomfort, like pulling away in a dentist's chair even when one has an overriding desire that the dental work be performed. Basically, although the circumstances of the family's claim about Mrs. Wanglie's statement of her views make the claim questionable, it is their word against nobody's. No one claims that she ever said she would prefer *not* to be kept alive, despite her months of conscious existence on a respirator.

It has also been argued that we should not allow patients to demand medically inappropriate care when the costs of that care are borne by others who have not consented to do so. I have already discussed the question of medical appropriateness. And a private health plan is paying for Mrs. Wanglie's care, a plan whose officials have publicly stated that cost should not be a factor in treatment decisions. The pool of subscribers to the plan, whose premiums are what indirectly subsidize Mrs. Wanglie's care, have, by being members of this plan, committed themselves to a practice of medicine that does not take cost into account. It would be unfair to make cost a factor in Mrs. Wanglie's treatment decision now. Public statements by health insurance plan officials are expected to be taken into account by consumers selecting health insurance and must not be reneged upon. Mrs. Wanglie's insurer is not seeking to renege. Instead, it is her *doctors* who have decided that her life is not worth prolonging.

Moreover, to say it would be the underlying disease rather than the act of removing the respirator that would cause Helga Wanglie's death is not helpful. If Mrs. Wanglie is, as the HCMC staff claims, irreversibly respirator-dependent, then saying that removing the respirator would cause her death is just as logical as saying that withdrawing a rope from a drowning man would cause his death, even if his death is to be "attributed" to his drowning. If the person in either case has an interest in living, one violates his interest by withdrawing the necessary means. This is what HCMC is seeking court permission to do to Mrs. Wanglie.

REFERENCES

1. For example, consider the case of seventy-eight-year-old Earl Spring, whose mental deterioration did not prevent him from saying that he did not want to die. The statement of this preference was not considered conclusive reason to keep him on dialysis over his family's objections. Similarly, the *New York Times Magazine* recently described the situation of a severely disabled, elderly woman whose explicit advance directive that she wanted everything possible done to keep her alive was apparently ignored by both her husband and the hospital's ethics committee (K. Bouton, "Painful Decisions: The Role of the Medical Ethicist," 5 August 1990).
2. This argument comes from an unpublished letter from Dr. Steven Miles, made available to me by the *Hastings Center Report* at his request.
3. The Coons case was widely reported in newspapers. For example, see C. DeMare, "'Hopeless' Hospital Patient, 86, Comes Out of Coma," *Albany Times Union*, 12 April 1989. Additional cases of this sort are cited in President's Commission for the Study of Ethical Problems in Medicine and Biomedical and Behavioral Research, *Deciding to Forego Life-Sustaining Treatment* (Washington, D.C.: U.S. Government Printing Office, 1983).
4. President's Commission, *Deciding to Forego Life-Sustaining Treatment*, p. 182.
5. President's Commission, *Deciding to Forego Life-Sustaining Treatment*, p. 183.
6. I have given this sort of argument in a letter to the *New York Times*, 4 November 1987, as well as in a short story about terminal illness, "The Forecasting Game, in *Prize Stories 1990: The O. Henry Awards*, ed. W. Abrahams (New York: Doubleday, 1990), pp. 315–35, and in an op-ed "No Thanks, I Don't Want to Die with Dignity," *Providence Journal-Bulletin*, 19 April 1990 (reprinted in other newspapers under various different titles).

POSTSCRIPT

Should Doctors Be Able to Refuse Demands for "Futile" Treatment?

Three days after the Minnesota court named Oliver Wanglie as his wife's legal conservator, thus preserving his right to make decisions about her treatment, Helga Wanglie died of multisystem organ failure. Her aggressive treatment had been continued throughout. Mr. Wanglie said, "We felt that when she was ready to go that the good Lord would call her, and I would say that's what happened." Her daughter said that her mother's care had been excellent; "We just had a disagreement on ethics."

A series of cases involving infants has extended the debate on medical futility. The most publicized case is that of "Baby K," who was born in 1992 with most of her brain missing. In most cases of this condition (anencephaly), babies die within a few days. Baby K's mother, however, insisted that Fairfax Hospital in Falls Church, Virginia, provide ventilator support to help the baby breathe, which kept her alive in a nursing home. In February 1994 the hospital's request to stop this treatment was denied by a federal appeals court, which extended to this case a federal law requiring hospitals to treat emergency patients even if they cannot pay. Payment was not an issue here, however, because the mother is a member of a Health Maintenance Organization, which paid the bills. Despite continued treatment, Baby K died in April 1995 at the age of three.

E. Haavi Morreim addresses the issue of how to preserve respect for moral diversity while preventing patients, families, physicians, and society from coercing one another into providing costly ineffective treatments in "Profoundly Diminished Life: The Casualties of Coercion," *Hastings Center Report* (January/February 1994).

John S. Paris and Frank E. Reardon provide a comprehensive overview of the cases in this area in "Physician Refusal of Requests for Futile or Ineffective Treatments," a chapter in *Emerging Issues in Biomedical Policy, vol. 2*, edited by Robert H. Blank and Andrea L. Bonnicksen (Columbia University Press, 1993). See also "Futility and Hospital Policy," by Tom Tomlinson and Diane Czlonka, *Hastings Center Report* (May–June 1995); *Wrong Medicine*, by Lawrence J. Schneiderman and Nancy Jecker (Johns Hopkins University Press, 1995); and "Religious Insistence on Medical Treatment: Christian Theology and Re-Imagination," by Russell B. Connors, Jr., and Martin L. Smith, *Hastings Center Report* (July–August 1996).

An additional source for information on the concept of futility is the following Web site of the University of Chicago's Center for Clinical Medical Ethics: http://ccme-mac4.bsd.uchicago.edu/CCMEDocs/Death.

PART 3

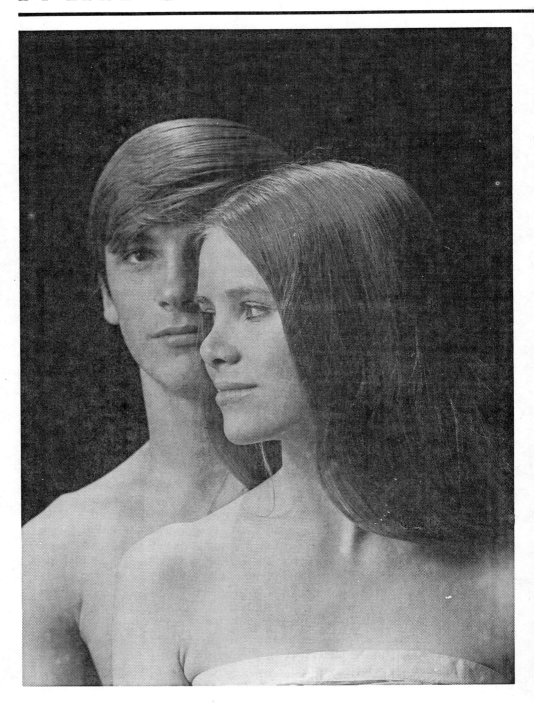

Choices in Reproduction

Few bioethical issues could be of greater significance than questions concerning reproduction. Advances in medical technology, such as in vitro fertilization and cloning human embryos, and changes in social mores that have made surrogate mothering more acceptable have opened new possibilities to infertile couples. Nevertheless, these practices challenge established family patterns. Our enhanced understanding of fetal development creates new pressures to control the mother's behavior. New long-acting forms of contraception seem tailor-made for situations in which courts or legislatures wish to limit a person's reproduction. The centuries-old debate about abortion takes on new significance in the modern era, when abortion is safe and legal but still highly controversial. The issues in this section come to grips with some of the most perplexing and fundamental questions that confront medical practitioners and society.

■ Should Courts Be Permitted to Order
  Women to Use Long-Acting Contraceptives?

■ Is There a Moral Right to Abortion?

ISSUE 8

Should Courts Be Permitted to Order Women to Use Long-Acting Contraceptives?

YES: Jim Persels, from "The Norplant Condition: Protecting the Unborn or Violating Fundamental Rights?" *The Journal of Legal Medicine* (vol. 13, 1992)

NO: Rebecca Dresser, from "Long-Term Contraceptives in the Criminal Justice System," *Hastings Center Report* (January–February 1995)

ISSUE SUMMARY

YES: Jim Persels, editor in chief of the *Southern Illinois University Law Journal,* contends that the use of long-acting but reversible contraceptive technologies as requirements for probation for women convicted of child abuse or drug use serves to guard the unborn while simultaneously limiting the intrusion on the individual's privacy rights and the state's burden of supervision.

NO: Law professor Rebecca Dresser argues that sentencing women to use contraceptives is unjust because it has a disproportionately coercive effect on women, especially low-income minority women, with a very small likelihood of reducing child abuse and neglect.

In December 1990 the Food and Drug Administration approved the use of Norplant as a contraceptive for American women. Although Norplant is the first long-acting contraceptive to be marketed and the first new birth control method developed in 25 years, in the future other products will undoubtedly be approved, some of them for men.

Norplant works in this way: Six small silicone tubes, each about the size of a matchstick, are inserted under the skin of a woman's upper arm with a local anesthetic. The procedure takes about 10 to 15 minutes. The tubes release a synthetic version of the hormone progestin, which suppresses ovulation. Because she does not produce ova (eggs), the woman is infertile. The hormones also act in other ways to inhibit fertilization. The hormones are released at a steady pace over five years. When the tubes are removed, also a relatively simple procedure, the woman again becomes fertile.

Norplant has been widely used around the world. It is extremely effective, with a failure rate of only 0.3 percent to 0.6 percent in one year and 1.5 percent over five years. It has several advantages over other contraceptive options, the primary one being the guaranteed compliance of the user while the tubes are in place. In addition, there are relatively few side effects, although headaches, acne, and irregular menstrual bleeding do occur among some women. Women with a history of diabetes, hypertension, cardiovascular disease, and some other diseases should not use Norplant because the additional hormones present some risks. Except for its high cost ($350 for the device, plus $150 to $650 for the insertion, counseling, and checkups), Norplant seems to be almost entirely a good-news story, and nearly 1 million American women have chosen this method of birth control over others that require either partner participation (condom), daily usage (oral contraceptives), or insertion before intercourse (diaphragm).

There is, however, a controversial aspect to this contraceptive. Because it does not require constant monitoring and is nearly foolproof, Norplant is an appealing candidate for use as a method of controlling the reproduction of women whom courts or others deem unfit to be mothers, either because they have been convicted of child abuse or because they are drug users. The use of Norplant could be required as a condition of probation. In addition, Norplant may be used as an incentive to women on welfare or as a condition of receiving further benefits to induce them to have fewer children and thus to lower welfare costs.

Mandatory sterilization of convicted criminals or other socially "undesirable" people has a long history in the United States. The case of *Buck v. Bell*, in which the Supreme Court upheld the sterilization of a young woman assumed to be retarded but later proved not to be, is a legal benchmark in this area. Decided in 1927, it has never been overturned. Other courts have upheld a fundamental right to procreate.

The question of whether or not Norplant can be used in the modern context arose in 1991 when Judge Howard Broadman suggested in his California court that Darlene Johnson, a woman convicted of abusing two of her children, might reduce her prison sentence if she agreed to accept Norplant. In Kansas that same year a legislator proposed a variation on this idea: drug-abusing fertile women could be placed on probation only if they accepted Norplant. The ethical question raised by these proposals is whether or not the interests of the state in reducing child abuse or welfare costs justifies the imposition of a temporary form of contraception.

In the following selections, Jim Persels argues that the Johnson case and the Kansas legislation are harbingers of more defensible uses of the imposition of Norplant and that under some conditions the state is justified in imposing this technology. Rebecca Dresser, on the other hand, asserts that sentencing that involves long-term contraceptives and other punitive measures to solve the problems of child abuse and neglect is shortsighted and raises real questions of injustice to the mostly poor and minority women who would be its primary targets.

YES

Jim Persels

THE NORPLANT CONDITION: PROTECTING THE UNBORN OR VIOLATING FUNDAMENTAL RIGHTS?

INTRODUCTION

The children are at risk. Approximately 1,727,000 cases of child abuse are reported annually. Studies show that more than 25 of each 1,000 children in the United States suffer some form of abuse or neglect. In addition, there has been a dramatic increase in the number of babies born to drug-abusing mothers. Some experts now estimate that as many as 375,000 infants affected by maternal drug use are born each year. The prevalence of crack cocaine has ignited this explosion. Crack cocaine is the drug of choice for many women of childbearing age because it is relatively inexpensive and can be smoked rather than injected. Infants born to mothers that are addicted to cocaine are subject to premature birth, low birth weight, and withdrawal symptoms. Furthermore, these infants demonstrate neurobehavioral problems, congenital disorders and deformities, and have a tenfold greater risk of dying of sudden infant death syndrome than babies not so affected.

This wholesale maiming of our children has recently motivated a judge in California and a legislator in Kansas in their attempts to use a newly approved medical technology to deal with the problem. That new technology is Norplant, a highly effective contraceptive implant that renders a woman infertile for up to five years or until the device is removed. A California appellate court is currently considering the case of *People v. Johnson,* in which a superior court judge ordered that Norplant be implanted in a convicted child abuser as a condition of probation. Similarly, during the 1990 session of the Kansas legislature, a legislator introduced a bill [House Bill 2255] that would mandate the implantation of Norplant as a condition of probation for drug-abusing fertile women.

From Jim Persels, "The Norplant Condition: Protecting the Unborn or Violating Fundamental Rights?" *The Journal of Legal Medicine,* vol. 13 (1992). Copyright © 1992 by Hemisphere Publishing Corporation. Reprinted by permission. Portions of this article and all footnotes have been omitted and are available upon request.

The defense in the *Johnson* case and the opponents of the Kansas Norplant bill claim that court-ordered contraception violates the individual's right of privacy. Specifically, they argue that the Norplant condition is an unconstitutional intrusion on the fundamental right of procreation. In contrast, the states argue that the condition is valid for two reasons. First, the implantation of Norplant in child-abusing and drug-using women facilitates achievement of the state's probationary goal of rehabilitation by greatly reducing the risk of an untimely childbirth. This factor has been identified as one of the key risk factors for child abuse and neglect. Second, Norplant furthers the states' compelling interest in protecting the welfare of their children.

The purpose of this commentary is to discuss whether the state has the power to use this new contraceptive technology to defeat an individual probationer's fundamental right of procreation. . . .

THE FUNDAMENTAL RIGHT OF PROCREATION

The seminal case that articulated a fundamental right of procreation was *Skinner v. Oklahoma*. Jack Skinner was a chicken thief and an armed robber. His crimes landed him in the Oklahoma penal system. His record of three felony convictions brought him under the heavy hand of the Oklahoma Habitual Criminal Sterilization Act.

This law defined an "habitual criminal" as one who was convicted three or more times for crimes "amounting to felonies involving moral turpitude." The law further provided that the Oklahoma attorney general could initiate proceedings against the habitual criminal for a judgment that such person be rendered sexually sterile. The issues in a proceeding under this act were narrow and well-defined. The trier of fact had to decide whether the defendant was an "habitual criminal" and, if so, whether he "may be rendered sexually sterile without detriment to his or her general health." If the answer to both inquiries were affirmative, the court could then "render judgment to the effect that said defendant be rendered sexually sterile" by vasectomy [a surgical procedure that prevents sperm from being ejaculated] for males or salpingectomy [surgical removal of the fallopian tubes] for females. Jack Skinner qualified under both criteria and was sentenced to be sterilized. The Oklahoma Supreme Court affirmed by a five to four decision, and the United States Supreme Court granted the petition for certiorari.

The Court found that Oklahoma's law was fatally flawed because it ran afoul of the Equal Protection Clause of the fourteenth amendment. Justice Douglas noted many inconsistencies in the act. For instance, under the law, a man that broke into a chicken coop and stole chickens was a felon. Therefore, he could be sterilized after his third conviction. Ironically, however, an embezzler that feloniously appropriated significant sums of money from a bailor could not be sterilized under the law regardless of the number of times he was convicted for that crime. The Court reasoned that because the two crimes were intrinsically the same, the availability of this most serious sanction for one crime and not the other was inequitable under the fourteenth amendment. Justice Douglas characterized the nature of the violated right by stating, "[w]e are dealing here with legislation which involves one of the basic civil rights of man. Marriage and procreation are fundamental to the very existence and survival of the race."

Later decisions of the Supreme Court expanded and shaped the fundamental right of procreation that was initially expounded in *Skinner*....

The Court has demonstrated its willingness to permit states to interfere with the fundamental right of procreation only when two criteria have been met. First, the state must be able to show a compelling interest. Second, the state must demonstrate that there are no more effective or less intrusive means than that chosen to protect the interest....

Against the backdrop of these precedents and the great national debate over abortion, the fundamental right of procreation has been steadily eroded during the past 10 to 15 years by the decisions of an increasingly conservative Supreme Court. It is in light of this hostile environment that the use of contraception as a condition of probation must be considered.

CONTRACEPTION AS A CONDITION OF PROBATION

Probationary conditions include a variety of restrictions on the liberty of convicted persons. In general, the restrictions are, or should be, tailored to relate to the crime for which the person was convicted. This section defines probation and its legitimate uses in the criminal justice system. Further, this section focuses on one probationary condition that has been considered in a few state courts, that of remaining childless or having no additional children during the probationary period. This discussion leads to consideration of the Norplant condition.

A. Nature and Goals of Probation

Probation is the suspension of a convicted defendant's sentence before its execution. In *Griffin v. Wisconsin*, the Court likened probation to imprisonment, stating it is "a form of criminal sanction imposed by a court upon an offender after verdict, finding, or plea of guilty."...

B. State Decisions Mandating Contraception as a Condition of Probation

People v. Johnson is the first case involving a probationary restriction on conception that mandated a specific contraceptive modality. Several other state cases, however, have ruled on probationary conditions that have generally required probationers to remain childless or have no additional children during the probationary period. In each of these cases, the courts have ruled that probationary conditions mandating that a probationer remain childless were void.

In *People v. Dominguez*, the trial court placed a woman who was convicted of second-degree robbery on probation. The woman was unmarried, had two illegitimate children, and was pregnant with a third. One probationary restriction was that she remain childless until she was married. Accordingly, when she later became pregnant again without being married, the trial court revoked her probation. On appeal, however, a California appellate court overturned the probationary condition, concluding that it was unreasonable. The court articulated a test that voided a condition of probation if it "(1) has no relationship to the crime of which the offender was convicted, (2) relates to conduct that is not in itself criminal, and (3) requires or forbids conduct that is not reasonably related to future criminality." Applying the test in this case, the court found no relation between the woman's future pregnancy and her crime. In addition, the court noted that there was no demonstrable evidence that unmarried, pregnant women were predisposed to commit crimes. Nor was there any rational basis for believing that poor, unmarried women tend to commit crimes upon becoming pregnant.

In sum, when the underlying crime is not child abuse, courts have generally struck down the probationary condition that the defendant remain childless, reasoning that the nexus between the crime and the condition is too tenuous. The nexus is more substantial, however, where the offense is related to abuse of a child.

In *State v. Livingston,* a woman allowed her seven-month-old child to be seriously burned when she placed him on a space heater. She was convicted of child abuse and placed on probation. As a condition of her probation, the trial court required that the defendant remain childless for five years. On appeal, however, an Ohio appellate court voided this condition of probation. The court said that a test of reasonableness should be applied in determining the validity of conditions of probation. While conceding that trial courts have considerable discretion in imposing probationary conditions, the court said that the condition failed here because it imposed arbitrary conditions that severely constrained the defendant's exercise of liberty. It also noted that the condition was unreasonable because it was only remotely related to the crime for which she was convicted and the rehabilitative goals of probation.

Similarly, in *Howland v. State,* a Florida appellate court held that a condition of probation that prohibited a man who was convicted of child abuse from fathering a child was void. The court admitted that the condition of probation could reasonably relate to future criminality in the form of further child abuse if the defendant were allowed to have custody of or to have contact with the child. In this case, however, those possibilities were foreclosed by other valid conditions of probation.

These concerns also arise in cases of child endangerment. In *State v. Mosburg,* a mother who abandoned her two-hour-old baby was convicted of endangering her child. As a condition of her probation, the trial court prohibited Ms. Mosburg from becoming pregnant during her probationary period. The appellate court found that the condition was an undue intrusion on her right to privacy, however, and remanded the case to the court below for deletion of the probationary condition.

In its analysis, the *Mosburg* court discussed some of the preceding cases but relied most significantly on the California case of *People v. Pointer. Pointer* helps focus the reasoning in this line of cases. In *Pointer,* Ruby Pointer was the mother of two young children. A strict adherent to a macrobiotic diet consisting only of grains, legumes, and vegetables, she imposed this dietary regime on her children. Despite repeated warnings by her physician and intervention by Children's Protective Services, Ms. Pointer continued to restrict the children's diet. As a result, the state removed the children to a foster home. Ms. Pointer later abducted the children and took them to Puerto Rico. Nearly a year later, the Federal Bureau of Investigation discovered Ms. Pointer and her children and subsequently returned them to California. Because of the macrobiotic diet, one of the children was seriously underdeveloped, and the other had suffered severe growth retardation and permanent neurological damage.

On these facts, Ms. Pointer was convicted of the felony of child endangerment and sentenced to five years probation. The conditions of probation included one year in county jail, participation in a counseling program, a ban on contact with her children or custody of any children without court approval, and a prohibition against conception during the probationary period. Ms. Pointer appealed the decision, claiming that the latter condition was an unconstitutional invasion of her fundamental right of procreation.

In applying the three-part *Dominguez* test, the *Pointer* court determined that the condition was reasonable because there was a direct nexus between the condition and the crime and possible future criminality. In arriving at that conclusion, the court distinguished *Pointer* from cases in other jurisdictions where courts had held that the challenged condition lacked the requisite relation to child abuse or to future criminality. The court noted that "those cases relied heavily upon the fact that the abuse could be entirely avoided by removal of any children from the custody of the defendant. This case is distinguishable, however, because of evidence that the harm sought to be prevented by the trial court may occur before birth." After concluding that the crime-condition nexus and the condition-future criminality nexus satisfied the *Dominguez* test, the court had to decide whether the condition was "impermissibly broad."

The court found that the condition clearly infringed on the fundamental right of procreation because it inhibited Ms. Pointer's power to choose to conceive and give birth to additional children.

The court further noted that it was equally clear that "the condition must be subjected so special scrutiny to determine whether the restriction is entirely necessary to serve the dual purposes of rehabilitation and public safety." It relied on *Parrish v. Civil Service Commission* to conclude that "[i]f available alternative means exist which are less violative of a constitutional right and are narrowly drawn so as to correlate more closely with the purpose contemplated, those alternatives should be used."

Applying the *Parrish* test, the court found that the condition was not designed to afford any rehabilitative purpose. Instead, it was designed to protect the public by preventing injury to an unborn child. According to the court, this purpose could be served by less intrusive means. It suggested that those means might include periodic pregnancy testing and, should Ms. Pointer become pregnant, close supervision by both her physician and her probation officer. In addition, if a child was born during her probation, the child could be removed to a foster home if necessary.

The appellate court further noted that the trial judge made it clear that he would uphold every condition of the probation and, if any was violated, Ms. Pointer would be sent to prison. It concluded that this threat posed a danger that Ms. Pointer might seek a clandestine abortion should she become pregnant during her probationary period. The potential for this result and the availability of less intrusive means of achieving the goals of probation led the court to reverse and remand the case for resentencing that would exclude the condition that prohibited conception.

Dominguez, Pointer, and their progeny provide the framework of precedent for the current initiatives....

FACTORING THE NORPLANT TECHNOLOGY INTO THE STATE INTEREST VERSUS INDIVIDUAL RIGHTS EQUATION

The underlying question in this privacy analysis is whether Norplant technology tips the scale in favor of state interests when balanced against the individual's fundamental right of procreation. In resolving this issue, *People v. Johnson* and H.R. 2255 must be considered separately because they address different behaviors. In the case of a drug-abusing pregnant woman, the fetus may be harmed in utero by the drugs that the woman ingests. Thus, there is a clear nexus between the crime of drug abuse and the welfare of any infant that may be born to the woman who ingests drugs during her pregnancy. In the case of a child-abuser, however, the nexus may not be so clear.

People v. Johnson
Darlene Johnson beat her children with a belt and electrical extension cord. She was subsequently convicted of child abuse. In applying the *Dominguez* test to these facts, the inclusion of Norplant as a probationary condition would seem to have little or no influence on the decision whether the prohibition on conception is unconstitutionally intrusive. The test makes a condition of probation invalid if it (1) has no relationship to the crime of which the offender was convicted, (2) relates to conduct that is not in itself criminal, and (3) requires or forbids conduct that is not reasonably related to future criminality and does not serve the statutory ends of probation.

Ms. Johnson sets forth four arguments to show that the condition fails the *Dominguez* test because it is neither directly related to child abuse nor to the prospect that she would engage in similar unlawful conduct in the future. First, she points out that there was no evidence that she inflicted similar treatment on her youngest child; nor was there any evidence that she mistreated any of them as infants. Second, she argues that the Norplant condition is unreasonable because it is unrelated to the rehabilitative goals of probation.... Third, she stresses that she is already required to undergo counseling and education that are specifically designed to help her cope with the stress of parenting and to teach her acceptable means of disciplining her children. Finally, she reasons that, should she become pregnant, the nine month gestation period would allow her time to complete her rehabilitation before another child is born. Thus, there would be no risk of an infant being born before she was fully rehabilitated....

Ms. Johnson also invokes her fundamental right of procreation as protected by the California and United States Constitutions. The trial court recognized the fundamental right but reasoned that it could be limited in certain circumstances. The court concluded that the defendant's constitutional rights should be balanced against the state's interests in protecting her unconceived children and ensuring that Ms. Johnson's rehabilitation was effective. In this case, the trial court held that the state's interests were more compelling than those of the individual. It is in the application of this balancing test that the unique characteristics of Norplant may have an impact in the outcome of the analysis.

1. Probationer's Reduced Expectation of Privacy

Before considering the impact of Norplant, the effect of probationary status in relation to fundamental rights should be examined. Ms. Johnson argues that "[a] probationer has the right to enjoy a significant degree of privacy, or liberty, under the Fourth, Fifth and Fourteenth Amendments to the federal Constitution." Ms. Johnson recognizes that a prisoner must forego some of her privacy rights because of the necessity for orderly administration of the prison system. She distinguishes probationers, however, on the basis that there is "[n]o parallel justification [that] supports depriving a defendant under the supervision of the probation system of fundamental human rights."

In contrast, the state argues that a probationer has an expectation of privacy that is less than that of an ordinary law abiding citizen. The Supreme Court has explicitly recognized a reduced expectation of privacy in probationers. "To a greater or lesser degree, it is always true of probationers... that they do not enjoy 'the absolute liberty to which every citizen is entitled, but only... conditional liberty properly dependent on observance of special [probation] restrictions.'" "Supervision, then, is a 'special need' of the State permitting a degree of impingement upon privacy that would not be constitutional if applied to the public at large." This reduced expectation of privacy must be considered in balancing state interests against individual rights.

2. The Balancing Test

Factoring in this reduced expectation of privacy, the scale tips slightly toward the state. The use of Norplant to enforce the probationary condition arguably could tip the scale further to the state's side. The probationer has been convicted of a crime. She could often be incarcerated for that crime. If incarcerated, the prisoner loses a wide array of rights, including not only the right of procreation but also the right of sexual expression. A probationer who has been ordered to practice contraception is in a significantly better position than the prisoner. Though she has temporarily given up the right of procreation, she has retained the right to associate with persons other than fellow criminals, to move freely in society, and to sexual expression.

Using standard contraceptive methods, this invasion of privacy could still be substantial. Periodic pregnancy checks or supervision of appropriate contraceptive use could seriously broaden the restraints on the probationer's liberty. In addition, the probationer must always be concerned that if her attempts at contraception fail, the court may revoke her probation and send her to prison. This is where the new technology may play a role. Once the Norplant was in place, the requirement for supervision would be obviated, and the probationer would not have to worry about being held in violation of probation. Courts would have to accept an inadvertent pregnancy as a failure of the technology for which the probationer is not responsible. Therefore, there would be no willful violation of the probation. In all likelihood, however, given the effectiveness of Norplant, this would happen only rarely. In addition, while the implantation does involve an invasion of bodily integrity, it is relatively minor because the procedure is required only once every five years. Further, it avoids the intrusiveness related to court monitoring that is required when other forms of contraception are used.

The intrusion would be great, however, on those women that could not medically tolerate the drug. This factor would make it imperative that any woman on whose behalf the Norplant condition is ordered receive a complete medical exam before implantation and ongoing medical care during her probation. No woman for whom Norplant was contraindicated or who had a major risk factor should be a candidate for a probationary condition mandating the implantation of Norplant.

The final factor that may make Norplant attractive as a condition of probation is its reversibility. When the probation ends and the Norplant capsules are removed, there is very little, if any, lingering restraint on the woman's ability to conceive if she so desires.

To win its argument for imposition of the Norplant condition, the state must first establish a reasonable nexus between the condition, child abuse, and the potential for future similar crimes. Once the state has demonstrated this nexus in a given case, the technological advantages of Norplant may become a factor in the analysis. Arguably, Norplant reduces the extent of the intrusion on the individual's fundamental rights because of its effectiveness, safety, ease of compliance, and reversibility. These unique characteristics tip the scale toward the state when this balancing test is applied in select cases.

3. Limiting the Probation Condition

The courts should be very selective in their application of the condition because it is an intrusion on the probationer's right of procreation. Norplant becomes the least invasive alternative only if the probationer is one who has been convicted of multiple offenses or particu-

larly egregious crimes that could result in her imprisonment. The woman who has failed at one or more previous courses of counseling, education, or other less intrusive measures may also fall into this category. The first time offender who may be rehabilitated by other means should not be a candidate for the Norplant condition. In addition to this limitation, all women should be medically evaluated before the condition is imposed. The condition should be ruled out for any woman for whom the drug is contraindicated. Additionally, any woman who receives the implant should receive medical supervision throughout the probationary period. Within the framework of these constraints, the Norplant condition may be an effective state tool in the battle against the problem of child abuse.

The Future for the Use of the Norplant Condition Against Child Abuse

The future of the Norplant condition in combating child abuse must be considered in light of three different factors. First, child abuse is gaining national attention as a major problem in society. Some legislators and judges have been proposing extremely serious sanctions for this crime. Similarly, courts have found that sterilization as an aspect of a plea bargain in child abuse cases is constitutional. Second, the Supreme Court has become increasingly active in restricting freedom of procreative choice. Third, the composition of the United States Supreme Court, with the retirement of Justices Brennan and Marshall and their replacement by the current administration's appointees, will be decidedly conservative for many years to come. Under these circumstances, it is not unreasonable to predict that the Norplant condition will become a viable weapon in the justice system's battle against child abuse at some point in the future. . . .

Kansas House Bill 2255

The purported intent of this bill is analogous to *People v. Pointer* in that both relate to situations where the newborn may be injured if the mother were to conceive. House Bill 2255 focuses on babies of mothers that use illegal drugs. The nexuses between the condition and the crime and the condition and future criminality in these cases are easy to identify. In *Pointer*, the nexus was that the mother persistently adhered to a macrobiotic diet, thereby putting any child that she may conceive at risk of in utero injury. For drug-abusing mothers, the nexus lies in the fact that the newborn is infused with the drugs that the mother uses during the pregnancy. Balancing the state interest against individual rights, it seems clear that the compelling state interest in protecting the newborn from maternal drug abuse outweighs the probationer's reduced expectation of privacy as it relates to the right of procreation.

House Bill 2255 is fatally flawed, however, because it is broadly drafted to include a wide range of drug-related crimes. A more narrowly drafted bill may well survive legislative scrutiny. Such a bill would limit imposition of the condition to drug-abusing fertile women and exclude nonusers such as possessors and traffickers. Again, considering the changing orientation of the Supreme Court and the high visibility of the "war on drugs," it is very possible that legislation of this type will become law in the future.

CONCLUSION

Child abuse and the terrible consequences of maternal drug abuse are at epidemic proportions in this country. In attempts to deal with this problem, a judge in California and a legislator in Kansas have proposed using a new contraceptive technology, Norplant. The use of this new drug delivery system to prevent probationers from conceiving during the probationary period runs headlong into the constitutionally protected fundamental right of procreation. The right is not absolute, however, and it has suffered significant erosion during the past decade. The increasingly conservative face of the United States Supreme Court means that this weakening of the fundamental right of procreation will likely continue.

Although these crimes against children have very high visibility with the public, it is improbable that either of the pioneering initiatives discussed above will succeed in gaining acceptance for the Norplant condition. The judge in California picked the wrong defendant on whom to impose the condition. Her conviction for child abuse was her first for that crime, and less intrusive alternative methods of rehabilitation had not been tried in her case. In addition, insufficient attention was given to a medical determination of whether she was an appropriate candidate for the implant. Similarly, the bill in the Kansas legislature is too broad to gain acceptance. It opens an expansive spectrum of drug-related crimes to the Norplant condition. A bill drafted to impose the condition only on drug users would have a much better chance of passage.

The issue, however, is not likely to die with these fledgling initiatives. Norplant and other contraceptive technologies on the research horizon are becoming increasingly appealing to lawmakers as tools to ensure compliance with conditions of probation that mandate contraception. They serve to safeguard the unborn while simultaneously limiting both the intrusion on an individual's privacy rights and the state's burden of probationary supervision. Accordingly, Norplant and the contraceptive technologies that will follow are likely to find their place as judicially imposed shields to help protect the children.

NO
Rebecca Dresser

LONG-TERM CONTRACEPTIVES IN THE CRIMINAL JUSTICE SYSTEM

Three weeks after Norplant® was approved by the U.S. Food and Drug Administration, it was incorporated into the sentence imposed on a woman convicted of child abuse. In a criminal justice system beset by inadequate financial resources, large numbers of child abuse and neglect cases, and a longing for easy answers to complex problems, one judge found Norplant a welcome addition to his array of sentencing options. In very short order, a device created to expand women's reproductive freedom was revealed as a potential instrument of state power.

Many commentators have discussed possible constitutional and statutory obstacles to including long-term contraceptive use as a condition of probation for women convicted of harming their children. Although the Illinois legislature has enacted a statute prohibiting contraceptive sentencing, the practice could be legally permissible in other jurisdictions. In the following analysis, I consider whether the approach can be justified on moral and policy grounds.

IS CONTRACEPTION JUSTIFIED PUNISHMENT?

To evaluate the merits and drawbacks of contraception as punishment, one must consider why any sort of punishment may be imposed on persons convicted of crime. Punishment is usually justified as a means of advancing four goals: retribution, deterrence, incapacitation, and rehabilitation. To what degree are orders to use contraceptives compatible with these aims?

Retributive principles have the strongest influence on contemporary punishment theory and practice. According to retributive theory, persons who commit crimes deserve punishment. Because such individuals have harmed their victim's and community's welfare, the state is in turn entitled to subject them to the burdens and stigma of punishment. On the retributive model, punishment must be proportionate to the offender's level of culpability and the harm produced by the criminal behavior. Serious crimes merit heavy sanctions, less serious offenses call for more moderate punitive measures.

From Rebecca Dresser, "Long-Term Contraceptives in the Criminal Justice System," *Hastings Center Report*, vol. 20, no. 1 (January–February 1995). Copyright © 1995 by The Hastings Center. Reprinted by permission.

Do contraceptive sentences fit this model? The retributivist would be receptive to such sentences as long as they met the general requirements for punishment. The retributivist would demand rough equivalence between any probation conditions proposed for a particular offense and the prison term that could otherwise be imposed. The intrusions on autonomy and the experiential burdens of the two types of punishment must be similar. Meeting this demand would require sentencing officials to evaluate the nature of the contraceptive measure—its benefits and burdens (including the length of required use)—and then to compare it to other sanctions deemed suitable for the defendant's specific offense. To qualify as a suitable punishment for murder or other severe forms of child abuse, the retributivist would probably demand at a minimum that contraceptive sentencing be supplemented by other significant burdens and restrictions; on the other hand, the retributivist might well reject the imposition of contraceptive sentences in less serious abuse and neglect cases.[1]

The remaining three justifications for punishment—deterrence, incapacitation, and rehabilitation—all seek to achieve future societal benefits through imposing criminal sanctions. Their overall aim is crime reduction, which may be promoted through actions directed at the individual offender or the broader society. Deterrence operates at both these levels. Specific deterrence focuses on preventing the punished individual from committing future crimes. Punishment is inflicted to impress on the offender the risks accompanying a decision to engage in wrongdoing. According to the specific deterrence model, sentences should be calibrated to the offender's individual characteristics and situation. Defendants who refuse to acknowledge responsibility, have prior criminal records, or evidence other characteristics suggesting that they will be relatively less responsive to corrective measures will receive heavier sentences than those who appear more easily deterred.

General deterrence is aimed at the broader community. Punishment of convicted individuals is justified on grounds that it will discourage other members of society who might be tempted to engage in criminal behavior. Would-be wrongdoers are more likely to abandon their plans for criminal activity if they recognize that they too could experience the burdensome restrictions imposed on convicted offenders.[2]

When judges encounter a woman whose parenting behavior appears persistently irresponsible, they might see court-ordered contraception as a burden that could effectively discourage her from such behavior in the future. Yet it is difficult to understand why enforced contraception would be a particularly effective deterrent in most cases. It is more likely that judges have in mind general deterrence when they invoke contraceptive sentences. The judges may intend through their actions to notify the public that they are serious about discouraging child abuse and neglect, and are ready to resort to strong measures to do so.[3] If general deterrence is indeed their aim, the ethical and policy questions concern whether contraceptive sentences will actually discourage potential offenders and whether the intrusion on the defendant's physical integrity and reproductive autonomy is justified to promote the greater good.

Incapacitation is another forward-looking punishment aim. Incapacitative punishment is designed to prevent future crime by removing the offender's opportunity to repeat her behavior. People in prison are removed from most of their potential victims and the means necessary to commit many crimes. Certain probation conditions have incapacitation as their goal, for example, house arrest, electronic monitoring, and other forms of close supervision. Incapacitation simply puts physical and other barriers in the way of persons who seek to persist in their criminal activities.[4]

Judges have sometimes explicitly invoked the goal of incapacitation to justify contraceptive sentences. They have expressed hope that a defendant's contraceptive use will prevent her from injuring future children. Preventing women from conceiving substantially reduces their access to new victims during the punishment period. When this measure is combined with removal of existing children from the home, the probation conditions create an effective obstacle to commission of future crimes.

Yet the underlying logic of the incapacitative rationale for contraceptive sentencing can be challenged on two grounds. First, this justification depends on the philosophically sticky idea that potential future children can be protected by preventing their very existence.[5] Second, it extends legal protection and concern to unborn, indeed, to unconceived children. Although there are a few other areas in which the law arguably seeks to confer such protection, such as through permitting sterilization of mentally disabled adults and restricting the practice of contract pregnancy, these laws are controversial and justifiable on alternative grounds as well.[6] A further issue concerns whether the hoped-for incapacitative effect could be achieved by more acceptable means.

A few appellate courts have rejected contraceptive sentences on grounds that this goal could be achieved through less intrusive means.[7]

Rehabilitation is the final of the four traditional punishment goals. Rehabilitative punishment seeks to change the individual offender into a law-abiding citizen through enhancing her chances for successful community life. Typical rehabilitative measures are education, job training, and counseling. Although at one time rehabilitation was the dominant goal of the U.S. punishment system, in the last quarter-century its appeal has diminished.[8] This is not to suggest that rehabilitative efforts have been completely abandoned, but simply to note their relatively minor role in contemporary punishment policy.

Contraceptive sentences have been justified as rehabilitative. For example, Judge Howard Broadman claimed a rehabilitative intent when he sentenced Darlene Johnson to three years of Norplant use:

> Invading a human being's body is a big step. But locking somebody up in prison is also a big step. Clearly, I could just have locked her up for four years, but I thought it would be better to try to keep the family together, to see if she could get her act together. I thought that not having more children in the next three years would help in her potential rehabilitation.[9]

Judge Broadman's rehabilitation claim rests on the belief that preventing future births would reduce stress and other impediments to Darlene Johnson's becoming a nonabusive parent. There is some evidence that large family size is one factor associated with maternal violence toward children, although no direct relationship has been established.[10] Yet parenting classes, counseling, and similar measures also offer less extreme alternatives to promote a defendant's rehabilitation.[11]

No form of punishment is perfectly justified in light of traditional punishment goals. Contraceptive sentencing joins other contemporary punishment practices in offering a possible means of advancing some of these goals. Thorough evaluation of contraceptive sentencing demands attention to two additional dimensions of the practice, however. These are its coercive elements and its likely disproportionate effect on low-income women, especially on low-income women of color.

COERCION AND DISPROPORTIONATE IMPACTS

Contraceptive sentencing occurs in a system which is itself highly coercive. A fundamental principle of the criminal justice system is that the state is morally authorized, indeed, is morally required, to deprive convicted offenders of substantial freedom and experiential comfort. It is in this coercive context, then, that the coercion entailed in contraceptive sentencing must be evaluated.

The most recent instances of contraceptive sentencing involved conditions of probation imposed on convicted defendants. Does the availability of another "choice"—the prison sentence she would otherwise receive—make a defendant's consent to probation sufficiently voluntary to survive moral scrutiny? On first examination, it might seem that a defendant faced with such a probation proposal has been given a freedom-enhancing opportunity to improve her baseline punishment situation.[12]

The calculation is a bit trickier than this, however, because the very availability of contraceptive sentencing could negatively influence the specific defendant's baseline situation. The danger is that the sentence would have involved fewer burdens than either of the two options now facing the defendant—probation conditioned on contraceptive use or a burdensome period of incarceration. If so, the very availability of easily monitored long-term contraceptives leaves such women worse off than they were in their baseline situations.

Contraceptive sentences thus could reduce the overall freedom of at least some women convicted of child abuse and neglect. At the same time, such sentences could enhance the freedom of offenders whose baseline situations include a substantial and burdensome prison term.

But perhaps it is something about the nature of the contraceptive probation condition that creates special concern about its coercive potential. The explicit entry of fertility control into the realm of punishment seems to conflict with the strong legal and ethical support for protecting individual autonomy in medical and reproductive decisionmaking.

At the same time, prison terms and conditions of probation typically impose restrictions on many of the rights and freedoms enjoyed by ordinary citizens. Convicted defendants often "consent" to give up legally protected rights to avoid going to prison. So the harsh context of the criminal justice system weakens the claim that contraceptive sentencing is extraordinarily coercive. The options presented to women in these cases are not distinctively different from those faced by other criminal offenders.

The disproportionate gender, race, and class effects of contraceptive sentencing constitute a second reason to be disturbed about the practice, however.

Feminist concern about potential gender bias in contraceptive sentencing is valid. The emergence of long-term implantable and injectable contraceptives supplies added reason for concern, because they are effective, easily monitored, and can be used only in women. As such, these methods could easily become vehicles for exercising control over women's lives in a variety of settings. If long-term contraceptives are adopted in the criminal justice system, their attractiveness as a means to promote or impose state policy in other areas could increase.[13]

Similar concerns exist regarding the kind of women who are likely to be the subjects of contraceptive sentencing. I have no doubt that they will be overwhelmingly poor, and many will be women of color.[14]

CONTRACEPTIVE SENTENCING: A PROPOSAL

One way to reconcile the competing concerns about potential abuses and possible benefits of contraceptive sentencing would be to adopt the following principle: whenever long-acting contraceptives are proposed as a probation condition, judges must also present to the defendant at least one nonincarcerative alternative sentence. If the defendant was convicted of an offense that would not ordinarily call for a prison term, then she should be given two alternatives: one including contraceptives as a probation condition, and one including a set of noncontraceptive probation conditions customarily applied to defendants in her situation.[15] If individuals convicted of the offense are eligible for a prison term, and the judge believes that probation with contraceptive use would be an appropriate alternative, the judge would be obligated to make three proposals: probation with contraceptive use, an alternative set of probation conditions, and the prison term the defendant would normally have to serve. Adherence to this principle would remove some of the pressure a defendant might feel to compromise her medical or reproductive preferences for the sake of avoiding confinement in a correctional institution.

The proposal fails to offer a perfect resolution. It may deter some judges from offering any probationary sentence at all. Yet by supplying a constraint that would discourage liberal judicial resort to contraceptive sentencing, the proposal reduces the ethically troubling aspects of the practice.

Contraceptive sentencing can have only the most minimal impact on the incidence of child abuse and neglect. I close with a reminder of all the other measures that would be incorporated into a governmental system that was truly serious about protecting children from this form of harm. Such a system would include a probation office with enough employees to implement all types of court-ordered probation conditions. It would include high-quality counseling and education for overwhelmed parents. It would include help for substance-abusing parents and job and educational training for those in need of employment. It would include a child protective services system that responded promptly to reports of abuse or neglect. It would include teacher training programs on detection of children at risk. It would include regular health care by professionals familiar with the signs of abuse and neglect. It would include good prenatal care and full family planning services for poor women.

We ought to direct our energies to developing and supporting a system like this. Seizing on long-term contraceptives and other punitive measures to solve the problems of abused and neglected children is shortsighted at best. We must not allow this strategy to divert our country from the real and pressing obligations we have to improve the lives of these children and those who care for them in very difficult circumstances.

REFERENCES

1. For a summary of the retributive rationale for punishment, see Andrew Ashworth, "Desert," in *Principled Sentencing*, ed. Andrew von Hirsch and Andrew Ashworth (Boston: Northeastern University Press, 1992), pp. 181–87. For an analysis of intermediate punishments and the retributive rationale, see Norval Morris and Michael Tonry, *Between Prison and Probation* (New York: Oxford University Press, 1990), pp. 84–108.
2. For a summary of general and specific deterrence issues, see Andrew Ashworth, "Deterrence," in *Principled Sentencing*, pp. 53–60.
3. Contraceptive sentencing is endorsed on general deterrence grounds in Thomas Bartrum, "Birth Control as a Condition of Probation—A New Weapon in the War against Child Abuse," *Kentucky Law Journal* 80, no. 4 (1991–92): 1037–53, at 1053.
4. For discussions of incapacitation, see Andrew von Hirsch, "Incapacitation," in *Principled Sentencing*, pp. 101–8; Morris and Tonry, *Between Prison and Probation*, pp. 13–14, 180–86, 212–18.
5. See John Robertson, *Hastings Center Report*, (January–February 1995).
6. See Stacey Arthur, "The Norplant Prescription: Birth Control, Woman Control, or Crime Control?" *UCLA Law Review* 40, no. 1 (1992): 1–101, at 47–48.
7. See Arthur, "Norplant Prescription," pp. 56–59, 66–67; American Medical Association Board of Trustees, "Requirements or Incentives by Government for the Use of Long-Acting Contraceptives," *JAMA* 267 (1992): 1818–21.
8. See Andrew von Hirsch, "Rehabilitation," in *Principled Sentencing*, pp. 1–6, at 3.
9. Quoted in Arthur, "Norplant Prescription," note 231.
10. Melissa Burke, "The Constitutionality of the Use of the Norplant Contraceptive Device as a Condition of Punishment," *Hastings Constitutional Law Quarterly* 20, no. 1 (1992): 207–46, at 229–30.
11. See Julie Mertus and Simon Heller, "Norplant Meets the New Eugenicists: The Impermissibility of Coerced Contraception," *St. Louis University Public Law Review* 11, no. 2 (1992): 359–83, at 374–76; AMA Board of Trustees, "Requirements or Incentives by Government," p. 1819.
12. See Alan Wertheimer, *Coercion* (Princeton: Princeton University Press, 1987), pp. 202–21.
13. See Arthur, "Norplant Prescription," pp. 22–24; Cheri Pies, "Creating Ethical Reproductive Policy," Education Programs Associates (1993), pp. 29–32, expressing these concerns.
14. See Dorothy Roberts, "Punishing Drug Addicts Who Have Babies: Women of Color, Equality, and the Right of Privacy," *Harvard Law Review* 104, no. 7 (1991): 1419–81, at 1432–33; Mertus and Heller, "Norplant Meets the New Eugenicists," pp. 376–83; Kristyn Walker, "Judicial Control of Reproductive Freedom: The Use of Norplant as a Condition of Probation," *Iowa Law Review* 78, no. 3 (1993): 779–812, at 807–10.
15. The usual legal standards for disclosure of the device's risks and benefits would also have to be met before a defendant's agreement to use Norplant could be accepted.

POSTSCRIPT

Should Courts Be Permitted to Order Women to Use Long-Acting Contraceptives?

At the time of her sentencing, Darlene Johnson agreed to the Norplant implantation but later changed her mind. In addition to the implantation, her sentence included one year in jail and three years probation. Two months after the decision, Judge Broadman was shot at in his courtroom by a man who claimed to be angry about the Johnson decision. As a result of this incident and the publicity surrounding his decision, Judge Broadman removed himself from the case. The district attorney's office then asked for an appeal on the grounds that Johnson did not voluntarily agree to the implantation. The appeal was dismissed in April 1992 at the request of her lawyers because she had violated the terms of her probation by testing positive for drug use and was sentenced to five years in prison. The Norplant order never became effective and was never adjudicated. The Kansas legislation was defeated, as were similar proposals introduced in other states.

In 1991 a Texas judge ordered the implantation of Norplant as part of a plea bargain agreement. A woman who pleaded guilty to injuring her hospitalized 10-month-old daughter was ordered to serve 10 years probation, including 5 years of using Norplant and participation in parenting classes. In addition, she was denied unsupervised visits with her other children for 10 years. In Baltimore a 1993 plan to offer Norplant in high school clinics has failed to attract many young women. Health officials believe that misinformation about side effects and accusations by some black leaders that the program is genocidal and would lead to promiscuity have contributed to its failure.

In 1994 a class action suit was filed by 400 women who had used Norplant and who claimed that removing the contraceptive when they wanted to become pregnant was painful and difficult. Some of the women said that they required surgery and that they have been left with extensive scars as a result.

Another long-acting contraceptive, Depo-Provera, was approved by the Food and Drug Administration in 1992. Depo-Provera is an injectable drug that prevents pregnancy for three months. Like Norplant, it has side effects for some women; but it does not require implantation or removal.

In "Norplant: The New Scarlet Letter?" *Journal of Contemporary Health Law and Policy* (vol. 8, 1992), Michael T. Flannery presents legal arguments for and against the use of Norplant and concludes, "Implantation of Norplant will remain a sentencing option available to the courts." Also see Anita Hardon,

"Norplant: Conflicting Views on Its Safety and Acceptability," in *Issues in Reproductive Technology (I): An Anthology* edited by Helen B. Holmes (Garland Publishing, 1992) and Madeline Henley, "The Creation and Perpetuation of the Mother/Body Myth: Judicial and Legislative Enlistment of Norplant," *Buffalo Law Review* (vol. 41, no. 2, 1993). *Norplant and Poor Women* edited by Sarah E. Samuels and Mark D. Smith (Henry J. Kaiser Family Foundation, 1992) contains essays on the potential for coercion and other issues relating to poor, minority women.

Finally, a broad survey of the many ethical and policy issues raised by long-term contraceptives can be found in the January–February 1995 special supplement of the *Hastings Center Report*, "Long-Acting Contraception: Moral Choices, Policy Dilemmas."

ISSUE 9

Is There a Moral Right to Abortion?

YES: Bonnie Steinbock, from *Life Before Birth: The Moral and Legal Status of Embryos and Fetuses* (Oxford University Press, 1992)

NO: Sidney Callahan, from "Abortion and the Sexual Agenda: A Case for Prolife Feminism," *Commonweal* (April 25, 1986)

ISSUE SUMMARY

YES: Philosopher Bonnie Steinbock argues for a pro-choice position based on two independent considerations: the moral status of the fetus, which she claims begins when the fetus has a capacity for conscious experience, and the pregnant woman's moral right to bodily self-determination.

NO: Psychologist Sidney Callahan asserts that a woman's moral obligation to continue a pregnancy arises from both her status as a member of the human community and her unique life-giving female reproductive power.

Abortion is the most divisive bioethical issue of our time. The issue has been a persistent one in history, but in the past 20 years or so the debate has polarized. One view—known as "pro-life"—sees abortion as the wanton slaughter of innocent life. The other view—"pro-choice"—considers abortion as an option that must be available to women if they are to control their own reproductive lives. According to the pro-life view, women who have access to "abortion on demand" put their own selfish whims ahead of an unborn child's right to life. According to the pro-choice view, women have the right to choose to have an abortion—especially if there is some overriding reason, such as preventing the birth of a child with a severe genetic defect or one conceived as a result of rape or incest.

Behind these strongly held convictions, as political scientist Mary Segers has pointed out, are widely differing views of what determines value (that is, whether value is inherent in a thing or ascribed to it by human beings), the relation between law and morality, and the use of limits of political solutions to social problems, as well as the value of scientific progress. Those who condemn abortion as immoral generally follow a classical tradition in which abortion is a public matter because it involves our conception of how we ought to live together in an ideal society. Those who accept the idea of abortion, on the other hand, generally share the liberal, individualistic ethos of contemporary society. To them, abortion is a private choice, and public policy ought to reflect how citizens actually behave, not some unattainable ideal.

This is what we know about abortion practices in America today: It has been legal since the 1973 Supreme Court decision of *Roe v. Wade* declared that a woman has a constitutional right to privacy, which includes an abortion. Abortion is seven times safer than childbirth, although there are some unknown risks—primarily the effect of repeated abortions on subsequent pregnancies. Abortion is common: Each year about 1.5 million abortions are performed. That is, one out of four pregnancies (and half of all unintended pregnancies) end in abortion. About 90 percent of all abortions are performed within the first 12 weeks of pregnancy by a method called suction aspiration. Eighty percent of the women who have abortions are unmarried, and nearly 63 percent are between the ages of 15 and 24. (In comparison, however, in 1965 there were between 200,000 and 1.2 million illegal abortions, and 20 percent of all deaths from childbirth or pregnancy were caused by botched abortions.) Although the number of abortions performed in 1990 was about 10 percent higher than in 1980, the number of live births increased by 16 percent. In 1992 the ratio of abortions to live births was lower than for any year since 1977, which means that a greater proportion of pregnancies ended with a live birth. The national fertility rate reached a peak in 1990 and is somewhat lower today.

If abortion today is legal, safe, and common, it undeniably involves the killing of fetal life, and so the question remains: Is it ethical? At the heart of the issue are two complex questions. Does the fetus have a moral status that entitles it to life, liberty, and the pursuit of happiness as guaranteed by the Constitution? And even if it does, does a woman's rights to the same freedoms outweigh those of the fetus?

The selections that follow are written from two different feminist perspectives. Bonnie Steinbock asserts that consideration of both the moral status of the fetus and a pregnant woman's right to bodily self-determination is necessary to establish the moral status of abortion. She places the beginning of a fetus's status as a potential human at the point when the capacity for conscious experience develops, sometime toward the end of the second trimester. Her criteria support a liberal stance on abortion. Sidney Callahan seeks to broaden what she sees as feminists' excessively narrow focus on "rights." She argues that women, as members of the human community with unique life-giving powers, have a moral obligation not to terminate a pregnancy and that society should provide the support that women need to enhance their lives.

YES

Bonnie Steinbock

ABORTION

Nearly two decades after the Supreme Court ruled in *Roe* v. *Wade*[1] that a woman has a constitutional right to terminate her pregnancy, abortion remains one of the most divisive and emotionally charged issues in America. Pro-lifers march with posters of macerated fetuses; pro-choicers use a bloody coat hanger as their symbol of the days of illegal abortions. But behind the drama and the emotion are claims that can be subjected to philosophical scrutiny. Is the unborn a human being, with a right to life like any other human being, as pro-lifers maintain? If it is, then very few abortions, if any, could be justified. For we do not generally think that it is morally permissible to kill children because they are unwanted or illegitimate or severely handicapped. On the other hand, if the fetus[2] is not a child, but only part of the pregnant woman's body, then restrictive abortion laws would be as difficult to justify in a pluralistic society as laws against contraception. For restrictive abortion laws impose enormous physical, emotional, and financial burdens on women. Even legal moralists, who hold that society has the right to enforce its moral beliefs through law, could not justify the imposition of such heavy burdens. Only the assumption that the unborn is a human being like any other, entitled to the law's protection, could justify the prohibition of abortion. Thus, the moral status of the unborn is central to the abortion debate....

Few writers on abortion come to the topic with a fully open mind, and I am no exception. I believe that the decision to have an abortion is one that belongs to the pregnant woman—not the state, not her doctor, not her husband. My pro-choice position is based on two independent considerations: the moral status of the fetus and the pregnant woman's moral right to bodily self-determination. I believe that both are necessary to an adequate treatment of abortion, yet many writers on abortion focus on only one aspect, while ignoring or downplaying the other. Thus, some opponents of abortion talk about the fetal right to live, or the wrongness of depriving a potential human being of its future life, without even mentioning the fact that a particular woman must carry and bear the fetus for it to have a future life.[3] On the other side, some feminists regard the inquiry into the status of the fetus as irrelevant to the problem of abortion.[4] The central questions, from a feminist perspective, are not about the abstract individual rights of fetuses but how to create the social conditions that make possible the fulfillment of reproductive responsibilities....

But these questions, important as they are, do not go "beneath the surface of the abortion dispute." *They change the subject.* The issue is whether abortion is a morally permissible choice. This question would remain, even if poverty, racism, or sexism were eliminated. In such a world, there would presumably still be contraceptive failures and unwanted pregnancies. It goes without saying that women ought to be recognized as fully autonomous choosers; the question is whether abortion is a choice that autonomous choosers are morally permitted to make. It is hard to see how one can answer this question without responding to the claim that abortion is the killing of a human being, with a right to life.

The interest view responds to this claim by arguing that embryos and early fetuses lack moral status. We are not morally required to consider their interests because, prior to becoming conscious and sentient, fetuses do not *have* interests. The defense of this claim requires some factual investigation as to when sentience occurs. More important, I will need to explain why sentience is essential to moral status. After all, if allowed to grow and develop, the nonconscious, nonsentient fetus will become conscious and sentient. It has been argued that its potential to acquire these characteristics gives the fetus a present interest in continued existence, and makes abortion seriously wrong....

CRITERIA FOR MORAL STATUS

The Conservative Position

...[T]here are two parts to the extreme conservative position. First, it attaches moral significance to the genetic humanity of the fetus; second, it argues that this humanity is present from conception onward. Either part can be challenged independently. For example, Baruch Brody takes what might be called a modified conservative position. Like Noonan, Brody bases the moral status of the unborn on its being human. However, he does not agree that humanity begins at conception. Brody argues that a functioning brain is essential for being human. When the brain stops functioning, the person dies and goes out of existence. On the same reasoning, the fetus "comes into humanity" when its brain begins to function.[5] In other words, the beginning of brain function marks a radical discontinuity in the life of the unborn. The human being who begins when brain function starts is not identical with the embryo whose brain has not yet begun to function.

Even if one accepts the thesis of radical discontinuity (a thesis that most conservatives would reject as inconsistent with the reality of continuous physical development), it is not clear why this should be marked by the emergence of brain waves. The beginning of brain function, taken as a physiological occurrence, is not different from any other change in the fetus. The significance of brain function lies rather in its connection with mental states such as conscious awareness. Brody suggests this when he says, "One of the characteristics essential to a human being is the capacity for conscious experience, at least at a primitive level. Before the sixth week, as far as we know, the fetus does not have this capacity. Thereafter, as the electroencephalographic evidence indicates, it does. Consequently, that is the time at which the fetus becomes a human being."[6]

The phrase "capacity for conscious experience" is ambiguous. It might refer to the physiological ability of a being to have conscious experiences *at some point* in its development. The fetus at six weeks after conception (eight weeks g.a. [gestation age]) certainly has the capacity for conscious experience in this sense, but so does the single-celled zygote. Obviously, this is not what Brody intends. In another sense of "capacity," a being has the capacity for an experience x if x occurs, given the appropriate stimulus. A frog has the capacity to feel pain if, on being subjected to certain kinds of stimuli, the frog feels pain. However, in this sense of "capacity," neither a zygote nor a 6-week-old fetus has the capacity for conscious experience. The emergence of brain waves is only a necessary, not a sufficient, condition of conscious experience.

What further development is necessary for the fetus to feel pain, arguably the most primitive form of conscious experience? ... Admittedly, the evaluation of pain in the fetus is difficult, both because pain is a subjective phenomenon and because we do not have access to the fetus *in utero* to perform behavioral tests. Nevertheless, from what we do know about the physiology of pain perception, it seems reasonable to conclude that the fetus during the first trimester, and probably well into the second trimester, is not sentient. The neural pathways are not sufficiently developed to transmit pain messages to the fetal cortex until 22 to 24 weeks of gestation. If the early fetus is not sentient, it is unlikely to have conscious awareness of any kind. Certainly the ability to feel pain would precede more highly developed cognitive states, such as thoughts, emotions, and moods.

To summarize, brain function has no significance if taken as a purely physiological development in the fetus. Brain function is significant only because it is a necessary condition for mental states, such as sentience, conscious awareness, beliefs, and memories. However, brain function is not a sufficient condition for even the most rudimentary mental states. Thus, Brody's claim that the emergence of brain waves marks the beginning of human life is not tenable. If the capacity for conscious experience is a necessary condition of humanity, the fetus does not become human until sometime toward the end of the second trimester. This criterion for moral status supports a liberal, rather than a conservative, stance on abortion....

A conscious, sentient newborn ordinarily has a life worth living, a life he enjoys, a life that is a good to him. Continuing to live is certainly *in* the baby's interest, because of the value to him of his life *right now*. A right to life protects his interest in his life. I conclude that there is no conceptual bar to ascribing to newborns a right to life.[7] Nor is there any conceptual bar to ascribing a right to life to the nearly born fetus. A late-gestation fetus is conscious and sentient. It is possible that it has pleasurable experiences. If so, it has an interest in continuing to live, an interest that can be protected by a right to life. By contrast, embryos and preconscious fetuses do not have lives that they value, lives that are a good to them. Life is no more a good to an embryo than it is to a plant or a sperm. Thus, the importance of sentience is not primarily that abortion causes pain to the sentient fetus. That problem might be taken care of with an anesthetic. The relevance of sentience is that a sentient being can have a life it values, and that we can protect for its own sake.

Some antiabortionists consider it callous and unfeeling to deny moral status to the preconscious fetus. But the charge of callousness makes sense only if we persist in thinking of embryos and fetuses as being just like babies, only smaller. In fact, I think that this is how many opponents of abortion do regard the fetus. For example, the film *The Silent Scream* purported to show a 12-week fetus struggling to get away from the abortionist's scalpel, and opening its mouth in "a silent scream." Critics of the film charged that normal fetal movements were speeded up to make it look as if the fetus were recoiling in pain. But even if the film was not doctored, such movements are not by themselves evidence of pain. A mimosa plant shrinks from touch, but no one claims that the mimosa feels pain. The reason is that a plant lacks the nervous system necessary for the experience of pain. Similarly, the fetal nervous system at 12 weeks is not sufficiently developed to carry and transmit pain messages. Insofar as opposition to abortion is based on factual error, or worse, deliberate misrepresentation of the facts, it must be rejected out of hand.

A more sophisticated conservative position acknowledges that zygotes, embryos, and early fetuses do not suffer from being aborted, nor does death deprive them of happy lives. Nevertheless, it maintains that even a zygote has an interest in not being killed. This interest in continued existence does not derive from the kind of life it has *now*, but rather on the kind of life it *will* have, if it is allowed to develop and grow. Such arguments are known as arguments from potential. If successful, they can support the conservative proposal that genetic humans ought to be treated as normative persons.

THE ARGUMENT FROM POTENTIAL

There are different versions of the argument from potential, but the basic idea is that it is wrong to kill, or otherwise prevent the development of, a human fertilized egg because it possesses the potential to be a descriptive person. As Stephen Buckle expresses it, "It is, potentially, just like us, so we cannot deny it any rights or other forms of protection that we accord ourselves."[8] A fertilized egg does not now have any of the properties of a person. It isn't even sentient. But this does not matter because, left alone and allowed to develop, the zygote will become a person. Buckle says, "The fertilized egg is not 'just like us' only in the sense that it is not *yet* just like us. Therefore, the argument concludes, we should not interfere with its natural development towards being a rational, self-conscious being. On its strongest interpretation, the argument is thought to establish that we should treat a potential human subject as if it were already an actual human subject."[9]

The Logical Problem

A standard objection to the argument from potential is that it involves a logical mistake. The mistake consists in thinking of a "potential person" as a kind of person, and, on this basis, ascribing to "potential persons" the rights of other persons. But potential persons are not persons; they do not now have the characteristics of persons....

It is a logical error to think that potential personhood implies possession of the rights of actual persons. However, the argument from potential need not be based on this logical mistake. Like the defender of the genetic humanity criterion, the defender of the argument from potential can be understood as making a normative proposal: that potential persons *ought* to have the same rights as actual persons. Understood this way, the argument is not based on a logical confusion, but is rather in need of defense. Why should beings who are potentially "just like us" be entitled to the same protection as we are?

A Future Like Ours

Don Marquis argues that abortion is seriously immoral, for the same reason that killing an innocent adult human being is immoral.[10] What makes killing wrong is not primarily the effects on other people, or the threat to the fabric of society. What makes killing wrong is the effect on the victim. The loss of one's life is one of the greatest losses one can suffer. The loss of one's life deprives one of all the experiences, activities, projects, and enjoyments that would otherwise have constituted one's future. When I am killed, I am deprived of all of the value of my future. Abortion deprives the fetus of its future, a future just like ours. Hence, abortion is prima facie seriously morally wrong.

Marquis maintains that this is not an argument based on the wrongness of killing potential persons, since the central category is not *personhood* at all, but the category of having a valuable future like ours. However, if we ask what it is that makes "a future like ours" valuable, the answer is likely to be in terms of our capacity to enjoy our lives and derive meaning from them, to envisage a future

and to make plans about it, to have relationships with others. In other words, the very capacities that make us people are what enable us to have a valuable future. So the notion of personhood, and the special wrongness of killing persons, is implicit in Marquis's account.

On the interest view, only beings that have already begun to experience their lives have an interest in the continuation of their lives. Only sentient beings can be harmed or wronged by being killed. Marquis calls this the *discontinuation account.* He concedes that it is intelligible, but holds that it is inferior to his "future-like-ours" account of the wrongness of killing. The value of one's present life is irrelevant, Marquis argues. What matters is the future of which one is deprived by death. Whether one has immediate past experiences or not does not work in the explanation of what makes killing wrong....

Contraception and the Moral Status of Gametes

The strongest objection to the argument from potential is that it seems to make contraception, and even abstinence, prima facie morally wrong. If the objection to abortion is that it deprives the zygote of "a future like ours," why, it may be asked, cannot the same complaint be made of contraceptive techniques that kill sperm, or prevent fertilization? Why don't gametes have "a future like ours"? Why aren't unfertilized eggs and sperm also potential people? John Harris makes the point this way:

> To say that a fertilized egg is potentially a human being is just to say that if certain things happen to it (like implantation), and certain other things do not (like spontaneous abortion), it will eventually become a human being. But the same is

also true of the unfertilized egg and the sperm. If certain things happen to the egg (like meeting a sperm) and certain things happen to the sperm (like meeting an egg) and thereafter certain other things do not (like meeting a contraceptive), then they will eventually become a new human being.[11]

So, if abortion is seriously wrong because it kills a potential person, then the use of a contraceptive is equally seriously wrong. In using a spermicide, one commits mass murder! Indeed, even abstinence is wrong, insofar as it prevents the development of a new human being. Very few defenders of the potentiality principle are willing to accept this conclusion.[12] They must then give reasons why a zygote, but not a sperm or ovum, is a potential person.

Defenders of the potentiality criterion sometimes appeal to an enormous difference in probabilities. John Noonan points out that the chances of any particular sperm becoming a person are remarkably low. There are about two hundred million spermatozoa in a normal ejaculate, of which only one has a chance of developing into a zygote. By contrast, he estimates the chances of a zygote developing into a person to be about 80 percent. The difference is still impressive, even if we adjust Noonan's estimate to reflect more recent information on the miscarriage rate. A 1988 study found that 31 percent of all conceptions end in miscarriage, usually in the early months of pregnancy and often before women even know they are pregnant. Even this study probably underestimated the miscarriage rate by an unknown amount, since some fertilized eggs are so defective that they never make chorionic gonadotropin, the hormone that pregnancy tests measure, and are miscarried within

days of fertilization.[13] This suggests that a given zygote's chance of becoming a person is about 50 percent, rather than the 80 percent chance Noonan gives it. Still, the zygote's one-in-two chance is a lot better than a sperm's one-in-two-hundred-million chance. The odds of an ovum's developing into a person are better than those of a sperm, but still much worse than those of a fertilized egg. If we think of potential in terms of statistical likelihood, a zygote has greater potential than a gamete. But it is not clear that the odds matter. Although the chances of any particular sperm becoming a person are infinitesimal, why should that prevent its being a potential person? Is not every entrant in a lottery a potential winner, even if the odds of winning are extremely low? Every gamete, it may be said, has the potential to develop into a person, even though very few do....

At this point, the debate seems to be at a standstill. Antiabortionists are convinced that there is an enormous moral difference between the product of conception and the ingredients of conception. Their opponents are convinced that the difference is one of degree, and lacking in moral importance. Neither side is obviously right or wrong. Yet the success of the argument from potential hinges on differentiating the zygote from its component gametes....

There is no question that abortion is for most women psychologically and emotionally different from contraception. Few women experience abortion as just another way to avoid motherhood. Abortion is the end of a specific pregnancy, and this termination can be psychologically distressing, even when it is felt to be necessary. Pregnancy affects a woman's body in concrete, noticeable ways, preparing her to carry and bear a child. The child she would have, if she did not abort, is thus likely to have for her a reality that no merely possible person can have. Some women are pleased at finding that they *can* bear a child, even if they realize that having a child at this point in their lives is unwise. In ending the pregnancy, they are likely to have mixed feelings. In addition, pregnancy is imbued with certain cultural meanings. It is ordinarily a joyous experience, and one that is associated with congratulations, gift-giving, and special treatment. As one woman expresses it, "Sadness at not being able to celebrate pregnancy, to enjoy the sense of specialness it brings, is an understandable response."[14] Once we understand this, we can see why so many women (and men) do not have the same attitude toward abortion as they do toward contraception. Unless one's religion forbids it, contraception is likely to be regarded as morally neutral, a sensible preventive health habit, like flossing your teeth. It has none of the sadness or sense of loss that often accompanies abortions. A view that equates abortion and contraception is remote from the experiences of most people.

Does this matter? Some philosophers deny that it does. They argue that people's intuitions or felt convictions have no moral significance. They remind us that some people "experience" blacks and women to be inferior to whites and men. They maintain that we should not try to account for such feelings in our moral theories. The appropriate response to feelings that do not accord with moral theory is, "So what?"

I do not agree with this total rejection of moral feelings. It *may* be that a feeling is mere prejudice, incapable of being supported by good reasons. I think that this can fairly easily be shown of racist

and sexist views. But from the fact that some strong convictions are indefensible, it does not follow that all are. A morality that is radically divorced from our deepest feelings, and disconnected from our experiences and emotions, cannot be practical or action-guiding. For all the reasons I have given above, I think we are justified in regarding abortion as morally more serious than contraception, and for thinking that abortion is a moral issue in a way that contraception is not. Still, I would not go so far as Rosalind Hursthouse, who argues that abortion is a choice that a completely wise and virtuous person would rarely make, because it usually displays a callous and light-minded attitude toward life.[15] This is unfair. A great many abortions occur because of contraceptive failure. A woman who is responsibly using a reliable contraceptive, and nevertheless gets pregnant, should not be labeled callous or light-minded. At the same time, this characterization might fit a woman who does not use contraceptives, repeatedly becomes pregnant, and has several abortions. I knew a sixteen-year-old girl who was about to have her third abortion. I asked her what seemed to be the problem. "Oh," she responded, "I can never remember to put in a diaphragm, and the pill makes me fat." We can acknowledge that her attitude toward sexuality, pregnancy, and potential human life is immature and superficial, without implying that the unborn has moral status. Abortion may be morally undesirable, in a way that contraception is not, without its being a *wrong to* the unborn. . . .

Sentient Fetuses

What is the moral status of sentient fetuses? They have begun to have experiences, and so it is at least possible that they enjoy their lives. Obviously, the range and nature of their enjoyment is not very great, but perhaps late fetuses, like babies, are capable of sensuous pleasure, from sucking their thumbs, from the warmth of the womb, from the sound of their mothers' heartbeats, from motion as the mother moves around. Certainly in newborn nurseries the temperature is kept quite high, on the ground that this is what the baby was used to before birth. The ability to calm infants by motion is often attributed to this being a replication of the uterine environment. Studies have been done correlating fetal activity with extrauterine sound, leading researchers to claim that fetuses can not only hear inside the womb, but that they enjoy some kinds of sounds more than others. If all of this is right, then it seems plausible to say that late fetuses have, or have begun to have, lives in the biographical sense. Death deprives them of their lives, and so is a harm to them. Thus, it seems that life is *in* the interest of the conscious fetus, and it, like a newborn, can have a right to life.

On the other hand, fetuses, unlike born babies, dwell inside pregnant women. This has been dismissed by conservatives as "mere geography," but the geography is not insignificant. Any attempt to protect the life of a fetus may conflict with, or even endanger, the interests of the pregnant woman, including her life or health. There is a possibility of conflict that simply does not exist in the case of the newborn. For this reason, we cannot simply extend the right to life possessed by all human newborns to sentient fetuses.

To summarize, sentience is sufficient for minimal moral status. The interests of all sentient beings—persons, animals,

conscious fetuses, and babies—must be considered. However, some sentient beings may have lives that are more valuable than others. They occupy a higher place on the moral-status scale. For example, we have good reasons for extending normative personhood, and a right to life, to human infants, stemming both from their relation to other human persons and from their potential personhood. We do not have these reasons to extend normative personhood to nonhuman animals. Conscious fetuses, though substantially similar to newborns, and thus entitled to some legal protection, are located inside the pregnant woman's body. This makes it impossible to give them full protection without violating her right to privacy or bodily self-determination.

Embryos and preconscious fetuses are admittedly potential persons, but they do not have interests. Therefore, their interests cannot be considered in making the decision to abort. A pregnant woman who wishes to be responsible and conscientious in making a decision about abortion is not required to consider the child who might have been born. In order to justify having an abortion, she does not have to claim that her child would be miserable. She can acknowledge that, if she does not abort, the resulting child might well have a very happy life. Pro-lifers are quite right to cast scorn on the notion that all unplanned pregnancies result in unwanted children, or that all unwanted children necessarily have unhappy lives.[16] Instead, pro-choicers should respond that the happiness of the potential child is not determinative— indeed, not even relevant to the decision to abort. There is no obligation to bring happy people into the world, only an obligation to try to give the children one decides to bring into the world a decent chance at happiness....

THE ARGUMENT FROM BODILY SELF-DETERMINATION

Thomson's Defense of Abortion

In 1971, Judith Jarvis Thomson published a genuinely novel defense of abortion.[17] She noted that most debates about abortion center on the moral status of the fetus: whether it is a person with a right to life. This is because people have generally thought that if we accept the premise that the fetus is a person, it follows that abortion is always wrong. The argument goes like this: All persons have a right to life. The fetus is a person, and so it has a right to life. The mother has the right to decide what happens in and to her body, but the right to life is stronger and more stringent than the mother's right to decide, and so outweighs it. So the fetus may not be killed; an abortion may not be performed.

It is this argument that Thomson wants to challenge. She argues that even if we grant the personhood of the fetus, abortion is not necessarily wrong. For it is possible that in at least some cases abortion does not violate the fetus-person's right to life. This is initially puzzling. If the fetus has a right to life, and abortion kills it, then how can abortion fail to violate its right to life? Thomson suggests that our perplexity stems from a failure to understand the nature of rights in general and the right to life in particular. In a nutshell, her argument is that having a right to life does not entitle a person to whatever he or she needs to stay alive, and in particular does not entitle him to the use of another person's body.

To illustrate this point, Thomson creates the following example:

> You wake up in the morning and find yourself back to back in bed with an unconscious violinist. He has been found to have a fatal kidney ailment, and the Society of Music Lovers has canvassed all the available medical records and found that you alone have the right blood type to help. They have therefore kidnapped you, and last night the violinist's circulatory system was plugged into yours, so that your kidneys can be used to extract poisons from his blood as well as your own.[18]

The director of the hospital, while acknowledging that it was very wrong of the Society to kidnap you, nevertheless refuses to unplug you, since to unplug you would be to kill him. Anyway, it's only for nine months. After that, the violinist will have recovered and can be safely unplugged. Thomson questions whether it is morally incumbent on you to accede to this situation. It would be very nice of you, of course, but do you *have* to stay plugged in to the violinist? What if it were not nine months, but nine years? Or longer still? What if the director were to maintain that you must stay plugged in forever, on the ground that the violinist is a person, and all persons have a right to life? Thomson suggests that you would regard this argument as "outrageous," and says that this suggests that something really is wrong with the plausible-sounding right-to-life argument presented above.

The violinist example, fantastic though it is, preserves some of the features of the pregnancy situation without making at all doubtful the personhood of the "victim." Given that the violinist is a person, with a right to life, do you murder him, do you violate his right to life, if you unplug yourself? If not, then we have, it seems, a case of terminating the life of an innocent person that is not a case of violating his right to life.

The violinist example is intended to demonstrate Thomson's central theme, that the right to life does not necessarily include getting whatever you need to live. To take a less fanciful example, I may need your bone marrow in order to live, but that does not give me a right to it. Even if you *ought* to be willing to donate, even if your refusal is selfish and mean, it does not follow that I have a right to your bone marrow, or that you may legitimately be compelled to donate.[19] The right to life does not imply a right to use another person's body.

However, it may be objected that the fetus *does* have a right to use the pregnant woman's body because she is (partly) responsible for its existence. By engaging in intercourse, knowing that this may result in the creation of a person inside her body, she implicitly gives the resulting person a right to remain. This argument would not apply in the situation most closely aligned with the violinist example—pregnancy due to rape. A woman who is pregnant due to rape does not voluntarily engage in sexual intercourse, and so cannot be said to have implicitly given the fetus permission to use her body.

On this analysis, even if abortion is ordinarily a grave wrong, it is permissible in the case of rape. Many antiabortionists wish to make such an exception, but they have been hard-pressed, on their own argument, to account for it. For antiabortionists maintain that the fetus is an innocent person. How can it be right to kill the fetus because its father is a rapist? The Thomson argument gives an answer: the fetus whose existence is caused by rape has no right to use the pregnant woman's body. Killing it does not violate its right to life.

But what about most pregnancies, which do not result from rape but from voluntary intercourse? Given that the presence of the fetus is due in part to the woman's own voluntary action, can she now eject it at the cost of its life? Thomson responds by saying that even where the woman voluntarily engages in sex, she may not be responsible for the presence of the fetus. She argues that responsibility for an outcome depends on what one has done to prevent it. She suggests that if a person has taken all reasonable precautions to prevent something from happening, then she has not been negligent, and should not be held responsible for its having occurred. So whether the woman can be said to have given the fetus a right to use her body would depend on such variables as whether she was using a reliable contraceptive that happened to fail.

Some critics of Thomson have taken her to task for concentrating exclusively on rights. The real question, they say, is not what constitutes giving the unborn person a right to use one's body, but rather the conditions that make aborting the fetus morally permissible. Thomson responds by saying that since her intention was to examine the right-to-life argument, she can hardly be faulted for concentrating on rights. However, she acknowledges that we can have moral obligations to help people, even when they do not have rights against us. Suppose that the violinist needed your kidneys only for an hour, and that this would not affect your health at all. Even though you were kidnapped, even though you never gave anyone permission to plug him into you, still you ought to let him stay: "it would be indecent to refuse."[20] Similarly, if pregnancy lasted only an hour, and posed no threat to life or health, the pregnant woman ought to allow the fetus-person to remain for that hour. She ought to do this even if the pregnancy was due to rape, and the fetus has no right to use her body. This conclusion is based on the principle (which Thomson calls "minimally decent Samaritanism") that if you can save a person's life without much trouble or risk to yourself, you ought to do it. In the real world, however, pregnancies do not last for only an hour, and they do involve considerable sacrifices.[21] Thomson concludes, "Except in such cases as the unborn person has a right to demand it—and we were leaving open the possibility that there may be such cases—nobody is morally *required* to make large sacrifices, of health, of all other interests and concerns, of all other duties and commitments, for nine years, or even for nine months, in order to keep another person alive."[22]

Thomson's analysis apparently justifies abortion only in a relatively narrow range of cases. Many unwanted pregnancies occur because contraception was not used at all, or only occasionally. In such cases, the woman *is* (partly) to blame, and so the resulting fetus may be said to have been given the right to use her body. If so, then abortion violates its right to life, and is impermissible. Mary Anne Warren writes, "This is an extremely unsatisfactory outcome, from the viewpoint of the opponents of restrictive abortion laws, most of whom are convinced that a woman has a right to obtain an abortion regardless of how and why she got pregnant."[23]

It seems to me that Warren is right. A successful defense of abortion cannot be based solely on the woman's moral right to decide what happens in and to her body. This yields a defense of abortion in a relatively narrow range of cases—namely, those in which the woman is absolved of responsibility for the presence of the unborn. By the same token, a defense of abortion based solely on the claim that presentient fetuses lack moral status is vulnerable to potentiality arguments. The strongest argument in favor of a liberal abortion policy combines both these approaches. This was the approach taken by the United States Supreme Court in *Roe v. Wade*.

NOTES

1. *Roe v. Wade*, 410 U.S. 113 (1973).
2. Technically, the term "fetus" refers to the unborn after eight weeks of gestation. Many writers on abortion use the term "fetus" to refer generally to the unborn throughout pregnancy. I will follow this convention except where necessary to distinguish the different phases of gestation.
3. A good example is Don Marquis, "Why Abortion is Immoral," *The Journal of Philosophy* 76:4 (April 1989), pp. 183–202.
4. See, for example, Sandra Harding, "Beneath the Surface of the Abortion Dispute," in Sidney Callahan and Daniel Callahan, eds., *Abortion: Understanding Differences* (New York and London: Plenum Press, 1984).
5. Baruch Brody, *Abortion and the Sanctity of Life* (Cambridge, Mass.: The MIT Press, 1975), p. 111.
6. Ibid., p. 83.
7. A similar argument is made by Carson Strong, "Delivering Hydrocephalic Fetuses," *Bioethics* 5:1 (January 1991), pp. 7–11.
8. Stephen Buckle, "Arguing from Potential," *Bioethics* 2:3 (July 1988), p. 227.
9. Ibid.
10. Don Marquis, "Why Abortion is Immoral," pp. 183–202.
11. John Harris, *The Value of Life: An Introduction to Medical Ethics* (London: Routledge & Kegan Paul, 1985), pp. 11–12.
12. R. M. Hare may be the only potentiality theorist who does not hinge his argument on a morally significant difference between embryos and gametes. On Hare's version of the argument from potential, abortion is *prima facie* morally wrong,

but so are contraception and abstention from procreation. See "Abortion and the Golden Rule," *Philosophy & Public Affairs* 4:3 (Spring 1975).

13. "Study Finds 31% Rate of Miscarriage," *The New York Times*, Wednesday, July 27, 1988, p. A14.

14. Angela Neustatter, with Gina Newson, *Mixed Feelings: the Experience of Abortion* (London: Pluto Press, 1986), p. 10.

15. I borrow this term from Rosalind Hursthouse, *Beginning Lives* (Oxford: Basil Blackwell in association with the Open University), 1987.

16. However, a recent study showed that more than a third of women denied abortions confessed to strongly negative feelings toward their children, and that children born to women whose requests for abortion were refused are much likelier to be troubled and depressed, to drop out of school, to commit crimes, to suffer from serious illnesses, and to express dissatisfaction with life than are the offspring of willing parents. See Natalie Angier, "Study Says Anger Troubles Women Denied Abortions," *The New York Times*, May 29, 1991, p. C10.

17. Judith Jarvis Thomson, "A Defense of Abortion," *Philosophy & Public Affairs* 1:1 (1971). Reprinted in Joel Feinberg, ed., *The Problem of Abortion*, 2nd edition (Belmont, Calif.: Wadsworth Publishing Company, 1984), pp. 173–187.

18. Ibid., p. 174.

19. The claim that individuals do not have a legal obligation to donate body parts to others, even when they are needed for life itself, has been upheld in several cases. The first recorded case, to my knowledge, is *Shimp* v. *McFall*, 10 Pa. D. & D.3d 90 (1978).

20. Thomson, "A Defense of Abortion," p. 182.

21. The burdens of even normal pregnancies are well detailed by Donald Regan, "Rewriting *Roe* vs. *Wade*," *Michigan Law Review* 77 (1979).

22. Thomson, "A Defense of Abortion," p. 184.

23. Mary Anne Warren, "On the Moral and Legal Status of Abortion," *The Monist* 57 (1973). Reprinted by Joel Feinberg, ed., *The Problem of Abortion*, p. 108.

NO   Sidney Callahan

ABORTION AND THE SEXUAL AGENDA:
A CASE FOR PROLIFE FEMINISM

The abortion debate continues. In the latest and perhaps most crucial development, prolife feminists are contesting prochoice feminist claims that abortion
rights are prerequisites for women's full development and social equality.
The outcome of this debate may be decisive for the culture as a whole. Prolife feminists, like myself, argue on good feminist principles that women can
never achieve the fulfillment of feminist goals in a society permissive toward
abortion.

These new arguments over abortion take place within liberal political circles. This round of intense intra-feminist conflict has spiraled beyond earlier
right-versus-left abortion debates, which focused on "tragic choices," medical judgments, and legal compromises. Feminist theorists of the prochoice
position now put forth the demand for unrestricted abortion rights as a *moral
imperative* and insist upon women's right to complete reproductive freedom.
They morally justify the present situation and current abortion practices.
Thus it is all the more important that prolife feminists articulate their different feminist perspective.

These opposing arguments can best be seen when presented in turn. Perhaps the most highly developed feminist arguments for the morality and
legality of abortion can be found in Beverly Wildung Harrison's *Our Right
to Choose* (Beacon Press, 1983) and Rosalind Pollack Petchesky's *Abortion and
Woman's Choice* (Longman, 1984). Obviously it is difficult to do justice to
these complex arguments, which draw on diverse strands of philosophy and
social theory and are often interwoven in prochoice feminists' own version
of a "seamless garment." Yet the fundamental feminist case for the morality
of abortion, encompassing the views of Harrison and Petchesky, can be analyzed in terms of four central moral claims: (1) the moral right to control
one's own body; (2) the moral necessity of autonomy and choice in personal
responsibility; (3) the moral claim for the contingent value of fetal life; (4) the
moral right of women to true social equality.

1. The Moral Right to Control One's Own Body

Prochoice feminism argues that a woman choosing an abortion is exercising a basic right of bodily integrity granted in our common law tradition. If she does not choose to be physically involved in the demands of a pregnancy and birth, she should not be compelled to be so against her will. Just because it is *her* body which is involved, a woman should have the right to terminate any pregnancy, which at this point in medical history is tantamount to terminating fetal life. No one can be forced to donate an organ or submit to other invasive physical procedures for however good a cause. Thus no woman should be subjected to "compulsory pregnancy." And it should be noted that in pregnancy much more than a passive biological process is at stake.

From one perspective, the fetus is, as Petchesky says, a "biological parasite" taking resources from the woman's body. During pregnancy, a woman's whole life and energies will be actively involved in the nine-month process. Gestation and childbirth involve physical and psychological risks. After childbirth a woman will either be a mother who must undertake a twenty-year responsibility for child rearing, or face giving up her child for adoption or institutionalization. Since hers is the body, hers the risk, hers the burden, it is only just that she alone should be free to decide on pregnancy or abortion.

The moral claim to abortion, according to the prochoice feminists, is especially valid in an individualistic society in which women cannot count on medical care or social support in pregnancy, childbirth, or child rearing. A moral abortion decision is never made in a social vacuum, but in the real life society which exists here and now.

2. The Moral Necessity of Autonomy and Choice in Personal Responsibility

Beyond the claim for individual *bodily* integrity, the prochoice feminists claim that to be a full adult *morally*, a woman must be able to make responsible life commitments. To plan, choose, and exercise personal responsibility, one must have control of reproduction. A woman must be able to make yes-or-no decisions about a specific pregnancy, according to her present situation, resources, prior commitments, and life plan. Only with such reproductive freedom can a woman have the moral autonomy necessary to make mature commitments, in the area of family, work, or education.

Contraception provides a measure of personal control, but contraceptive failure or other chance events can too easily result in involuntary pregnancy. Only free access to abortion can provide the necessary guarantee. The chance biological process of an involuntary pregnancy should not be allowed to override all the other personal commitments and responsibilities a woman has: to others, to family, to work, to education, to her future development, health, or well-being. Without reproductive freedom, women's personal moral agency and human consciousness are subjected to biology and chance.

3. The Moral Claim for the Contingent Value of Fetal Life

Prochoice feminist exponents like Harrison and Petchesky claim that the value of fetal life is contingent upon the woman's free consent and subjective acceptance. The fetus must be invested with maternal valuing in order to become human. This process of "humanization" through personal consciousness and "sociality" can only be bestowed by the woman in whose body and psychosocial system a new life must mature. The meaning and value of fetal life are constructed by the woman; without this personal conferral there only exists a biological, physiological process. Thus fetal interests or fetal rights can never outweigh the woman's prior interest and rights. If a woman does not consent to invest her pregnancy with meaning or value, then the merely biological process can be freely terminated. Prior to her own free choice and conscious investment, a woman cannot be described as a "mother" nor can a "child" be said to exist.

Moreover, in cases of voluntary pregnancy, a woman can withdraw consent if fetal genetic defects or some other problem emerges at any time before birth. Late abortion should thus be granted without legal restrictions. Even the minimal qualifications and limitations on women embedded in *Roe v. Wade* are unacceptable —repressive remnants of patriarchal unwillingness to give power to women.

4. The Moral Right of Women to Full Social Equality

Women have a moral right to full social equality. They should not be restricted or subordinated because of their sex. But this morally required equality cannot be realized without abortion's certain control of reproduction. Female social equality depends upon being able to compete and participate as freely as males can in the structures of educational and economic life. If a woman cannot control when and how she will be pregnant or rear children, she is at a distinct disadvantage, especially in our male-dominated world.

Psychological equality and well-being is also at stake. Women must enjoy the basic right of a person to the free exercise of heterosexual intercourse and full sexual expression, separated from procreation. No less than males, women should be able to be sexually active without the constantly inhibiting fear of pregnancy. Abortion is necessary for women's sexual fulfillment and the growth of uninhibited feminine self-confidence and ownership of their sexual powers.

But true sexual and reproductive freedom means freedom to procreate as well as to inhibit fertility. Prochoice feminists are also worried that women's freedom to reproduce will be curtailed through the abuse of sterilization and needless hysterectomies. Besides the punitive tendencies of a male-dominated health-care system, especially in response to repeated abortions or welfare pregnancies, there are other economic and social pressures inhibiting reproduction. Genuine reproductive freedom implies that day care, medical care, and financial support would be provided mothers, while fathers would take their full share in the burdens and delights of raising children.

Many prochoice feminists identify feminist ideals with communitarian, ecologically sensitive approaches to reshaping society. Following theorists like Sara Ruddick and Carol Gilligan, they link abortion rights with the growth of "maternal thinking" in our heretofore patriarchal society. Maternal thinking is loosely defined as a responsible commitment to the loving nature of specific human beings as they actually exist in socially embedded interpersonal contexts. It is a moral perspective very different from the abstract, competitive, isolated, and principled rigidity so characteristic of patriarchy.

* * *

How does a prolife feminist respond to these arguments? Prolife feminists grant the good intentions of their prochoice counterparts but protest that the prochoice position is flawed, morally inadequate, and inconsistent with feminism's basic demands for justice. Prolife feminists champion a more encompassing moral ideal. They recognize the claims of fetal life and offer a different perspective on what is good for women. The feminist vision is expanded and refocused.

1. From the Moral Right to Control One's Own Body to a More Inclusive Ideal of Justice

The moral right to control one's own body does apply to cases of organ transplants, mastectomies, contraception, and sterilization; but it is not a conceptualization adequate for abortion. The abortion dilemma is caused by the fact that 266 days following a conception in one body, another body will emerge. One's own body no longer exists as a single unit but is engendering another organism's life. This dynamic passage from conception to birth is genetically ordered and universally found in the human species. Pregnancy is not like the growth of cancer or infestation by a biological parasite; it is the way every human being enters the world. Strained philosophical analogies fail to apply: having a baby is not like rescuing a drowning person, being hooked up to a famous violinist's artificial life-support system, donating organs for transplant—or anything else.

As embryology and fetology advance, it becomes clear that human development is a continuum. Just as astronomers are studying the first three minutes in the genesis of the universe, so the first moments, days, and weeks at the beginning of human life are the subject of increasing scientific attention. While neonatology pushes the definition of viability ever earlier, ultrasound and fetology expand the concept of the patient *in utero*. Within such a continuous growth process, it is hard to defend logically any demarcation point after conception as the point at which an immature form of human life is so different from the day before or the day after, that it can be morally or legally discounted as a nonperson. Even the moment of birth can hardly differentiate a nine-month fetus from a newborn. It is not surprising that those who countenance late abortions are logically led to endorse selective infanticide.

The same legal tradition which in our society guarantees the right to control one's own body firmly recognizes the wrongfulness of harming other bodies, however immature, dependent, different looking, or powerless. The handicapped, the retarded, and newborns are legally protected from deliberate harm. Prolife feminists reject the suppositions that would except the unborn from this protection.

After all, debates similar to those about the fetus were once conducted about feminine personhood. Just as women, or blacks, were considered too different, too underdeveloped, too "biological," to have souls or to possess legal rights, so the fetus is now seen as "merely" biological life, subsidiary to a person. A woman was once viewed as incorporated into the "one flesh" of her husband's person; she too was a form of bodily property. In all patriarchal unjust systems, lesser orders of human life are granted rights only when wanted, chosen, or invested with value by the powerful.

Fortunately, in the course of civilization there has been a gradual realization that justice demands the powerless and dependent be protected against the uses of power wielded unilaterally. No human can be treated as a means to an end without consent. The fetus is an immature, dependent form of human life which only needs time and protection to develop. Surely, immaturity and dependence are not crimes.

In an effort to think about the essential requirements of a just society, philosophers like John Rawls recommend imagining yourself in an "original position," in which your position in the society to be created is hidden by a "veil of ignorance." You will have to weigh the possibility that any inequalities inherent in that society's practices may rebound upon you in the worst, as well as in the best, conceivable way. This thought experiment helps ensure justice for all.

Beverly Harrison argues that in such an envisioning of society everyone would institute abortion rights in order to guarantee that if one turned out to be a woman one would have reproductive freedom. But surely in the original position and behind the "veil of ignorance," you would have to contemplate the possibility of being the particular fetus to be aborted. Since everyone has passed through the fetal stage of development, it is false to refuse to imagine oneself in this state when thinking about a potential world in which justice would govern. Would it be just that an embryonic life—in half the cases, of course, a female life—be sacrificed to the right of a woman's control over her own body? A woman may be pregnant without consent and experience a great many penalties, but a fetus killed without consent pays the ultimate penalty.

It does not matter... whether the fetus being killed is fully conscious or feels pain. We do not sanction killing the innocent if it can be done painlessly or without the victim's awareness. Consciousness becomes important to the abortion debate because it is used as a criterion for the "personhood" so often seen as the prerequisite for legal protection. Yet certain philosophers set the standard of personhood so high that half the human race could not meet the criteria during most of their waking hours (let alone their sleeping ones). Sentience, self-consciousness, rational decision-making, social participation? Surely no infant, or child under two, could qualify. Either our idea of person must be expanded or another criterion, such as human life itself, be employed to protect the weak in a just society. Prolife feminists who defend the fetus emphatically identify with an immature state of growth passed through by themselves, their children, and everyone now alive.

* * *

It also seems a travesty of just procedures that a pregnant woman now, in effect, acts as sole judge of her own case, under the most stressful conditions. Yes, one can acknowledge that the pregnant woman will be subject to the potential burdens arising from a pregnancy, but it has never been thought right to have an interested party, especially the more powerful party, decide his or her own case when there may be a conflict of interest. If one considers the matter as a case of a powerful versus a powerless, silenced claimant, the prochoice feminist argument can rightly be inverted: since hers is the body, hers the risk, and hers the greater burden, then how in fairness can a woman be the sole judge of the fetal right to life?

Human ambivalence, a bias toward self-interest, and emotional stress have always been recognized as endangering judgment. Freud declared that love and hate are so entwined that if instant thoughts could kill, we would all be dead in the bosom of our families. In the case of a woman's involuntary pregnancy, a complex, long-term solution requiring effort and energy has to compete with the immediate solution offered by a morning's visit to an abortion clinic. On the simple, perceptual plane, with imagination and thinking curtailed, the speed, ease, and privacy of abortion, combined with the small size of the embryo, tend to make early abortions seem less morally serious—even though speed, size, technical ease, and the private nature of an act have no moral standing.

As the most recent immigrants from nonpersonhood, feminists have traditionally fought for justice for themselves and the world. Women rally to feminism as a new and better way to live. Rejecting male aggression and destruction, feminists seek alternative, peaceful, ecologically sensitive means to resolve conflicts while respecting human potentiality. It is a chilling inconsistency to see prochoice feminists demanding continued access to assembly-line, technological methods of fetal killing—the vacuum aspirator, prostaglandins, and dilation and evacuation. It is a betrayal of feminism, which has built the struggle for justice on the bedrock of women's empathy. After all, "maternal thinking" receives its name from a mother's unconditional acceptance and nurture of dependent, immature life. It is difficult to develop concern for women, children, the poor and the dispossessed—and to care about peace—and at the same time ignore fetal life.

2. From the Necessity of Autonomy and Choice in Personal Responsibility to an Expanded Sense of Responsibility

A distorted idea of morality overemphasizes individual autonomy and active choice. Morality has often been viewed too exclusively as a matter of human agency and decisive action. In moral behavior persons must explicitly choose and aggressively exert their wills to intervene in the natural and social environments. The human will dominates the body, overcomes the given, breaks out of the material limits of nature. Thus if one does not choose to be pregnant or cannot rear a child, who must be given up for adoption, then better to abort the pregnancy. Willing, planning, choosing one's moral commitments through the contracting of one's individual resources becomes the premier model of moral responsibility.

But morality also consists of the good and worthy acceptance of the unexpected events that life presents. Responsiveness and response-ability to things unchosen are also instances of the highest human moral capacity. Morality is not confined to contracted agreements of isolated individuals. Yes, one is obligated by explicit contracts freely initiated, but human beings are also obligated by implicit compacts and involuntary relationships in which persons simply find themselves. To be embedded in a family, a neighborhood, a social system, brings moral obligations which were never entered into with informed consent.

Parent-child relationships are one instance of implicit moral obligations arising by virtue of our being part of the interdependent human community. A woman, involuntarily pregnant, has a moral obligation to the now-existing dependent fetus whether she explicitly consented to its existence or not. No prolife feminist would dispute the forceful observations of prochoice feminists about the extreme difficulties that bearing an unwanted child in our society can entail. But the stronger force of the fetal claim presses a woman to accept these burdens; the fetus possesses rights arising from its extreme need and the interdependency and unity of humankind. The woman's moral obligation arises both from her status as a human being embedded in the interdependent human community and her unique lifegiving female reproductive power. To follow the prochoice feminist ideology of insistent individualistic autonomy and control is to betray a fundamental basis of the moral life.

3. From the Moral Claim of the Contingent Value of Fetal Life to the Moral Claim for the Intrinsic Value of Human Life

The feminist prochoice position which claims that the value of the fetus is contingent upon the pregnant woman's bestowal—or willed, conscious "construction"—of humanhood is seriously flawed. The inadequacies of this position flow from the erroneous premises (1) that human value and rights can be granted by individual will; (2) that the individual woman's consciousness can exist and operate in an *a priori* isolated fashion; and (3) that "mere" biological, genetic human life has little meaning. Prolife feminism takes a very different stance toward life and nature.

Human life from the beginning to the end of development *has* intrinsic value, which does not depend on meeting the selective criteria or tests set up

by powerful others. A fundamental humanist assumption is at stake here. Either we are going to value embodied human life and humanity as a good thing, or take some variant of the nihilist position that assumes human life is just one more random occurrence in the universe such that each instance of human life must explicitly be justified to prove itself worthy to continue. When faced with a new life, or an involuntary pregnancy, there is a world of difference in whether one first asks, "Why continue?" or "Why not?" Where is the burden of proof going to rest? The concept of "compulsory pregnancy" is as distorted as labeling life "compulsory aging."

In a sound moral tradition, human rights arise from human needs, and it is the very nature of a right, or valid claim upon another, that it cannot be denied, conditionally delayed, or rescinded by more powerful others at their behest. It seems fallacious to hold that in the case of the fetus it is the pregnant woman alone who gives or removes its right to life and human status solely through her subjective conscious investment or "humanization." Surely no pregnant woman (or any other individual member of the species) has created her own human nature by an individually willed act of consciousness, nor for that matter been able to guarantee her own human rights. An individual woman and the unique individual embryonic life within her can only exist because of their participation in the genetic inheritance of the human species as a whole. Biological life should never be discounted. Membership in the species, or collective human family, is the basis for human solidarity, equality, and natural human rights.

4. The Moral Right of Women to Full Social Equality from a Prolife Feminist Perspective

Prolife feminists and prochoice feminists are totally agreed on the moral right of women to the full social equality so far denied them. The disagreement between them concerns the definition of the desired goal and the best means to get there. Permissive abortion laws do not bring women reproductive freedom, social equality, sexual fulfillment, or full personal development.

Pragmatic failures of a prochoice feminist position combined with a lack of moral vision are, in fact, causing disaffection among young women. Middle-aged prochoice feminists blamed the "big chill" on the general conservative backlash. But they should look rather to their own elitist acceptance of male models of sex and to the sad picture they present of women's lives. Pitting women against their own offspring is not only morally offensive, it is psychologically and politically destructive. Women will never climb to equality and social empowerment over mounds of dead fetuses, numbering now in the millions. As long as most women choose to bear children, they stand to gain from the same constellation of attitudes and institutions that will also protect the fetus in the woman's womb—and they stand to lose from the cultural assumptions that support permissive abortion. Despite temporary conflicts of interest, feminine and fetal liberation are ultimately one and the same cause.

Women's rights and liberation are pragmatically linked to fetal rights because to obtain true equality, women need (1) more social support and changes in the structure of society, and (2) increased self-confidence, self-expectations, and self-esteem. Society in general, and men in particular, have to provide women more support in rearing the next generation, or our devastating feminization of poverty will continue. But if a woman claims the right to decide by herself whether the fetus becomes a child or not, what does this do to paternal and communal responsibility? Why should men share responsibility for child support or child rearing if they cannot share in what is asserted to be the woman's sole decision? Furthermore, if explicit intentions and consciously accepted contracts are necessary for moral obligations, why should men be held responsible for what *they* do not voluntarily choose to happen? By prochoice reasoning, a man who does not want to have a child, or whose contraceptive fails, can be exempted from the responsibilities of fatherhood and child support. Traditionally, many men have been laggards in assuming parental responsibility and support for their children; ironically, ready abortion, often advocated as a response to male dereliction, legitimizes male irresponsibility and paves the way for even more male detachment and lack of commitment.

For that matter, why should the state provide a system of day care or child support, or require workplaces to accommodate women's maternity and the needs of child rearing? Permissive abortion, granted in the name of women's privacy and reproductive freedom, ratifies the view that pregnancies and children are a woman's private individual responsibility. More and more frequently, we hear some version of this old rationalization: if she refuses to get rid of it, it's her problem. A child becomes a product of the individual woman's freely chosen investment, a form of private property resulting from her own cost-benefit calculation. The larger community is relieved of moral responsibility.

With legal abortion freely available, a clear cultural message is given: conception and pregnancy are no longer serious moral matters. With abortion as an acceptable alternative, contraception is not as responsibly used; women take risks, often at the urging of male sexual partners. Repeat abortions increase, with all their psychological and medical repercussions. With more abortion there is more abortion. Behavior shapes thought as well as the other way round. One tends to justify morally what one has done; what becomes commonplace and institutionalized seems harmless. Habituation is a powerful psychological force. Psychologically it is also true that whatever is avoided becomes more threatening; in phobias it is the retreat from anxiety-producing events which reinforces future avoidance. Women begin to see themselves as too weak to cope with involuntary pregnancies. Finally, through the potency of social pressure and the force of inertia, it becomes more and more difficult, in fact almost unthinkable, *not* to use abortion to solve problem pregnancies. Abortion becomes no longer a choice but a "necessity." ...

New feminist efforts to rethink the meaning of sexuality, femininity, and reproduction are all the more vital as new techniques for artificial reproduction, surrogate motherhood, and the like present a whole new set of dilemmas. In the long run, the very long run, the abortion debate may be merely the opening round in a series of far-reaching struggles over the role of human sexuality and the ethics of reproduction. Significant changes in the culture, both positive and negative in outcome, may begin as local storms of controversy. We may be at one of those vaguely realized thresholds when we had best come to full attention. What kind of people are we going to be? Prolife feminists pursue a vision for their sisters, daughters, and granddaughters. Will their great-granddaughters be grateful?

POSTSCRIPT

Is There a Moral Right to Abortion?

Although the Supreme Court consistently upheld the legality of abortion in a series of cases in the early and mid-1980s, that trend was reversed in the last several years. The 1989 decision in *Webster v. Reproductive Health Services* upheld the constitutionality of Missouri's restrictive abortion statutes, thus giving more power to state legislatures and courts in regulating abortion. In 1991, in *Rust v. Sullivan*, the Court affirmed a Department of Health and Human Services regulation prohibiting federally funded family planning clinics from counseling or referring women for abortions. In March 1992 the Bush administration changed the regulation to allow physicians, but not nurses or counselors, to discuss abortion under some circumstances. And three days after he became president in 1992, Bill Clinton reversed restrictive federal policies on abortion—the ban on abortion counseling at federally financed clinics was lifted, as was a prohibition on aid to international family planning programs that are involved in abortion-related activities.

Planned Parenthood of Southeastern Pennsylvania v. Casey, the most significant of the more recent Supreme Court cases on abortion, was decided in June 1992. The ruling reaffirmed the constitutionality of *Roe v. Wade*, but it also declared that a woman's legal right to an abortion was not unduly restricted by the provisions of Pennsylvania's law. The law requires physicians to provide information about the nature, risks, and alternatives to abortion, as well as the gestational age of the fetus. It also imposes a 24-hour waiting period after the information is given before the abortion is performed. Finally, it requires the consent of a parent or a court when women under age 18 seek abortion. For two articles critical of the *Casey* decision, see R. Alta Charo, "Life after *Casey*: The View from Rehnquist's Potemkin Village," *The Journal of Law, Medicine and Ethics* (Spring 1993) and Janet Benshoof, "Planned Parenthood v. Casey: The Impact of the New Undue Burden Standard on Reproductive Health Care," *Journal of the American Medical Association* (May 5, 1993).

In May 1994 President Clinton signed the Freedom of Access to Clinic Entrances Act, which makes it a crime to obstruct or threaten anyone who is seeking or performing an abortion. The penalty for violating the law may be a fine or imprisonment. For a history of the political and ethical issues surrounding abortion in the United States, see Eva R. Rubin's *The Abortion Controversy: A Documentary History* (Greenwood, 1994). Abortion technology may change if mifepristone, also known as RU-486, becomes widely used. This drug provides a nonsurgical technique for terminating early pregnancies. Long used in Europe, it was approved for use in the United States by the Food and Drug Administration in 1996.

PART 4

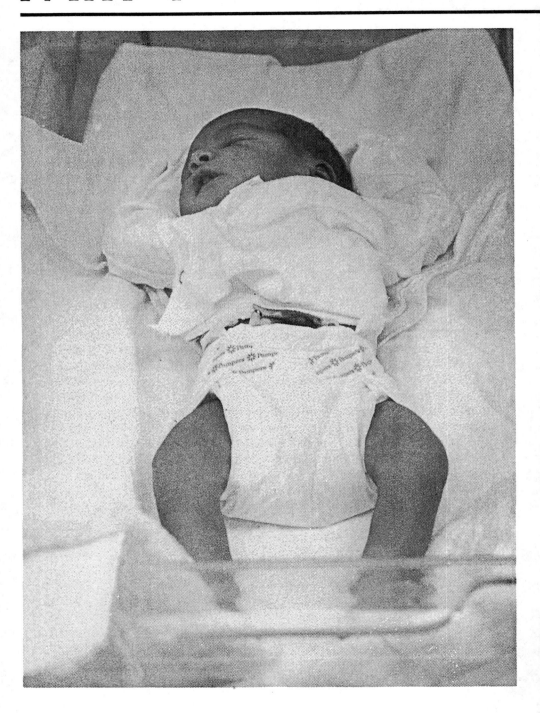

Children and Bioethics

Children are often the subjects of controversies in biomedical ethics. Too young to make fully autonomous decisions, vulnerable to the pressures and interests of adults (including parents and health care providers), children are nonetheless persons in their own right with clear interests and a need for guidance and protection. Unless proven otherwise, parents are presumed to be the primary decision makers for their children. The common belief is that parents know and love their children, have a family history of values and choices, and can make informed choices about the best interests of their children. Yet this ideal does not always hold true, and in many cases what parents find acceptable, physicians or public health officials see as medical negligence. In other cases parents whose own child is born dying want to donate that child's organs to another child; this requires an exception from adult standards. This section presents some of the most vexing dilemmas in medical ethics.

- Should Newborns Be Screened for
  HIV Infection?

- Should Newborns Without Brains Be
  Used as Organ Donors?

- Do Parents Harm Their Children
  When They Refuse Medical Treatment
  on Religious Grounds?

ISSUE 10

Should Newborns Be Screened for HIV Infection?

YES: Mark S. Rapoport, from "Mandatory Newborn Screening for HIV: Long Overdue, but Not Nearly Enough," *The AIDS Reader* (September/October 1994)

NO: Alan R. Fleischman, from "Mandatory Newborn Screening for HIV: The Wrong Answer to the Wrong Question," *The AIDS Reader* (September/October 1994)

ISSUE SUMMARY

YES: Pediatrician and county health commissioner Mark S. Rapoport argues that the knowledge that a baby may be HIV-infected benefits the baby's health and that parents should have this information—even if they do not want it.

NO: Pediatrician Alan R. Fleischman argues against mandatory testing because universal counseling for women and voluntary testing will best develop the trusting relationship that is essential for providing services to both mother and child.

The first cases of what is now called AIDS (acquired immunodeficiency syndrome) were seen in 1981 and, in retrospect, probably as early as the mid-1970s. The retrovirus that most scientists believe causes the disease—human immunodeficiency virus, or HIV—was discovered in 1984, and a laboratory test that recognizes antibodies to HIV was approved for marketing in 1985. Clinical and ethical justifications for the use of the HIV antibody test have been controversial ever since. Except for some settings (admission to the military, job corps, immigration, and some prisons), HIV testing is voluntary. There is an uneasy compromise between those who would institute compulsory, widespread testing without consent and those who would restrict the use of the test to clinical and research settings under strict consent procedures.

In 1987 the Centers for Disease Control and Prevention (CDC)—the federal agency that monitors disease—established a "family of serosurveys" in selected hospitals, drug treatment centers, and sexually transmitted disease clinics. In these settings, discarded blood was tested without any links to the patient. This method was designed to give an unbiased picture of HIV infection. Because no one in the surveys could be identified, no consent was necessary, and no one could opt out of participating.

Newborn nurseries were among the settings chosen by the CDC. Positive results on newborns give a reasonably accurate picture of the incidence of infection in women giving birth in a certain geographic area. Positive tests for the babies themselves are only suggestive of HIV infection because at least three-quarters of the newborns who test positive are not actually HIV-infected and lose their maternal antibodies in the first 15 months of life. A newborn's positive test result, however, almost certainly indicates HIV infection in the mother.

Pediatricians treating babies with HIV infection began to challenge this study design. As they gained more experience with HIV infection, they found that the leading cause of death in the first year of life was Pneumocystis carinii pneumonia (PCP). Prophylaxis (or preventive medicine) was proving successful in adults in forestalling PCP. Other medical benefits are also possible, although nothing so far can cure the disease or guarantee long-term survival. Pediatricians frustrated by their inability to identify potentially HIV-infected babies called for "unblinding" the serosurveys, that is, linking the positive test results to individual mothers so that they could be informed about their babies' HIV status (and by implication, their own infection).

The controversy erupted in New York State in 1993–1994 when a member of the legislature proposed that the serosurveys be unblinded and mothers be told of their infants' HIV status, even though they had not consented to the test for themselves. While the debate was raging, another study—known by its AIDS Clinical Trial Group number 076—was released. This showed that pregnant women treated with the antiviral drug zidovudine (AZT) during the last stages of pregnancy and during delivery had a much lower rate of HIV transmission to their newborns (8.3 percent compared to 25 percent in the untreated group). The newborns were also treated with AZT in the first weeks of life. This further complicated the focus and shifted the issue to screening pregnant women as well as newborns.

The following selections summarize the debate. Mark S. Rapoport declares that the benefits of mandatory testing to the baby's health are compelling and that voluntary HIV testing programs do not achieve high enough rates of participation. Mothers, he believes, will see in retrospect (if not at the time) that testing was the right thing to do. Alan R. Fleischman argues that it is critical that the testing of women be done with their permission and full understanding of the benefits and risks. Treatment for themselves and their babies requires trust and full cooperation, which are unlikely to be achieved with mandatory testing.

YES

Mark S. Rapoport

MANDATORY NEWBORN SCREENING FOR HIV: LONG OVERDUE, BUT NOT NEARLY ENOUGH

The very fact that New York State and New York City have been actively grappling for more than a year with the question of mandatory HIV antibody screening of all newborns tells a great deal. Multiple benefits accrue from knowing that a baby is HIV-seropositive (with actual infection easily verifiable). These include better diagnosis of febrile and pulmonary illness; antibiotic prophylaxis for pneumocystis infection and modified immunization for the baby; counseling on the risks of breast feeding and a host of other medical interventions for the mother; potential location of other cases, especially the child's father; education for prevention of additional transmission by any and all recognized routes; and a broad range of social services (especially those available via the Ryan White Care Act) for the family. None of these benefits are disputed.

For most people, in New York State and elsewhere, the case for screening is straightforward and compelling. It serves the HIV-seropositive baby's health for the data to be known, and parents should want to do well by their children. Parents should have this information, even if they do not want it. The headline on the cover of the February 21, 1994, issue of *New York* magazine may have captured that feeling. It said, "Should It Be a Crime to Treat This Baby for AIDS? The Rising Storm Over the Law That Keeps HIV-Positive Newborns from Early Treatment."

The view of the majority of people most deeply involved in AIDS policy and AIDS care, however, is very different. While they agree that real benefits accrue to both baby and mother and from knowing a baby's serostatus, other considerations take precedence. First, "coercion" is the key issue, with analogy sometimes made to testing Federal prisoners. Second, decade-old fears arise of losing insurance, spouses, and jobs (although the testing would be strictly confidential). Third, there is the unsubstantiated fear that state-mandated testing would forever estrange HIV-seropositive women from their doctors and "the system," and "drive them underground."

I find none of these arguments convincing. The evidence for these fears being realized is very weak. Furthermore,
all the perceived difficulties can be mini-
mized by good counseling, good follow-
up, and strong safeguards on confidentiality. All of these things are possible and
are already being done to a substantial
degree. The record of the public health
enterprise in maintaining confidentiality
is especially good.

A strong sense of the history of discrimination (against women, people of
color, and gay men) underlies many of
these fears. These sensibilities may be acknowledged, but should not be considered an eternal bar to progress in the ways
we combat the plague of AIDS. AIDS is
in many ways different from tuberculosis, hepatitis, and syphilis, but it is also
similar in many ways. All have some
stigma associated with them, nonetheless
we have mounted credible efforts against
them. In the course of these efforts, we
often encounter suspicion, distrust, and
fears, but usually we can overcome them.
This has direct relevance to the arguments relating to undermining the trust
of women who are indirectly tested by a
newborn screening program. I think we
give these women too little credit if we
assume that they will be unable to see
the benefits of screening (in retrospect,
if not prospectively) and that this failure
on their part will translate to a distrust
of and unwillingness to cooperate with
their doctors, nurses, and social workers.
The law would emanate from the state
government, not the professional at the
bedside, and this distinction is not difficult to discern. Mandating testing programs for hepatitis B and syphilis has
not had the feared effects and I do not
believe that an HIV newborn-screening
program would either. From our efforts

with these diseases, we should learn to
improve our strategies and to bring AIDS
care and AIDS policies closer to the norm
for public health problems. Mandatory
newborn screening is one such step and
is long overdue.

Having said that, we must address
the ACTG 076 study showing the clear
benefit of giving zidovudine prenatally
and intrapartum to pregnant women, and
then to the newborn. The beneficial results are truly exciting. Taken together,
the 3 interventions cut the rate of vertical
transmission by about two-thirds, from
26% to 8%. If all HIV-infected women received the entire "package," perhaps 400
lives would be saved annually in New
York State alone. There is a consensus that
our emphasis now must be to identify
and treat infection in pregnant women at
the earliest possible time. Further, there
is widespread agreement that a voluntary program would be the best first effort. I concur with this, since in the prenatal context, we confront the likelihood
that substantial numbers of women (especially those with the most risk-laden
medical history and social circumstances)
might be deterred from seeking early prenatal care, or might be more likely to drop
out of care. However, I believe that such
a program would have to be well designed and continually evaluated, with
a mandatory prenatal testing program as
a true alternative if a voluntary program
did not achieve and maintain high rates
of participation.

Although a prenatal effort at testing
and treatment must be the first priority, the issue of testing newborns is by
no means moot. Some women will not
seek prenatal care, and women at highest risk for HIV infection are likely to
be over-represented in that group. Also,
some women will refuse prenatal testing.

What should our response be to the needs of these women and their newborns? I believe that although the absolute number of infected babies will be lower (hopefully, a great deal lower) than under present circumstances, society's obligation to those babies remains unchanged. It is not difficult, I think, to make a case for considering the refusal to accept testing, and the attendant inability to act on the results of that testing, a form of the true "medical neglect."

As a society, we do not tolerate medical neglect of children's needs in regard to conditions other than AIDS, many of which are not nearly as lethal. We certainly need to develop a voluntary prenatal HIV program, incorporating mandatory counseling and minimizing barriers to participation; a mandatory testing program for the already-born child would not be at odds with such a program. In fact, it would reinforce it, just as it would reinforce our commitment to valuing the life of every child, and preserving and caring for those lives in the best way we know how.

NO

Alan R. Fleischman

MANDATORY NEWBORN SCREENING FOR HIV: THE WRONG ANSWER TO THE WRONG QUESTION

Pediatricians responsible for the care of children infected with the human immunodeficiency virus (HIV) increasingly voice concern that the earliest indication of HIV disease in a child is a fatal infection during the first months of life. Some of these health professionals believe that early identification of children at risk for HIV infection and the initiation of prophylactic therapies will greatly enhance the quality and quantity of children's lives. This has resulted in the recommendation that the standard newborn screening test done on all babies right after birth, which currently identifies several genetic and metabolic disorders, be utilized to find children who are infected with HIV. At first glance this recommendation seems both well-meaning and reasonable, in that the goal of protecting children from unnecessary illness is certainly laudable. However, there are many questions to be raised about the basic assumptions upon which this recommendation is made, as well as serious concerns about the consequences of universal, nonconsensual screening of newborns for HIV.

Ironically, this debate is occurring at a time when exciting new data are emerging about the prevention of transmission of HIV from pregnant women to their fetuses through the administration of zidovudine (ZDV) to the woman during pregnancy and intrapartum, and to the newborn for 6 weeks after birth. The possibility of pharmacologic primary prevention of HIV transmission during pregnancy creates a far more important question: How can we educate the entire population about the importance of knowing their HIV status in order to reduce HIV transmission from one person to another? With particular emphasis on women, how can we create a general standard of medical practice so that every woman who is of reproductive age or is at her first prenatal visit is counseled concerning the benefits of knowing her HIV status and offered appropriate comprehensive services for herself and her family?

A program of counseling and voluntary testing before or early in pregnancy can result in the identification of women who would be offered the option of antiretroviral treatment in an attempt to block HIV transmission to the fetus. Even though all of the questions concerning the use of ZDV in pregnancy have not been answered, the compelling nature of the data demands that we make this option available to women who want this intervention.

It is critically important that the testing of women be done with their permission and full understanding of the benefits and risks of the test. The health care establishment must foster an atmosphere of trust between patients and their providers that can be translated into the delivery of comprehensive services over a long period of time. The treatment of HIV disease and the potential prevention of transmission requires the full cooperation of a knowledgeable and committed patient. Mandatory programs based on coercion will only lead to greater distrust and result in patients who are appropriately reluctant to favorably consider therapeutic options presented by well-meaning health care professionals.

Knowing and accepting all of this, some legislators and health care leaders continue to press for mandatory screening of newborns for HIV. They argue that there is a need for a "safety net" to identify newborns whose mothers have not received prenatal care or who have refused to be tested. Of course, they realize that only a small proportion of the babies who test positive for antibody at birth actually will be infected (15% to 30%) while 100% of these infants' mothers will be infected. They also must be aware that the goal of a screening program is not merely the identification and labeling of a potential patient, but also the provision of needed services to that patient and family.

It is incredible to me that some physicians and politicians would consider a program that would combine voluntary testing during the prenatal period and mandatory testing after birth. Can we, as professionals, in good faith counsel women about the importance of knowing their HIV status during pregnancy and accept their voluntary decision about testing, only to test them involuntarily after birth? This seems duplicitous and inappropriate. Of course, all women who have not been tested previously should be counseled at the time of birth about the importance of testing, and we should encourage as many mothers as possible to know their and their newborns' HIV status.

We have the potential to ask the right question and create the right answer. The right question is: How can we offer appropriate counseling to all women and engage them voluntarily to learn their HIV status? If they are HIV-positive, how do we ensure that they receive needed care for themselves and potential interventions to prevent transmission to their fetus and, finally, that they provide care for their infants? This can only be accomplished through a new standard of medical practice that counsels women on the importance and appropriateness of knowing their HIV status before, during, and after pregnancy. Pregnant women should be counseled about the benefits and potential risks of HIV testing while receiving prenatal care and at the time of delivery. Testing should be linked to services and a positive test should result in referral to a program that provides comprehensive care for families.

Perhaps most critically important in the analysis of this complex problem is the issue of trust and respect among health care professionals, their patients, and the public at large. We need not create an atmosphere of fear and coercion when we have the opportunity to develop a program of screening and care that is both voluntary and comprehensive and will likely benefit the vast majority of those in need. We have available today a potential method to identify virtually all of the infants who are at risk for HIV infection through mandatory counseling and encouraged testing of women. With appropriate resources given to education and health care delivery, the desired goal of early identification and treatment of HIV-infected infants can be accomplished without mandatory newborn screening. The right question is how to develop a trusting relationship in order to provide services to those in need. The right answer is universal counseling and voluntary testing.

POSTSCRIPT

Should Newborns Be Screened for HIV Infection?

In July 1995 the Centers for Disease Control and Prevention (CDC) issued guidelines that reaffirmed its support for voluntary, not mandatory, HIV counseling and testing of pregnant women. In the event that the mother's HIV status is unknown, the CDC rejected mandatory newborn testing, asserting that "testing is not the intervention." Instead, it recommended policies that "foster trust, thereby creating the best opportunity for compliance with complex medical procedures."

Nevertheless, federal and state legislators continued to debate the issue. In May 1996 Congress passed amendments to the Ryan White Care Act—which funds much community-based care for people with AIDS—authorizing $10 million to assist states in implementing the CDC guidelines. To continue to receive Ryan White funding, states will have to prove that nearly all pregnant women agree to be counseled and tested, that new cases of transmission from mother to fetus have been reduced by 50 percent, or that the state has introduced a mandatory newborn screening program. Shortly after the amendments were passed, a mandatory newborn screening bill was passed in New York State.

In November 1996 the CDC reported that the number of perinatally acquired AIDS cases had declined 27 percent from 1992 to 1995. The decrease was attributed to increased voluntary counseling and testing and the use of zidovudine (AZT) during pregnancy to prevent HIV transmission.

For legal arguments against mandatory screening of newborns, see Jean R. Sternlight, "Mandatory Non-Anonymous Testing of Newborns for HIV: Should It Ever Be Allowed?" *The John Marshall Law Review* (Winter 1994) and Kevin J. Curnin, "Newborn HIV Screening and New York Assembly Bill No. 6747-B: Privacy and Equal Protection of Pregnant Women," *Fordham Urban Law Journal* (vol. 21, no. 3, 1994). An argument for mandatory screening of newborns is found in Margaret C. Heagarty and Elaine J. Abrams, "Caring for HIV-Infected Women and Children," *The New England Journal of Medicine* (vol. 326, 1992), pp. 887–888.

Three articles in *The New England Journal of Medicine* (November 3, 1994) discuss the impact of the results of the AIDS Clinical Trial Group number 076, which showed decreased maternal-fetal HIV transmission with AZT therapy. See "Reduction of Maternal-Infant Transmission of HIV-1 with Zidovudine Treatment," by E. M. Connor et al.; "Reducing the Risk of Maternal-Infant Transmission of HIV: A Door Is Opened," by Martha F. Rogers and Harold

W. Jaffe; and "Ethical Challenges Posed by Zidovudine Treatment to Reduce Vertical Transmission of HIV," by Ronald Bayer.

Also see Howard Minkoff and Anne Willoughby, "Pediatric HIV Disease, Zidovudine in Pregnancy, and Unblinding Heelstick Surveys," *Journal of the American Medical Association* (October 11, 1995). In it, the authors argue that, on balance, preserving consent will "best preserve the woman's role as fetal champion and the clinician's role as patient advocate." Ruth R. Fade and Nancy E. Kass are the editors of *HIV, AIDS, and Childbearing: Public Policy, Private Lives* (Oxford University Press, 1996), which offers a broad view of HIV testing in the context of other issues affecting women's lives.

ISSUE 11

Should Newborns Without Brains Be Used as Organ Donors?

YES: Michael R. Harrison, from "Organ Procurement for Children: The Anencephalic Fetus as Donor," *The Lancet* (December 13, 1986)

NO: John D. Arras and Shlomo Shinnar, from "Anencephalic Newborns as Organ Donors: A Critique," *Journal of the American Medical Association* (April 15, 1988)

ISSUE SUMMARY

YES: Pediatric surgeon Michael R. Harrison asserts that if anencephalic newborns were treated as brain-dead rather than as brain-absent, their organs could be transplanted and their families could be offered the consolation that their loss provided life for another child.

NO: Philosopher John D. Arras and pediatric neurologist Shlomo Shinnar argue that the current principles of the strict definition of brain death are sound public policy and good ethics.

There are too few organs for donation for all categories of persons in need, but one of the most poignant situations occurs in newborns and infants. Only small organs are suitable for these young patients, and appropriate organs become available only when other young patients die.

Today several thousand children could benefit from transplants. Those on dialysis regimens could be given the chance to lead more normal lives with kidney transplants. Those suffering from liver failure face certain death without transplants. Others are born with heart defects so severe that only new hearts can save their lives.

The technical problems in transplanting small organs are rapidly being overcome, but the ethical problems persist. Anencephalic babies are one potential source of organs for pediatric patients. These are babies who are born without brains or with large portions missing; they may survive for a few hours or days, or even weeks, but (except in rare cases) no longer. This condition occurs about once in every 1,000 to 2,000 births and can be detected through screening of the mother's blood and confirmed through sonograms, which reveal the baby's organs in utero. About 2,000 such babies are detected each year.

The parents of these babies are faced with a difficult choice: they can choose abortion (even in the third trimester) or they can carry the pregnancy to term, knowing that their baby is doomed to die. A few parents in this situation have asked for a third option: to donate the organs of their baby so that they can feel that some good for another family has come out of their personal tragedy.

If these babies had no brain activity at all, that is, if they were brain-dead, there would be no ethical problem. Their parents could consent for the removal of their organs, just as the next of kin of a brain-dead adult can consent to organ donation. But these babies, though lacking higher brain activity, do have some rudimentary brain-stem activity. Though doomed to die, they are not yet dead. If physicians wait until the babies are brain-dead, their organs may not be suitable for transplantation.

The ethical questions thus center around the justifiability of treating anencephalic newborns as if they were brain-dead in order to achieve the goal of salvaging their organs. Is the distinction between brain-absent and brain-dead a legal technicality, or does it go to the essence of human existence?

In the selections that follow, Michael R. Harrison declares that the ability to transplant fetal organs may now give us the chance to recognize the contribution of the doomed anencephalic fetus to mankind. He favors treating anencephalics as legally brain-dead. John D. Arras and Shlomo Shinnar argue that the attempt to reconcile the use of anencephalic newborns as organ donors with the current principles of brain death violates principles of ethics and public policy. They argue that the strict criteria for whole-brain death must be satisfied and that vital organs may not be taken from the living to benefit others.

YES

Michael R. Harrison

ORGAN PROCUREMENT FOR CHILDREN: THE ANENCEPHALIC FETUS AS DONOR

Organ transplants could give an increasing number of children with fatal childhood diseases the chance of a full life.[1,2] However, most children die waiting for an appropriate donor organ.

THE DYING CHILD: PROMISE AT A PRICE

The need for small organs is acute and the demand is likely to grow. In the United States 300–450 children with end-stage renal disease could be taken off dialysis regimens if they received renal transplants.[3,4] The only hope for the 400–800 children with liver failure (biliary atresia, cholestatic syndromes, and inherited metabolic defects) is liver transplantation;[5,6] for the 400–600 children with certain forms of congenital heart disease such as hypoplastic left heart syndrome it may be cardiac transplantation;[7,8] and for an increasing number with childhood haemopoietic and malignant diseases, it is bone-marrow transplantation.[9,10] Finally, enzymatic, immunological, and endocrine deficiencies may be corrected by the use of cellular (rather than whole-organ) grafts.[11,14]

For many childhood diseases, biological tissue replacement may be the only satisfactory solution because the transplant must be able to grow and adapt to increasing functional demand over the potentially long life span of the recipient. But the logistics of organ transplantation are very demanding for the young recipient, in whom rapid organ failure and lack of interim support measures make the "time window" for transplantation narrow.

The present system of obtaining vital organs from "brain-dead" accident victims cannot meet the demand for small organs. It is also logistically complex and very expensive. The cost of a new heart or liver often exceeds $100,000. Unless donor material becomes simpler and less costly to procure and transplant, these life-saving procedures will have to be rationed.

AVAILABILITY OF ANENCEPHALIC ORGANS AND TISSUES

Fetuses with defects so hopeless that they meet the requirements for pregnancy termination at any gestational age may be ideal donors. With anencephaly termination is justifiable even in the third trimester,[15] and vital organs other than the brain are usually normal. It occurs once in every 1000–2000 births,[16] is easily detected by screening for raised alphafetoprotein levels in maternal serum and amniotic fluid, and can be confirmed by sonography. When screening programmes capable of detecting 90% of all anencephalic fetuses are instituted, we can expect to detect around 2000 anencephalic fetuses in the United States each year. Even if only a small proportion proves suitable as source of donor material, it could go a long way towards satisfying estimated needs.

CAN IMMATURE ORGANS WORK?

It is unlikely that a functionally immature fetal organ can immediately replace and sustain vital organ function in a child; continued partial function of the native organ or availability of interim external support for organ function will be crucial. With support by dialysis, kidneys transplanted from newborn babies with anencephaly can show remarkable growth in size and function.[17] Technical difficulties with small-vessel anastomoses are now surmountable. Since there is no method of providing good interim support for failing liver and cardiac function, total orthotopic replacement with fetal heart or liver would be limited to neonatal recipients and nearterm donors. The fetal organ would have to be large enough to fit the recipient and functionally mature enough to immediately replace life-sustaining function. But traditional whole-organ orthotopic replacement may not be necessary or even desirable. Auxiliary transplantation of immature organs that can develop until they take over the life-sustaining function of the failing native organ may prove safer, simpler, and less expensive.

Fetal liver has tremendous potential for growth and functional adaptation. We have shown experimentally that auxiliary heterotopic liver transplantation is technically feasible and physiologically sound.[18, 19] A small liver allows auxiliary placement without the elaborate manoeuvres required for enlarging a child's abdomen or reducing donor liver size.[20] And the obvious disadvantage of small vessels may be offset by circulatory peculiarities of fetal liver—eg, portal inflow can be provided via the large umbilical vein, which carries all the fetal cardiac output, rather than via the small and delicate portal vein, which carries only 20% of liver blood flow in utero.[21] Also, the ductus venosus is patent for a short time after birth and this may help to adjust the haemodynamic pressure gradient across the grafted fetal liver.[18]

Orthotopic replacement of the fetal heart, like that of the liver, is limited to late-gestation donors and neonatal recipients. But use of the small immature fetal heart as a heterotopic assist device is a promising prospect. We have developed a simple way of inserting a fetal heart in neonatal animals as a right ventricular assist (vena cava to pulmonary artery) to bypass congenital right ventricular outflow obstruction, and as a left ventricular assist (left atrium to aorta) to correct hypoplastic left heart syndrome (unpublished). Thus auxiliary heterotopic placement, which has been effective in adults,[22] may be simpler and safer than orthotopic replacement for treating both right and left hypoplastic heart syndromes in children.

FETAL TISSUES AND "SELECTIVE" TRANSPLANTATION

Perhaps the most promising use of fetal tissue is for selective cellular grafts, which do not require surgical revascularisation.[2] Suspensions of fetal thymus have been used to correct immunodeficiencies,[23] and bone-marrow grafting can restore immunocompetence and haemopoietic function.[9, 10] However, the rejection and graft-versus-host disease seen with grafts from mature donors are less likely with immature haemopoietic stem cells harvested from fetal marrow or liver. Since many inherited defects (eg, thalassaemia) that may be correctable by cellular grafts can be diagnosed in the first half of gestation, it may be advantageous to reconstitute a deficient cell-line by in-utero transfusion.[11] We have shown experimentally that haemopoietic stem cells given by intraperitoneal injection in the first trimester can produce lasting haemopoietic chimerism.[24]

The difficulty of separating islets from exocrine pancreatic tissue and the rejection encountered with islet-cell transplantation, which can lead to cure of experimentally induced diabetes mellitus, may be ameliorated by the use of fetal pancreas.[13, 25] Transplantation of immature pituitary tissue[21] is also promising. Furthermore, there is the possibility that a functioning organ can be "grown" in a recipient by implanting a very primitive fetal organ as a non-vascularised free graft; fetal intestine, for example, may one day be used to treat infants with the short bowel syndrome.[26] Corneal grafts may restore sight, and fetal ventricular outflow tract has been used as a homograft valved conduit.[27]

ADVANTAGES OF USING FETAL ORGANS AND TISSUES

If fetal organs prove suitable, transplantation for children may be greatly simplified biologically, technically, and logistically. But the most important potential advantage is that use of fetal organs may need less immunosuppression than will use of mature organs. Fetal organs are not less "antigeneic" and thus less subject to rejection than mature organs because histocompatibility antigens are expressed early in fetal life. However, fetal grafts in general survive longer than do more mature grafts,[28, 29] and the use of fetal donors allows the immunological manipulations that improve graft survival. The fetus can be tissue-typed by examining amniotic fluid or fetal blood,[30] so the best possible recipient can be chosen by cross-matching. In addition, recipients can be pre-treated with donor cells (amniotic fluid or blood) by the same strategy that has led to improved graft survival in clinical renal transplantation.[31]

In the future, perhaps the unique immunological relation between mother and fetus can be exploited to facilitate graft acceptance. When the need for transplantation can be predicted before birth (eg, hypoplastic left heart, thalassaemia) it may be possible to induce specific unresponsiveness in the potential recipient antenatally, for transplantation either before or after birth. Although transplantation immunity develops early in all mammals, in early gestation the fetus is uniquely susceptible to induction of tolerance by donor cell suspensions.[32]

Also, graft rejection and graft-versus-host disease may be less likely if grafting is done before the recipient becomes immunocompetent and/or the donor organ becomes populated by "passenger" leucocytes.

RISKS AND BENEFITS OF ALLOWING FETAL ORGAN DONATION

The diagnosis of fetal anencephaly is always devastating. Once the family has worked through their grief and decided how the pregnancy will be managed, the possibility of organ donation may be brought up. In my experience families are surprisingly positive about donation; they clutch at any possibility that something good might be salvaged from a seemingly wasted pregnancy. Sometimes families even bring up the subject themselves, or they become upset when organs cannot be donated because of a legal ambiguity (see below).

Would allowing organ procurement from an anencephalic fetus increase maternal risk? To be successfully transplanted, the organs must be oxygenated and perfused until harvest. If labour were induced by the usual techniques (for example, by cervical dilatation and ripening, pitocin) rather than by the more violent techniques often used in late abortions (for instance, prostaglandin injection), most anencephalic fetuses can be delivered vaginally without increased risk to mother.[33] Caesarean delivery would ordinarily not be considered except for maternal indications, even when labour is difficult to induce, or when the anencephalic fetus seems to be in distress.

ETHICAL AND LEGAL ISSUES

If further research and clinical experience shows that use of fetal organs is a biologically sound and cost-effective treatment for otherwise hopeless childhood diseases, society will have to decide what attitude to adopt towards the anencephalic fetus.

One attitude is that the anencephalic baby is a product of human conception incapable of achieving "personhood" because it lacks the physical structure (forebrain) necessary for characteristic human activity; and thus can never become a human "person". The idea that a product of human conception is biologically incapable of achieving "humanness" seems radical until we consider the many products of conception lost by early miscarriage or stillbirth because of gross abnormalities. Although this approach makes organ procurement simple by denying the anencephalic baby the legal rights of personhood, there are compelling reasons for avoiding this stance. First, it is difficult to reach a consensus about personhood and what constitutes humanness. Secondly, denying personhood denigrates the pregnancy itself and may lead to a less respectful approach to the grieving family and to medical care of the fetus and newborn. Finally, there is the possibility of abuse; other fetuses or newborn babies, possibly with less severe handicaps, might be denied personhood.

Another attitude is that the anencephalic fetus is a dying person and that death is inevitable at or shortly after birth because of brain absence. The first point in favour of this attitude is that brain absence can be clearly defined and limited only to anencephalics, so individuals with less severe anomalies or injuries cannot be classed with anencephalic babies as exceptions for brain-death guidelines. Another point in favour of this attitude is that the anencephalic fetus is considered a person, albeit one doomed to death at birth. To consider the anencephalic baby as a person who is brain absent is to recognise his devastating anatomical and functional deficiency without demeaning his existence. He has rights and deserves respect, so removal of organs must not cause suffering, detract from the dignity of dying, or abridge the right to die. This is best done in the operating theatre as is currently being done for brain-dead subjects. This approach also provides a sound ethical rationale for the present practice of allowing the family to choose termination of an anencephalic pregnancy at any gestational age, and would eliminate potential incongruities, such as insisting on care of aborted anencephalic subjects.

Current laws seem to forbid removal of organs from an anencephalic subject until vital functions cease, by which time the organs and tissues are irreparably damaged. This is because anencephalic babies are not brain dead by the widely accepted whole-brain definition of death which requires "irreversible cessation of all functions of the entire brain, including the brain stem";[34] anencephalics may have lower-brain-stem activity capable of maintaining vital functions, although precariously, for hours after birth.

The whole-brain definition of death was drafted to protect the comatose patient whose injured brain might recover function. However, failure of the brain to develop is clearly different from injury to a functioning brain, and it was simply not considered when the brain-death definition was formulated. The extreme caution and safeguards needed in pronouncing brain death after brain injury should not apply to anencephaly, in which the physical structure necessary for recovery is absent. If failure of brain development, or brain absence, is recognised as the only exception to present brain-death statutes, society and the courts can then concentrate on the legal implications of regarding the anencephalic subject as being brain absent. I believe that brain absence will come to have the same medicolegal implications as brain death, but this will have to be recognised by society and confirmed by the courts.

If the anencephalic fetus is considered to be equivalent to brain-dead subjects for legal purposes, the family should be able to allow organ donation after delivery and to arrange the timing and place of delivery to facilitate transplantation.[35] Obstetrical decisions about how and when to end the pregnancy must be independent of plans to use the organs for transplantation. Members of the transplant team should not be involved in counselling or perinatal management, and the diagnosis of anencephaly should be confirmed by a panel independent of the transplant team and include a neurologist, a bioethicist, and a neonatologist. The family should also be able to decide before delivery whether they wish to see and hold the newborn.

Because many fetal disorders can now be diagnosed and even treated antenatally, we are learning to accept the fetus as an unborn patient.[30] We are also identifying fetuses so fatally damaged that survival outside the womb is impossible. The ability to transplant fetal organs may now give us the chance to recognise the contribution of this doomed fetus to mankind. If organs from prenatally diagnosed anencephalic fetuses can be obtained with safety for mother and respect for the fetus, the family should be allowed to salvage from their tragedy the consolation that their loss can provide life to another child.

I thank Dr John C. Fletcher, Dr Albert Jonsen, Professor John A. Robertson, Dr Mitchell Golbus, and colleagues at the Fetal Treatment Program, UCSF, for suggestions and review.

REFERENCES

1. Lum CT, Wassner SJ, Martin DE. Current thinking in transplantation in infants and children. *Ped Clins North Am* 1985; 32: 1203–32.
2. Russell PS. Selective transplantation: An emerging concept. *Ann Surg* 1985; 201: 255–62.
3. So SKS, Nevine TE, Chang PN, et al. Preliminary results of renal transplantation. *Transpl Proc* 1985; 17: 182–83.
4. Eggers PW, Connerton R, McMullan M. The medicare experience with end-stage renal disease: Trends in incidence, prevalence, and survival. *Hlth Care Financing Rev* 1984; 5: 69–88.
5. Lloyd-Still JD. Mortality from liver disease in children: Implications for hepatic transplantation program. *Am J Dise Child* 1985; 139: 381–84.
6. Gartner JC, Zatelli, BJ, Starzl TE. Orthotopic liver transplantation. Two year experience with 47 patients. *Pediatrics* 1984; 74: 140–45.
7. Baily LL, Jang J, Johnson W, Jolley WB. Orthotopic cardiac xenografting in the newborn goat. *J Thorac Cardiovasc Surg* 1985; 89: 242–47.
8. Penkoske PA, Freidman RM, Rowe RD, Trusler GA. The future of heart and heart-lung transplantation in children. *Heart Transplant* 1984; 3: 233–38.
9. Thomas ED. Marrow transplantation for nonmalignant disorders. *N Engl J Med* 1985; 312: 46–47.
10. Barranger JA. Marrow transplantation in genetic disease. *N Engl J Med* 1984; 311: 1629–30.
11. Simpson TJ, Golbus MS. In utero fetal hematopoietic stem cell transplantation. *Sem Perinatol* 1985; 9: 68–74.
12. Prummer O, Raghavachar A, Werner C, et al. Fetal liver transplantation in the dog. *Transplantation* 1985; 39: 349–55.
13. Brown J, Danilovs JA, Clark WR, Mullen YS. Fetal pancreas as a donor organ. *World J Surg* 1984; 8: 152–57.
14. Tulipan NB, Zacar HA, Allen GS. Pituitary transplantation: Part I. Successful reconstitution of pituitary dependent hormone levels. *Neurosurgery* 1985; 16: 331–35.
15. Chervenak FA, Farley MA, Walters LR, et al. When is termination of pregnancy during the third trimester morally justifiable? *N Engl J Med* 1983; 310: 501–04.
16. Elwood JM, Elwood JH. Epidemiology of anencephalus and spina bifida. New York: Oxford University Press, 1980: 253–99.
17. Kinnaert P, Persign G, Cohen B, et al. Transplantation of kidneys from anenephalic donors, *Transplant Proc* 1984; 16: 71–72.
18. Flake AW, Laberge JM, Adzick NS, et al. Auxiliary transplantation of the fetal liver I. Development of a sheep model, *J Pediatr Surg* 1986; 21: 515–20.
19. Flake AW, Harrison MA, Sauer L, et al. Auxiliary transplantation of the fetal liver II. Functional evaluation of an intra-abdominal model. *J Pediatr Surg* (in press).
20. Bismuth H, Houssin D. Reduced-sized orthotopic liver graft in hepatic transplantation in children. *Surgery* 1984; 95: 367–70.
21. Rudolph AM. Hepatic and ductus venosus blood flow during fetal life. *Hepatology* 1983; 3: 245–58.
22. Barnard CN, Cooper DKC. Heterotopic versus orthotopic heart transplantation. *Transplant Proc* 1984; 16: 886–92.
23. Thong YH, Robertson EF, Rischbieth GH, et al. Successful restoration of immunity in the DiGeorge Syndrome with fetal thymic epithelial transplat. *Arch Dis Child* 1978; 53: 580–84.
24. Flake AW, Harrison MR, Adzick NS, Zanjani ED. Transplantation of fetal lamb hematopoietic stem cells *in utero:* The creation of hematopoietic chimeras, *Science* (in press).
25. Mandel TE. Transplantation of organ-cultured fetal pancreas: Experimental studies and potential clinical application in diabetes mellitus. *World J Surg* 1984; 8: 158–68.
26. Bass BL, Schweitzer EJ, Harmon JW, et al. Anatomic and physiologic characteristics of transplanted fetal rat intestine. *Ann Surg* 1984; 200: 734–41.
27. Fontan F, Choussat A, Deville C, et al. Aortic valve homografts in the surgical treatment of complex cardiac malformations. *J Thorac Cardiovasc Surg* 1984; 87: 649–57.
28. Miller I. The immunity of the human foetus and newborn infant. Boston: Martinus Nijhoff, 1983.
29. Foglia RP, LaQuaglia M, DiPreta, J, et al. Can fetal and newborn allografts survive in an immunocompetent heart? *J Pediatr Surg* 1986; 21: 608–12.
30. Harrison MR, Golbus, MS, Filly RA. The unborn patient. New York: Grune & Stratton, 1984.
31. Monoco AP. Clinical kidney transplantation in 1984. *Transplant Proc* 1985; 17: 5–12.
32. Billingham RE, Brent L, Medawar PB. Actively acquired tolerance of foreign cells. *Nature* 1967; 214: 179.

33. Lawson J. Delivery of the dead or malformed fetus. Intrauterine death during pregnancy with retention of fetus. *Clins Obs Gynecol* 1982; 9: 745–56.

34. President's Commission for the Study of Ethical Problems in Medicine and Biomedical and Behavioral Research: Defining Death. US Government Printing Office, Washington DC. July 1981.

35. Harrison MR. Commentary. *Hastings Rep* 1986; 16: 21–22.

NO

**John D. Arras and
Shlomo Shinnar**

ANENCEPHALIC NEWBORNS AS ORGAN DONORS: A CRITIQUE

The debate over whether anencephalic newborns should be used as organ donors has entered a new phase with the... announcements from West Germany and California (*New York Times*, Oct 19, 1987, p A1) of kidney and heart transplants from anencephalic newborns. As we move from deliberation and debate to action, there is an urgent need to reflect on the ethical implications of this controversial procedure.

THE ISSUES

The case for taking hearts, paired kidneys, and other vital organs from anencephalic newborns is based on two distinct needs. First, there are many chronically ill infants, children, and adults who may benefit from organ transplant, and there is a relative scarcity of available donors. Second, there is the need of the parents of an anencephalic infant to salvage some good from a tragic situation. Allowing the infant to be used as an organ donor may help satisfy this need.

An important feature of anencephaly is the relative certitude of diagnosis and prognosis. Ultrasonography can now detect anencephaly in utero with relative certainty. The prognosis for these infants is death within hours, days, or weeks from birth, although there is some controversy over their exact life span. In view of the need for organs and the alleged uniqueness of anencephaly, it has been proposed that society consider such infants as persons who are born "brain absent." Anencephaly would be declared the *only* legitimate exception to our current insistence that all vital organ donors meet the criteria for whole-brain death. This would be useful in procuring neonatal organs, especially since the diagnosis of whole-brain death in the neonate is extremely difficult and fraught with uncertainty. The lack of established brain death criteria in the first week of life also poses additional problems for those who would use "brain dead" neonates as organ donors (*New York Times*, Oct 19, 1987, p A1).

From John D. Arras and Shlomo Shinnar, "Anencephalic Newborns as Organ Donors: A Critique," *Journal of the American Medical Association*, vol. 259, no. 15 (April 15, 1988), pp. 2284–2285. Copyright © 1988 by The American Medical Association. Reprinted by permission. References omitted.

Advocates of the brain absent approach specifically decline to view anencephalic newborns as "nonpersons" and insist that these infants are "persons" deserving of respect. However, they state that since they are also brain absent, they should be functionally equivalent to brain dead insofar as vital organs might be harvested from them. Another approach for justifying the use of anencephalic newborns as organ donors would be to regard them as nonpersons—ie, as biologically human entities that nevertheless lack the prerequisites of "personal" life and thus lack full moral status. This perspective provides the most direct route to salvaging their organs at the expense of redefining society's views of "personhood."

Despite the manifest importance of the "gift of life" to organ recipients and the laudable desire to help parents salvage some good from a tragedy, society must consider whether allowing anencephalic infants to be used as organ donors before they meet the traditional criteria for brain death is a morally acceptable and legitimate act. We believe it is not.

BRAIN ABSENT THEORY

Let us first address the issues posed by the brain absent theory. By insisting on the personhood of these infants, proponents of this scheme commit themselves to treat the anencephalic infant as a full member of the moral community, ie, one who has rights and is worthy of respect. The question is whether prolonging the infant's life by mechanical ventilation and then abruptly terminating it by harvesting vital organs is compatible with the minimum respect due to all persons. In Kantian philosophy, which is the source of many contemporary moral theories based on the concept of personhood, using one person merely as a means to benefit another constitutes a paradigmatic violation of moral law. As "ends in themselves," persons have an intrinsic worth that cannot be reduced to their instrumental value to others. The investigators' claims notwithstanding, it is difficult to reconcile the treatment of anencephalic newborns outlined in the... reports (*New York Times,* Oct 19, 1987, p A1) with the notion of respect for personhood.

One response to this objection is to claim that if the anencephalic infant could (miraculously) reflect on his plight, he would consent to organ donation, since losing vital organs would not deprive him of anything he would desire. Similar arguments can be made using the social contract theory of Rawls, in which the decision maker is unbiased because he does not know what role (parent, recipient, anencephalic infant, or physician) he would have in the societal drama and therefore tries to minimize the worst outcome, which may be a person in need of an organ with no available donor. However, these arguments are by no means unique to anencephalic newborns. They are equally applicable to other severely damaged infants as well as to adults in permanent vegetative states. We do not believe society is willing to harvest organs from living patients who have permanently lost the capacity for intelligent thought.

PERSONHOOD THEORY

Justifying the use of anencephalic newborns as organ donors by labeling them "nonpersons" creates the same uniqueness problem. In this philosophical theory, only beings capable of sapient life, whatever that means, have the rights and privileges of "personhood." If anencephalic newborns are nonpersons, one could perhaps justify using them as a mere means for the benefit of persons. Again, if the theory is carried out to its logical conclusion, other infants with conditions such as holoprosencephaly, hydranencephaly, and certain trisomies as well as adults in permanent vegetative states should be considered as potential organ donors.

Those who justify using anencephalic newborns as organ donors based on the fact that they will all die soon after birth must deal with two objections. First, even a dying person is still a person and is entitled to a full measure of dignity and respect as discussed above. Second, there is nothing special in this respect about anencephaly. If the crucial issue is uniform early mortality, then a number of other conditions, such as Potter's syndrome and trisomy 13, would qualify.

The availability of reliable prenatal diagnosis has led some authors to conclude that abortion of anencephalic fetuses is justified even in the third trimester. If we are willing to terminate a viable fetus just prior to term, why not terminate life just after delivery? However, the moral justification for third-trimester abortion is based on the certitude of both diagnosis and prognosis and not on any inherently unique feature of anencephaly. Many other conditions would meet the authors' criteria if reliable antenatal diagnosis were available.

BRAIN DEATH

Another fundamental objection to the proposals for amending the brain death statutes to define anencephalic infants as "dead" or "brain absent" is that this violates the spirit of our present brain death statutes regarding the definition of death. Although anencepahlic infants lack a cerebral cortex, they certainly have a brain stem that sustains and regulates a wide variety of vital bodily functions, including spontaneous respiration. Thus, it would be more accurate to describe them as "higher-brain absent" than as "brain absent." According to the present definition of brain death, ie, complete and irreversible cessation of all brain functions, including those of the brain stem, anencephalic infants are indisputably living human beings. Indeed, no one with spontaneous respirations meets the current criteria for brain death. Permitting the use of anencephalic newborns as organ donors by defining them as legally dead requires a radical reformulation of our current definition of death.

One way to accomplish this would be to reinterpret the original intent of the whole-brain definition of death. One advocate of this approach has argued that the stringent safeguards built into the current brain death statutes were put there to protect comatose patients who might eventually recover some higher cortical functions. Since anencephalic infants lack the capacity ever to achieve such a level of existence, there is no need to protect them with such rigorous definitions of brain death. Consequently, it is argued that taking organs from brain absent anencephalic newborns is ethically compatible with the spirit if not the letter of the laws governing brain death. Although the argument sounds plausible, it confuses a necessary condition for the definition of brain death with a sufficient condition. Of course, any adequate definition of brain death must preclude the possibility of meaningful recovery. However, it is one thing to note that a person is incapable of recovery of higher cortical functions and/or is imminently dying but quite another to say that he or she is dead.

Why should irreversible cessation of activity of the entire brain be necessary for a definition of death? According to the President's Commission, the brain, including the brain stem, performs an irreplaceable function in sustaining and regulating the physiological systems that keep us alive. Once it ceases to perform these vital tasks, modern technology can continue to oxygenate other organs, for a time creating a simulacrum of life, but cannot substitute for the spontaneous integrative functions that the Commission identified as the sine qua non of human life. The Commission insisted on a rigorous definition of brain death not solely to protect comatose patients, but because it believed that anything short of whole-brain death was not equivalent to the death of the human being. The Commission also specifically insisted that organ donors be *dead,* not just irrevocably brain damaged or imminently dying. This position has been cogently reiterated ... by the former executive director of the Commission. Thus, the attempt to reconcile the use of anencephalic newborns as organ donors with current principles of brain death founders on a flawed account of the rationale for accepting whole-brain death as death of the human being.

CONCLUSIONS

Current public policy and practice embody two fundamental principles: first, that vital organs may not be taken from the living for the benefit of others and, second, that for brain death to be considered the moral and legal equivalent of the death of the person, the strict criteria for whole-brain death must be satisfied. The second principle is accepted as sound public policy even by many, including one of us (J.D.A.), who do not fully agree with the President's Commission's philosophical rationale for choosing whole-brain death. The use of anencephalic newborns as organ donors is incompatible with both of these generally accepted principles. Advocates of using these infants as organ donors can invoke the more controversial "higher brain" definitions of either death or personhood to justify their proposal. However, to be consistent, infants with other severe brain malformations as well as adults in chronic vegetative states should then also be candidates for use as organ donors. We believe that the current principles of the strict definition of brain death are sound public policy and good ethics. We hope that, after careful scrutiny and debate, the use of anencephalic infants as organ donors is rejected. Admirable goals should not be advanced by improper means.

POSTSCRIPT

Should Newborns Without Brains Be Used as Organ Donors?

In the 1994 edition of its *Code of Medical Ethics*, the American Medical Association (AMA) made a limited exception to its general standard of organ transplantation because an anencephalic infant "has never experienced, and will never experience, consciousness." The AMA stated that it is ethically permissible to consider anencephalic infants as potential organ donors, "although still alive under the current definition of death," under three conditions: (1) the diagnosis of anencephaly is confirmed by two physicians who are not part of the transplant team; (2) the parents indicate in writing their desire to donate their baby's organs; and (3) there is compliance with other AMA guidelines on organ transplantation. Alternatively, the family wishing to donate may choose to support the infant with mechanical respiration until a determination of death can be made. In this case, the family must be advised that the organs might deteriorate in the process. This policy was published in the *Journal of the American Medical Association* (May 24/31, 1995). In December 1995 the AMA reversed this opinion with no comment.

Two articles in *Journal of Law, Medicine and Ethics* (vol. 23, 1995), pp. 398–402, focus on the AMA's policy: In "Ethics Consultation: Anencephaly and Organ Donation," James E. Reagan reports on a case in which although a hospital ethics committee was willing to comply with the AMA's May 1995 recommendations, they were vetoed by the hospital administration. David Orentlicher, formerly with the AMA, in "Commentary: Organ Retrieval from Anencephalic Infants: Understanding the AMA's Recommendations," responds that the AMA only gave ethical justifications; before any retrieval from a live infant was possible, state laws would have to be changed.

In March 1992 a Florida couple sought to have their newborn anencephalic daughter declared legally dead so that her organs could be transplanted to other infants. The baby was born with a partially formed brain stem but no brain cortex, the largest part of the brain. A lower court refused their request, and the Florida Supreme Court refused to hear the parents' appeal on an emergency basis. Theresa Ann Campo Pearson died 10 days after birth, with only her eyes donated for research. The family continued its legal battle before the Florida Supreme Court, which denied the appeal.

Robert M. Arnold and Stuart J. Youngner consider the question of whether or not the moral framework of organ donation is outdated because it still holds to the "dead donor rule" (persons must be dead before their organs are taken) in "The Dead Donor Rule: Should We Stretch It, Bend It, Or Abandon It?" *Kennedy Institute of Ethics Journal* (vol. 3, no. 2, 1993).

ISSUE 12

Do Parents Harm Their Children When They Refuse Medical Treatment on Religious Grounds?

YES: Ruth Macklin, from "Consent, Coercion, and Conflicts of Rights," *Perspectives in Biology and Medicine* (Spring 1977)

NO: Mark Sheldon, from "Ethical Issues in the Forced Transfusion of Jehovah's Witness Children," *The Journal of Emergency Medicine* (vol. 14, no. 2, 1996)

ISSUE SUMMARY

YES: Philosopher Ruth Macklin argues that Jehovah's Witness parents forfeit their rights to control their children when their refusal to permit blood transfusion—even when it is based on religious conviction—will result in the death of or severe harm to the children.

NO: Professor of philosophy Mark Sheldon assesses the case of Jehovah's Witness parents who refuse to allow their children to undergo blood transfusions and concludes that they cannot be said to be truly harming or neglecting their children. Rather, they are placing their children's spiritual interests above worldly ones.

On May 6, 1989, an 11-year-old Minnesota boy named Ian Lundman complained of stomach pains. Acting in accordance with her beliefs as a lifelong Christian Scientist, his mother, Katherine McKown, prayed for Ian but did not call a doctor. When the boy had not improved the following day, Ms. McKown sought the healing prayers of two Christian Science practitioners. Three days later, Ian was dead.

Christian Scientists believe that healing through prayer is scientific and effective and that if a patient dies, it is because the prayers had not been strong enough. Based on a state law that allows parents to rely on spiritual treatment for their children, Minnesota courts dismissed manslaughter charges against Ian's mother, stepfather, and the Christian Science practitioners. In 1993 Ian's father, Douglass Lundman, filed a civil suit against the four people that were involved in his son's death. A doctor testified that Ian had diabetes that could easily have been treated with insulin, while representatives of the First Church of Christ, Scientist (the official name of the church) testified that many people have been healed through prayer. The jury awarded Mr. Lundman $1.5

million in damages and assessed the Christian Science Church $9 million. An appeals court upheld the judgment against the four defendants but dismissed the punitive damages against the Church. In January 1996 the U.S. Supreme Court turned down a petition to restore the punitive damages, leaving the $1.5 million award intact.

Although few such cases reach the Supreme Court, they occur with troubling frequency and place some of the most cherished values in American society into conflict. Religious freedom and family privacy are pitted against society's obligation, through the medical profession and the courts, to protect the health and welfare of all children. In the most extreme cases, such as Ian's, honoring one value inevitably means violating the other.

Some of the debate turns on what constitutes child abuse and neglect. The legal picture is neither clear nor consistent. The federal Child Abuse Prevention and Treatment Act of 1974 defines abuse and neglect as "the physical and mental injury, negligent treatment, or maltreatment of a child under the age of 18 by a person who is responsible for the child's welfare under circumstances which indicate that the child's health and welfare is harmed or threatened thereby." However, state interpretations of the federal definition vary.

Cultural and religious differences clearly influence the interpretation of abuse and neglect statutes, especially where medical neglect is involved. Christian Scientists have been leaders in convincing many state legislatures to exclude religiously based refusals of medical treatment from child abuse and neglect statutes, and more than 40 states have passed laws recognizing spiritual treatment as an acceptable form of health care for children. In the past decade, however, some states have revoked these laws.

In general, the perspective of Jehovah's Witnesses differs from those of Christian Science and other religions that offer alternatives to modern medical care. Jehovah's Witnesses refuse only one intervention: the transfusion of whole blood and blood products. This refusal reflects a core belief in their religion. Jehovah's Witnesses take biblical bans on "eating" blood literally. Blood transfusion is held to violate this ban, and those who accept blood in this manner face loss of eternal life. Because blood transfusion is a common procedure in surgery and in the treatment of some diseases, cases involving refusal by Jehovah's Witnesses arise relatively frequently.

The following selections probe these dilemmas. In a classic article, written in 1977 but still relevant today, Ruth Macklin asserts that parents who withhold efficacious treatment harm their children and that refusal to allow blood transfusion when the result will be death or severe health consequences is a failure of parental duty. She concludes that the state is justified in such cases in taking control away from parents and allowing the administration of blood to children against the parents' wishes. Mark Sheldon asserts that the concept of harm is not appropriately applied to cases involving Jehovah's Witnesses because parents are sincerely acting in what they believe to be the child's higher interests—protecting the possibility of eternal life.

YES

Ruth Macklin

CONSENT, COERCION, AND
CONFLICTS OF RIGHTS

Cases of conflict of rights are not infrequent in law and morality. A range of cases . . . centers around the autonomy of persons and their right to make decisions in matters affecting their own life and death. This paper will focus on a particular case of conflict of rights: the case of Jehovah's Witnesses who refuse blood transfusions for religious reasons and the question of whether or not there exists a right to compel medical treatment. The Jehovah's Witnesses who refuse blood transfusions do not do so because they want to die; in most cases, however, they appear to believe that they will die if their blood is not transfused. Members of this sect are acting on what is generally believed to be a constitutionally guaranteed right: freedom of religion, which is said to include not only freedom of religious belief, but also the right to act on such beliefs.

This study will examine a cluster of moral issues surrounding the Jehovah's Witness case.... The focus will be on the case as a moral one rather than a legal one, although arguments employed in some of the legal cases will be invoked. This is an issue at the intersection of law and morality—one in which the courts themselves have rendered conflicting decisions and have looked to moral principles for guidance. As is usually the case in ethics, whatever the courts may have decided does not settle the moral dispute, but the arguments and issues invoked in legal disputes often mirror the ethical dimensions of the case. The conflict—in both law and morals—arises out of a religious prohibition against blood transfusions, a prohibition that rests on an interpretation of certain scriptural passages by the Jehovah's Witness sect....

TRANSFUSING MINOR CHILDREN OF JEHOVAH'S WITNESSES

The moral principles involved in the case of minor children of Jehovah's Witnesses differ in some important respects from principles that enter into the case of adult Witnesses who refuse transfusions for themselves.... In one case in Ohio the court argued as follows:

> It is true that parents exercise a dominion over their child so mighty and yet so minute as to be sometimes frightening. For example, they determine whether and

whom the child may marry...; whether and where he goes to school or college; which, if any, religious faith he may espouse; where he shall live; whether and where he may work, find his recreation, and so on; even whether he wears his rubbers, his pink tie, or she has her hair bobbed. Parents may, within bounds, deprive their child of his liberty and his property.

But there are well-defined limitations upon this appalling power of parent over child.... No longer can parents virtually exercise the power of life or death over their children.... Nor may they abandon him, deny him proper parental care, neglect or refuse to provide him with proper or necessary subsistence, education, medical or surgical care, or other care necessary for his health, morals, or well-being.... And while they may, under certain circumstances, deprive him of his liberty or his property, under no circumstances, with or without religious sanction, may they deprive him of his life! [1, p. 131]

In this and other legal decisions, the religious right of the parents is seen as secondary to the right to life and health on the part of the child. Indeed, in the above-quoted argument, relatively little weight is accorded the parents' claims of religious rights, and the court appears to view the issue as one that involves religious freedom only as a minor consideration. This is in sharp contrast to the situation where adult Jehovah's Witnesses are involved....

The chief moral issue appears to be as follows: Is it morally justifiable to take control of a child away from its parents and act contrary to their wishes concerning their own child? However one might attempt to answer this question when the medical treatment concerns an adult person, competent to make decisions and grant consent, the answer may differ significantly when the person requiring treatment is an infant or a child.

What considerations are relevant in making such decisions? First, there are factual considerations. The parents are denying permission to engage in procedures that are necessary to preserve the life or health of the child—in this case, the giving of blood. Without this treatment, the medical and scientific facts indicate that the child would die or fail to thrive. Next, there are ethical considerations concerning the rights of parents. There is a generally held moral assumption that parents have the right to make decisions about, and retain control over, their own minor children. But this right must be viewed as a prima facie right— one that is generally assumed to exist but may fail to exist or be overridden in some circumstances.

In spite of the fact that the parents are not engaging in some *positive* action that is harmful or detrimental to the child, it is, nevertheless, an intentional act of omission that the parents insist upon, and failure to act in the medically recognized way is, in this case, harmful and detrimental to the health and the life of the child. Other acts of omission—for example, failure to feed a normal, healthy infant—constitute legal and moral grounds for taking control of children away from the parents. The case of a child in need of transfusions appears similar in relevant respects. Having rights almost always goes hand in hand with having duties and responsibilities. So if there are parental rights with respect to children, there are also parental duties and responsibilities. It is surely the case that not all prima facie rights that people have constitute *actual* rights. This does not mean that we question the assumption that, *in general*, parents have such a right to retain control. It does mean, however, that there are cases in which, with good reason, a person's prima facie right to something can justifiably be taken away.

It might be argued that Jehovah's Witness parents, in refusing permission for blood to be given to their child, are acting in accordance with their perceived duty to God, as dictated by their religion, and that this duty to God overrides whatever secular duties they may have to preserve the life and health of their child. Here it can only be replied that when an action done in accordance with perceived duties to God results in the likelihood of harm or death to another person (whether child or adult), then the duties to preserve life here on earth take precedence. The duties of a physician are to preserve and prolong life and to alleviate suffering. These duties are not in the least mitigated by considerations of God's will, the possibility of life after death, or a view that God at some later time rewards those who suffer here on earth. Freedom of religion does not include the right to act in a manner that will result in harm or death to others.

If the parents refuse to grant permission for blood to be given to their child when failure to give blood will result in death or severe harm to the child, their prima facie right to retain control over their child no longer exists. Whatever the parents' reasons for refusing to allow blood to be given, and whether the parents believe that the child will survive or not, the case sufficiently resembles that of child neglect (in respect to harm to the child); in the absence of fulfillment of their primary duties, it is morally justifiable to take control of the child away from parents and administer blood transfusions against the parents' wishes and contrary to their religious convictions.

RIGHTS AND THE CONFLICT OF RIGHTS

It is evident that the case of the adult Jehovah's Witness who refuses blood transfusions for himself is a good deal more complicated than that of minor children of Jehovah's Witness parents. The arguments—both moral and legal—in the case of children rest largely on the moral belief that no one has the right or authority to make life-threatening decisions for persons unable to make those decisions for themselves. If this analysis is sound, it supplies a principle for dealing with the case of the adult patient who is not in a position to state his wishes at the time the treatment is medically required. This principle is avowedly paternalistic but is intended to be applied in those cases where a measure of paternalism seems morally justifiable. To the extent that a person is unable or not fully competent to decide for himself at the time transfusion is needed, it seems appropriate for medical personnel to decide in favor of life-saving treatment. Whatever a person may have claimed prior to an emergency in which death is imminent, and regardless of what relatives may claim on his behalf, it is morally wrong for others to act in a manner that will probably result in his death.

REFERENCES

1. *In re* Clark, 185 N.E. 2d 128, 1962.

NO   Mark Sheldon

ETHICAL ISSUES IN THE FORCED TRANSFUSION OF JEHOVAH'S WITNESS CHILDREN

BELIEFS OF JEHOVAH'S WITNESSES

Jehovah's Witnesses are Christians who believe the Bible is the Word of God in its entirety. Their name is taken from a statement that appears in the book of Isaiah: "Ye are my witnesses, saith Jehovah" (Isa. 43:10).... Presently, there are estimated to be approximately 2.2 million Jehovah's Witnesses in more than 200 countries around the world, with about 554,000 Witnesses in the United States (1).

As a group, Jehovah's Witnesses have faced numerous challenges. In the 1930s and 1940s, when their right to make home visitations was challenged, the courts affirmed their right to freedom of speech. Jehovah's Witnesses comply with most modern medical and surgical procedures, and a number of Witnesses are physicians and surgeons (2). They do not smoke, use recreational drugs, or have abortions. They view life as sacred. Why, then, do Witnesses appear to contradict this commitment to the idea that life is sacred, and reject blood transfusions at critical moments when it is a matter of life and death? In their pamphlet, *Jehovah's Witnesses and the Question of Blood* (3), they make the following statement:

> The issues of blood for Jehovah's Witnesses... involves the most fundamental principles on which they as Christians base their lives. Their relationship with their creator and God is at stake.

The seriousness of the question of blood for Witnesses can be compared to the seriousness of idolatry for Jews....

It is the Acts of Apostles, in particular, which serves most centrally as the basis for the rejection of blood transfusions. After listing those things from which believers should abstain, it reads: "... from which if ye keep yourselves, ye shall do well" (Acts 15:28–29).

Therefore, Jehovah's Witnesses take literally the numerous passages which proscribe the consumption of blood. They believe that the violation of this

From Mark Sheldon, "Ethical Issues in the Forced Transfusion of Jehovah's Witness Children," *The Journal of Emergency Medicine*, vol. 14, no. 2 (1996), pp. 251-257. Copyright © 1996 by Elsevier Science, Inc. Reprinted by permission.

proscription will result in loss of eternal life. Witnesses do not reject this world. To the contrary, they value and seek bodily health. Still, they do not think "physical life is limited to this present, temporal existence" (4). They believe that it is wrong to contrast "physical life" with "eternal life." Rather, Witnesses believe that God will, in the future, destroy life on earth, ending both personal life and conscious spiritual life. Eventually, they believe, God will resurrect the bodies of the faithful, and a limited number "will reign with God in heaven, while the remainder will live a life without end on a renewed earth" (4). They believe that life in the future, therefore, will be physical, earthly, and eternal....

THE LEGAL FRAMEWORK

... When adults are concerned, the courts generally have determined that the competent adult Jehovah's Witness, who has no dependent minor children, has a right to refuse blood transfusion (5). When children are concerned, however, the situation is very different. Interestingly enough, the decision that appears to have set the major precedent, *Prince v. Massachusetts* (1944), was not a case dealing with medical treatment, but with child labor laws (5). An aunt, who was the legal custodian of a 9-year-old, had the child on the street with her selling Jehovah's Witness magazines. Although this was in violation of child labor laws, the defense claimed that Jehovah's Witnesses were required by their religion to spread the gospel. The little girl indicated that she wanted to sell the magazines to avoid eternal damnation. Defense, therefore, claimed that this was a violation of her right to freedom of religious belief. In response, the Supreme Court ruled that

the state has authority as *parens patriae* to act in the interest of the child's well being, and that, on this basis, parental control can be restricted. While this particular decision had nothing to do with transfusion, the court (6) reached this conclusion:

> Neither the rights of religion nor the rights of parenthood are beyond limitation.... Parents may be free to make martyrs of themselves, but they are not free to make martyrs of their children before they have reached the age when they can make that choice for themselves.

A series of court decisions followed upholding *Prince*, but also dealing with the legitimacy of state intervention in matters that do or do not involve life-or-death situations. Again, it is interesting to note that *Prince* did not involve a life-and-death situation (5).

WITNESSES' VIEWS REGARDING CHILDREN

In their pamphlet, *Jehovah's Witnesses and the Question of Blood* (3), the Witnesses make the following statement:

> Jehovah's Witnesses are sure that obeying the directions from their Creator is for their lasting good....

The Witnesses then make the point that their refusal of blood transfusion cannot rightfully be construed either as suicide or as an exercise of the right to die, but it must be seen as respect for God's word (3).

In addressing the issue of children, Witnesses (3) make the following argument:

> Likely the aspect of this matter that is most highly charged with emotion involves the treating of children. All of us realize that children need care and protection. God-fearing parents particu-

larly appreciate this. They deeply love their children and keenly feel their God-given responsibility to care for them and make decisions for their lasting welfare. —Ephesians 6:14.

Society, too, recognizes parental responsibility, acknowledging that parents are the ones primarily authorized to provide for and decide for their children. Logically, religious beliefs in the family have a bearing on this. Children are certainly benefited if their parents' religion stresses the need to care for them. That is so with Jehovah's Witnesses, who in no way want to neglect their children. They recognize it as their God-given obligation to provide food, clothing, shelter and health care for them. Moreover, a genuine appreciation of the need to provide for one's children also requires inculcating in them morality and regard for what is right....

Parents who are Jehovah's Witnesses show great love for their children as well as their God by using the Bible to become moral persons. Thus, when these children are old enough to know what the Bible says about blood, they themselves support their parents decision to abstain from blood.—Acts 15:29.

... Witnesses indicate that they are fully aware of the significance of their refusal of blood transfusion for their children. However, they state that they do this out of devotion to God and out of love for their children. They claim that they cherish their children and are concerned for their children's future welfare. They do not believe that their actions should be construed as neglect. Rather, they believe that they probably are better parents than many parents in the larger society. They point to society's toleration for loose parenting, which leads to children growing up without respect for life, morality, or themselves. They hold up as examples the early Christian families who died at the hands of the Romans as models. Further, Witnesses claim to have evidence that as their children grow, they made the same choices that their parents previously made for them.

The aspect of the quote that should be emphasized is that Jehovah's Witness parents perceive themselves as acting in their children's best interest. They do not want their children to be "cut off" from the possibility of obtaining eternal life. They do not believe that it is in any way appropriate to describe their actions as involving neglect or disregard for their children. It is true, of course, that their belief that they may be better parents than others does not provide support for their right to deny blood transfusion to their children. Also, it is not clear what evidence they have to support their claim that their children will, when grown, reach the same decision as they have. But it seems clear that to describe their actions as neglectful is problematic....

THE ETHICS LITERATURE

Uniformly, the ethics literature expresses the view that it is right for the state to take temporary custody of a child to force it to undergo a blood transfusion in cases 1) when the lack of transfusion will lead to the child's death and 2) when the child is too young to give assent. However, I also believe that the basis upon which the state takes such action is not well defended in the existing ethics literature. This section consists of a review of representative arguments supporting state intervention, along with criticism of these arguments.

In 1977, Ruth Macklin (7) wrote, in an article still much referred to and often anthologized, the following:

It might be argued that Jehovah's Witness parents, in refusing permission for blood to be given to their child, are acting in accordance with their perceived duty to God, as dictated by their religion, and that this duty to God overrides whatever secular duties they may have to preserve the life and health of their child.

Macklin (7) criticized this belief:

Here it can only be replied that when an action done in accordance with perceived duties to God results in the likelihood of harm or death to another person (whether child or adult), then the duties to preserve life here on earth take precedence. The duties of a physician are to preserve and prolong life and to alleviate suffering.... Freedom of religion does not include the right to act in a manner that will result in harm or death to another.

A few points in response to Macklin's argument are in order. The first and fundamental question is: from whose perspective is "harm" being defined? Second, she identifies "harm" with "death." These are not necessarily the same. She (7) states:

If the parents refuse to grant permission for blood to be given to their child when failure to give blood will result in death or severe harm..., their prima facie right to retain control over their child no longer exists.... the case [at this point] sufficiently resembles that of child neglect [in respect to harm to the child].... in the absence of fulfillment of their duties, it is morally justifiable to take control of the child away from the parent.

From Macklin's point of view, the act "sufficiently resembles child neglect." However, on what basis is this determined to be child neglect? This is only possible to claim if the religious perspective of the parents is set aside. What makes this move acceptable? The vague comment "sufficiently resembles child neglect" does not seem to provide such a basis.

Another interesting discussion of this issue appears in a 1983 article (8) that appeared in *Hospital Progress*. The article states: "The basic ethical principle involved is beneficence: One is obliged to do whatever good one reasonably can for another person" (8). The argument is different from Macklin's in that duty is seen positively (doing good) rather than negatively (avoiding harm). The article indicates a certain concern for the family and recognizes that it is "especially dangerous today, when society tends increasingly to allow the state to take over parents' functions" (8). However, it makes the following point (8):

When the person is a minor, the obligation of beneficence falls primarily on the parents. When the parents for whatever reasons, even sincerely held religious beliefs, fail in this regard, then society, usually through its legal processes, must step in and provide for the child's good. Certain members of society, such as physicians or hospital administrators, are in a position to detect parental failure in these matters and therefore have a moral obligation to call the child's plight to civil authorities attention.

Two comments are necessary. The first is that the use of the language "parental failure" is heavily condemnatory, and not clearly appropriate. Second, while there may not be a problem, as there was above, in defining "harm," there is the problem of defining "good."

Another document that addresses the issue of state intervention is "Religious Exemptions From Child Abuse Statutes," produced by the Committee on Bioethics of the American Academy of Pediatrics in 1988 (9). This document is essentially a recommendation to change child abuse and neglect statutes that exempt parents on the basis of religious freedom....

Again, as in the Macklin article, the problem exists concerning the fact that whether harm is present depends on the perspective from which it is identified. Also, what truly constitutes the "welfare" of the child is a matter of perspective.

Another representative approach in the ethics literature appears in an article by Gary Benfield, MD, published in *Legal Aspects of Medical Practice* (10). He attempts, he points out, to address the human side of the issue, and he does, one can argue, make a sincere effort to try to understand the feelings of the Jehovah's Witness parents. He describes one of his cases that involved a young Rh-positive mother who gave birth to an Rh-positive male. He quotes (10) the mother:

Three days after the birth of our son, we were told that on the very day of his birth he was taken from us, by a simple dial of the phone, and given blood.... You have touched the very depth of my being. The pain I felt is the same pain had I been told of my son's death.... I realize it is difficult to understand how two people claiming to love their child are willing to let that child die. We as Jehovah's Witnesses believe in that promised kingdom of God's as a real ruling power, and when that kingdom that we all pray for does come to this earth, our son will be given back to us. We would just have to wait a little

longer to watch him grow and to give him all the love we stored up for him in our hearts over the last few months.... Jehovah's Witnesses do not reject blood for their children due to lack of love.... If we violate God's law on blood and the child dies, we have endangered his opportunity for everlasting life in God's new world.

Benfield's comments, in response to the mother's statement, are interesting and revealing. He remarks that after he considered all the options, he chose the one that "would best benefit my innocent patient" (10), a description which seems to impute something negative and possibly exploitative to the mother's relationship with the child. Second, he explains the basis for his choice. This consists of him asking himself, "Can I live with this decision?" (10). His answer is, "Yes." One can argue, however, that there is a problem in resolving an ethical dilemma on this basis. Such a criterion allows for anything that human beings "can live with." It is probably the case that Benfield is a sensitive and caring person, but this is a dangerous way to proceed. Presumably (this comment is not meant to reflect on Benfield but on the methodology he employs to resolve ethical dilemmas), Nazi doctors could "live with" their decisions.

Benfield (10) continues:

The parents felt that, by giving blood, I would compromise their son's chances for everlasting life. I disagreed. I felt that Jehovah, a loving God, would welcome their child in "God's new world" were he to die having received blood or not. Who was right?

In this passage, Benfield ventures beyond the basis justifying intervention expressed in the ethics literature quoted above. He does not focus on the issue of "harm" or "good" or "welfare." Instead, he is engaged in theological debate. This, of course, prompts a question concerning the expertise a physician must have in order to engage in such commentary, to make a judgment concerning the validity of another's religious belief. The question is not what Benfield does, but why. What legitimately entitles him to force a transfusion on the child? A claim to possess a more valid religious insight than the mother is not available to him simply by virtue of being a physician. Nothing about being a physician provides a basis for his conviction that he understands better than the mother does how God works. In addition, she does not make a decision on the basis of what she "can live with." She acts on the basis of scripture. For her, this is not a matter of speculation or theological debate. She acts in a way that is prescribed for her by her religious tradition.

OBSERVATIONS AND CONCLUSIONS

The following observations and conclusions should be viewed as preliminary thoughts in response to the issues raised in this article. They are preliminary in the sense that more discussion is warranted. . . .

- The criticism of the ethics literature, contained in this paper, does not imply that there is no basis for the existence of statutes concerned with child abuse and neglect. This is a different question. The state, on this issue, appropriately takes guidance from scientists (psychiatrists and psychologists) who do studies, determine consequences, and measure pain and adverse reaction related to abuse and neglect. The state can de-velop expertise in this area and can claim knowledge of what constitutes child welfare, benefit, best interest, and harm. But where the issue is ultimately spiritual and where obtaining eternal life is the objective, it is clear that the state can make no claim to any sort of knowledge. Undergoing a blood transfusion may, in fact, cut off one from obtaining eternal life, and the state simply does not have the expertise and knowledge that would enable it to judge the merits of such a claim.

- Given this lack of expertise in such ultimate questions, the state, it seems to me, must accede that all talk of harm, benefit, best interest, and martyrdom amounts to what appears to be rhetoric and not argument. Jehovah's Witness parents, in refusing blood transfusion, cannot be said to be truly harming or neglecting their children. It is simply not the case that knowledge, which would make such a judgment legitimate, is available. That refusing a transfusion is harmful can certainly be believed, and one can argue that such is the case, but it cannot be known. Therefore, the state, in taking temporary guardianship to transfuse the child, cannot be said, with certainty, to be doing this for the child's welfare. It is simply not known whether this is the case.

What, therefore, makes it legitimate to order transfusions for the children of Jehovah's Witness? The most defensible argument is that the state's weakness is also its strength. That is, while the state does not know truly what is in the child's best interest, neither does anyone else. What the parents believe is in the child's best interest may be mistaken. Given that no one knows what is in the child's best interest, the role of the state is to ensure that children ultimately become adults, able to decide, independently, what is in their own best interest. It is not even that the state assumes that it knows it to be in the child's best interest to become an adult. It may not be. It is simply that no one knows what is in the child's best interest, and the responsibility of the state is to make certain that persons who make decisions which are irrevocable do so when they are competent. A source of disquiet is that many people believe, with good reason, that parents know what is in their child's best interest. This is a belief that is not easily dismissed. And, in fact, it is not dismissed here. Ideally, the family is a very significant moral institution. More than any other institution in society, the family, properly focused, values human beings simply because they *are*, not because of any use to which they can be put. And, for this reason, it is probably in a child's best interest (and society's best interest, as well) that the family be maintained to the extent that it is, as a unit, consistent with this objective of such nurturance.

REFERENCES

1. Mead FS. Handbook of denominations in the United States. Nashville: Abingdon Press; 1980:148.

2. Dixon JL, Smalley MG. Jehovah's Witnesses: the surgical/ethical challenge. JAMA. 1981;246(27): 2471–2.

3. Jehovah's Witnesses and the question of blood. Brooklyn, NY: Watchtower Bible and Tract Society; 1977.

4. Studdard PA, Greene JY. Jehovah's Witnesses and blood transfusion: toward the resolution of a conflict of conscience. Ala J Med Sci. 1986;23(4):455.

5. Hirsh HL, Phifer H. The interface of medicine, religion, and the law: religious objections to medical treatment. Med Law. 1985;4(2):121–39.

6. *Prince v. Massachusetts.*

7. Macklin R. Consent, coercion and conflict of rights. Perspect Biol Med. 1977;20(365):365–6.

8. Editorial. May a Catholic hospital allow bloodless surgery for children? Hosp Prog. 1983;64(9): 58, 60.

9. Committee on Bioethics of the American Academy of Pediatrics. Religious exemptions from child abuse statutes. Pediatrics. 1988;81(1): 169–71.

10. Benfield DG. Giving blood to the critically ill newborn of Jehovah's Witness parents: the human side of the issue. Leg Aspects Med Pract. 1978;6(6):19–22.

POSTSCRIPT

Do Parents Harm Their Children When They Refuse Medical Treatment on Religious Grounds?

One solution to the problem posed by the refusal of Jehovah's Witnesses to undergo blood transfusions is to use alternative treatment methods, such as nonblood replacement fluids and surgical techniques that reduce the need for blood. Under many circumstances, these management alternatives allow even major surgery to be performed without additional risk. Another way to circumvent the religious prohibition is to choose medical, rather than surgical, treatment. In "Accommodating Jehovah's Witnesses' Choice of Nonblood Management," *Perspectives in Health Care Management* (Winter 1990), Donald Ridley, an attorney, argues that the sometimes inappropriate or unproven use of blood transfusions—as well as the lingering danger of transfusion-related infectious diseases, such as hepatitis—means that it may be reasonable to view Jehovah's Witnesses as "people making an informed choice between alternative courses of management." See also J. K. Vinicky et al., "The Jehovah's Witness and Blood: New Perspectives on an Old Dilemma," *Journal of Clinical Ethics* (Spring 1990).

Some of the most difficult situations arise when the patient is an adolescent. Determining whether or not an adolescent has the capacity to refuse blood transfusions is fraught with hazards. Some states have a provision for declaring an adolescent a "mature minor," that is, a person under the legal age of consent who has the capacity to make medical and other decisions. In 1994 a court of appeals in New Brunswick, Canada, set aside the order of a lower court that a 15-year-old Jehovah's Witness with leukemia be made a ward of the Crown in order that he may be given blood transfusions, if necessary. In that case, two doctors testified that the boy understood the consequences of his refusal. In a 1990 Texas case, however, the court ruled against a 16-year-old Jehovah's Witness who refused blood transfusions after he was hit by a train and severely injured. His doctor claimed that he would need transfusions during surgery to save his arm. The lower court supported the doctor and made the county child protective agency a temporary managing conservator. The Texas Court of Appeals upheld the decision, declaring that the parents' right to religious freedom did not include exposing their child to ill health or death. Moreover, because Texas law (like federal law) does not recognize the "mature minor" standard, the appeals court said that the district court was within its discretion in appointing the agency as conservator.

In "Religious Freedom and Forced Transfusion of Jehovah's Witness Children," *Journal of Emergency Medicine* (vol. 14, no. 2, 1996), Peter Rosen addresses the issue of the competency of youthful patients and advises physicians and ethicists to look at the circumstances of individual cases, rather than to seek a general ethical principle. Also of interest is "Suffering Children and the Christian Science Church," *The Atlantic Monthly* (April 1995), a highly critical account of the spiritual treatment of children's illnesses written by Caroline Fraser, the daughter of Christian Scientists.

PART 5

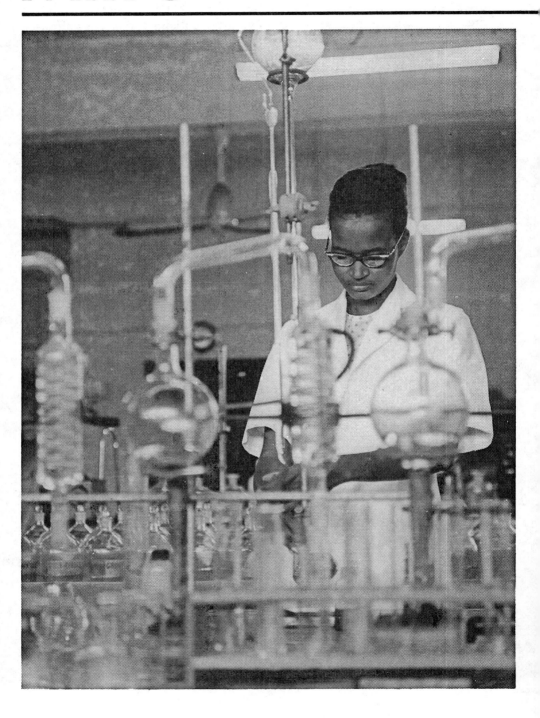

Genetics

The explosion of technology for unraveling the mysteries of human genetics has created enormous possibilities for the future in terms of understanding heredity and its influence on disease, of identifying people who are at risk for genetic diseases, and eventually of treating at-risk people. All scientific and technical breakthroughs, however, bring unresolved problems. Earlier abuses of genetic information (much of it misinformation) haunt efforts today to use this information wisely and compassionately. Also, although genetic information is intensely private, many people and institutions want to know, for their own reasons, whether or not a person has a genetic profile for a future disease. Adults may want to know their genetic structure before making reproductive choices or other future planning. Parents, on the other hand, may wish to test their children to determine whether or not they are susceptible to some adverse conditions far into the future. What impact will this knowledge have on their lives? These are some of the challenging issues raised in this section.

- Will the Human Genome Project Lead to Abuses in Genetic Engineering?

- Should Health Insurance Companies Have Access to Information from Genetic Testing?

- Should Parents Always Be Told of Genetic-Testing Availability?

ISSUE 13

Will the Human Genome Project Lead to Abuses in Genetic Engineering?

YES: Evelyn Fox Keller, from "Nature, Nurture, and the Human Genome Project," in Daniel J. Kevles and Leroy Hood, eds., *The Code of Codes: Scientific and Social Issues in the Human Genome Project* (Harvard University Press, 1992)

NO: Daniel J. Kevles and Leroy Hood, from "Preface" and "Reflections," in Daniel J. Kevles and Leroy Hood, eds., *The Code of Codes: Scientific and Social Issues in the Human Genome Project* (Harvard University Press, 1992)

ISSUE SUMMARY

YES: Professor of history and philosophy of science Evelyn Fox Keller warns that the Human Genome Project's beneficent focus on "disease-causing genes" may lead to a "eugenics of normality," in which inherently ambiguous standards of normality and individual responsibility may be abused.

NO: Professor of humanities Daniel J. Kevles and professor of biology Leroy Hood discount fears of a resurgence of negative eugenics because enlightened public opinion and contemporary political democracies, as well as technological difficulties, make it unlikely.

The Human Genome Project is big science, the first venture in biology that compares to huge projects in space exploration or astrophysics. This international project began in 1988, will take 15 years, and will cost somewhere between $300 million and $3 billion. A genome refers to all the genetic material contained within the chromosomes of a particular organism.

The origins of such a vast undertaking spans the twentieth century. In 1900 the earlier work of Gregor Mendel in explaining the scientific laws of heredity was resurrected by botanists and biologists. In 1953 James Watson (now director of the Human Genome Project) and Francis Crick discovered the double-helix structure of deoxyribonucleic acid (DNA), the long molecule that is the building block of human life. In 1973 the technology of recombinant DNA made it possible to take a fragment of DNA from one genome and splice it (recombine it) with another. Using recombinant DNA, scientists began to isolate single human genes and discover their function. Proposals to characterize the entire human genome began in the 1980s.

To comprehend the scale of the human genome project, consider these numbers: Each human cell is made up of 23 chromosome pairs (rod-like structures composed of proteins and cellular DNA). The chromosomes are believed to contain 100,000 or more genes (the fundamental unit of heredity). Each gene is an ordered sequence of nucleotides (subunits of DNA or RNA, which are designated by the four letters of the DNA alphabet—A [adenine], T [thymine], G [guanine], and C [cytosine]). These subunits are paired as A and T or G and C, and it is the bonds between these base pairs that hold together the double strands of DNA. The size of a genome is generally given as the number of its base pairs, in the human about 3 billion. According to Walter Gilbert, a molecular biologist, the amount of information contained in these base pairs is equal to a thousand thousand-page telephone books.

The Human Genome Project has been enthusiastically hailed and vigorously criticized. Professor Gilbert calls the project "a vision of the Grail," a reference to the plate from which Jesus ate at the Last Supper and a central object of medieval Christian pursuits and legends. Some geneticists and physicians look to the project as an unprecedented resource that will aid in understanding the genes involved in human biology and eventually in diagnosing and treating some of the approximately 4,000 known human genetic diseases as well as some diseases that may have genetic factors.

Some critics, on the other hand, have pointed out that only a minor percentage of DNA, perhaps less than 10 percent, represents genes and their regulatory sequences. The rest are repetitive or have an unknown function. In this view, the map of the human genome would be incredibly detailed but not much of a guide to major landmarks. Another view is that the millions that will be spent on the Human Genome Project might be more fruitfully allocated to other areas of basic or clinical research.

The most serious criticisms, however, concern not the possibility of failure but the probability of success. What will happen to individual rights and freedoms if genetic information is readily available to employers, insurers, schools, courts, and others who might make decisions based on prejudice, risk-avoidance, or misunderstanding of the limits of genetic data? At its best genetic information is usually only one factor in determining a particular individual's development of disease, intelligence, skills, or behavior.

Another, even more far-reaching concern, is discussed in the following selections. That is the possibility that the Human Genome Project might bring back eugenics. Eugenics (literally "good in birth"), involving efforts to alter human heredity by selective breeding, reached its most repressive form in the Nazi attempts to establish their superiority in their campaign of "racial hygiene," which involved mass murders of so-called inferior people. Evelyn Fox Keller warns that today's version of eugenics is more sophisticated but still dangerous. In her view the Human Genome Project fails to appreciate the complexity of human development and promotes an ambiguous definition of "normality." Daniel J. Kevles and Leroy Hood, on the other hand, look to today's political democracies and informed public opinion as protection against the authoritarian abuses of eugenics that characterized earlier decades.

YES

Evelyn Fox Keller

NATURE, NURTURE, AND THE HUMAN GENOME PROJECT

Genes became big business in the 1980s, and they are likely to become even bigger business in the decades to come. Plant genes, mouse genes, bacterial genes, and human genes are all in the news, but over the last couple of years it is human genes that have become the focus of particular interest. Daily, we are told—by Barbara Walters, by newspaper journalists, and above all, by proponents of the human genome project—that it is our genes that make us "what we are," that make some of us musical geniuses, Olympic athletes, or theoretical physicists and others alcoholics, manic-depressives, schizophrenics—even homeless. The Office of Technology Assessment concludes that "one of the strongest arguments for supporting human genome projects is that they will provide knowledge about the determinants of the human condition"; that, especially, the human genome project promises to illuminate the determinants of human disease, even of those diseases "that are at the root of many current societal problems."[1]

Some may worry about the "desirability of using genetic information to control and shape the future of human society," but others worry, perhaps equally, about a possible failure of courage.[2] To withhold support for this ambitious and expensive undertaking, writes Daniel Koshland, the editor of *Science* magazine, is to incur "the immorality of omission—the failure to apply a great new technology to aid the poor, the infirm, and the underprivileged."[3]

Thanks largely to the remarkable progress of molecular biology, it is claimed that the controversy between nature and nurture that has plagued us for so long has finally been resolved. To quote Koshland again, we now know what "may seem obvious to a scientist, but our judges, journalists, legislators, and philosophers have been slow to learn"—namely, that if we want to induce children to behave, to rehabilitate prisoners, to prevent suicides, we must recognize that

> we are dealing with a very complex problem in which the structure of society and chemical therapy will [both] play roles. Better schools, a better environment, better counseling, and better rehabilitation will help some individuals, but not all.

From Evelyn Fox Keller, "Nature, Nurture, and the Human Genome Project," in Daniel J. Kevles and Leroy Hood, eds., *The Code of Codes: Scientific and Social Issues in the Human Genome Project* (Harvard University Press, 1992). Copyright © 1992 by Daniel J. Kevles and Leroy Hood. Reprinted by permission of Harvard University Press. Some notes omitted.

Better drugs and genetic engineering will help others, but not all. It is not going to be easy for those without scientific training to cope with these complicated relationships even when all the factors are well understood.[4] ...

Most responsible advocates are of course careful to acknowledge the role of *both* nature and nurture, but rhetorically, as well as in scientific practice, it is "nature" that emerges as the decisive victor....

The shifts that Plomin, Koshland, and others note are real, and the usual assumption is that they are a direct consequence of developments in our scientific understanding of genetics. It is important to note, however, that our beliefs in nature and nurture have a cultural as well as a scientific history. There is indeed something new in the current configuration of our beliefs, and if we are to understand that novelty properly we must examine both histories, their mutual entwinement and their interdependence....

* * *

Of signal importance in the transfiguration of genetic determinism is the fact that, in the late 1960s, molecular biologists began to develop techniques by which they themselves could manipulate the "Master Molecule." They learned how to sequence it, how to synthesize it, and how to alter it. Out of molecular biology emerged a technological knowhow that decisively altered our historical sense of the immutability of "nature." Where the traditional view had been that "nature" spelled destiny and "nurture" freedom, now the roles appeared to be reversed. The technological innovations of molecular biology invited

a vastly extended discursive prowess, encouraging the notion that we could more readily control the former than the latter—not simply as a long-term goal but as an immediate prospect. This notion, though far in excess of the actual capabilities of molecular biology of that time, transformed the very terms of the nature-nurture debate; eventually, it would transform the terms of molecular biology as well.

For the first twenty years of molecular biology, research focused on organisms at the opposite end of the phylogenetic scale from humans, and to most people the implications for human beings seemed remote. For some, however, the distance from *Escherichia coli* to *Homo sapiens* had never seemed very large, and certainly by the late 1960s, with the development of new techniques for working with eukaryotic genes and mammalian viruses, that gap began to close. It was perhaps inevitable that the prospects of control invited by the new research would soon extend into the reaches of human nature. The first explicit formulations of such ambitions by molecular biologists began to appear around 1969. Even then, however, when molecular biology was just beginning to move into the domain of higher organisms, the kinds of control envisioned were already presented as crucially distinct from those of the older eugenics.

Whereas the eugenics programs of the earlier part of the century had had to rely on massive social programs, and hence were subject to social control, molecular genetics seemed to enable what Robert Sinsheimer called "a new eugenics"—a eugenics that "could, at least in principle, be implemented on a quite individual basis."[5] Sinsheimer added,

> The old eugenics was limited to a numerical enhancement of the best of our existing gene pool. The new eugenics would permit in principle the conversion of all the unfit to the highest genetic level.[6]

In short, in the vision inspired by the successes of molecular biology, "nature" became newly malleable, perhaps infinitely so; certainly it was vastly more malleable than anyone had ever imagined "nurture" to be....

The themes in these scientific/utopian scenarios that had particular influence on popular belief are (1) the newly acclaimed malleability of "nature"; (2) the reach across the divide between biology and culture that had been at least tacitly in place since World War II; and (3) the emphasis on the role of individual choice in the kinds of interventions the new genetics would make possible. In turn, of course, the influence of such arguments on popular belief would prove critical for making available the resources and support required for these aspirations to exert a practical influence over the future course of research in molecular biology....

Without doubt, the 1970s was a decade of extraordinary expansion for molecular biology: technically, institutionally, culturally, and economically. My aim is not to question that expansion per se, but rather to question the conventional understanding that the institutional, cultural, and economic expansion of molecular biology proceeded directly, and as a matter of course, from its technical successes. In particular, I want to focus on the ideological expansion of molecular biology into both popular culture and

medicine, and at least to raise a question about the effect of this ideological expansion on subsequent technical developments. To this end, the historian Edward Yoxen's exploration of the construction of the idea of "genetic disease" provides an absolutely essential starting point, for it is this concept which both has provided the ground for the cultural and medical expansion of molecular genetics and, at the same time, distinguishes current formulations of genetic determinism from those of the earlier part of the century.[7]

As Yoxen points out, one need not dispute the fact that "many of the phenomena of genetic disease are grounded in material reality" in order to ask "why we isolate or delineate certain phenomena for analysis, why we say that they constitute diseases, and why we seek to explain their nature and cause in genetical terms."[8] Although an earlier generation of geneticists may not have doubted the power of genes to determine (and thus ultimately to transform) human well-being, they did not (except in isolated instances) link their claims to a concept of genetic disease, and their medical colleagues, failing to see any direct relation between genes and treatment even for those diseases that were understood to be genetic, regarded genetics as being of little relevance to medical practice. Today, however, the relation between genetics and the medical sciences has dramatically changed. Even though, in actuality, genetics remains of quite limited practical relevance to the healing arts, the concept of disease—now extended throughout the domain of human behavior—has increasingly come to be understood by health scientists in terms of genetics. Indeed, the volume of medical literature on genetic disease has increased exponentially over the past decade,* and much of this literature suggests a conceptual shift that one commentator describes as follows:

> [In the past,] most physicians and investigators have perceived that deleterious influences on human health are of two kinds: either a deficiency of a basic resource such as food or vitamins, or exposure to hazards that may be either natural... or man-made... Genetics is now showing that this view of the determinants of health as being external is too simplistic. It neglects a major determinant of disease—an internal one. Far from being a rare cause of disease, genetic factors are a very important determinant of health or illness in developed countries.[9]

But as Yoxen points out, in the course of this conceptual shift "genetic disease" has become an extremely large category, encompassing not only genetic disorders that are thought of as diseases but also genetic abnormalities associated with no known disorder as well as disorders that may be neither genetic nor diseases.[10]

Many factors (both technical and cultural) have contributed to the expansion of the concept of genetic disease and, with it, the domain of clinical genetics. Among these one might note: increasingly general acceptance of the explanatory framework of molecular biology; the postwar diminution of the burden of acute disease; intensification of scientific training for medical practice; changing expectations for health in the general public; and patterns of resource distribution for scientific research. For example, Yoxen notes

that, in the early 1970s, the National Institute of General Medical Sciences (a subdivision of the NIH) sought

> to mobilize support for its programs by representing genetic disorders as a significant cause of ill health. Here, genetics offers a strategy of territorial expansion through the redefinition of the causes of disease to a relatively low status institution.[11]

Yoxen's main point, however, is to indicate the many social, economic, political, and technical issues that must be taken into account if we are to understand how the "basic explanatory form of a 'genetic disease' has been constructed to fit the contemporary context."[12]

My point is an even more general one. It is to note that the concept of genetic disease, enthusiastically appropriated by the medical sciences for complex institutional and economic reasons, represents an ideological expansion of molecular biology far beyond its technical successes. I also want to argue that the general acceptance of this concept has, in turn, proved critical for the direction that subsequent technical developments in molecular biology have now begun to take. Without question, it was the technical prowess that molecular biology had achieved by the early 1980s that made it possible even to imagine a task as formidable as that of sequencing what has come to be called "the human genome." But it was the concept of genetic disease that created the climate in which such a project could appear both reasonable and desirable.

* * *

I want to focus on two arguments that surfaced early in the advocacy of the human genome project. First is the startling

---

*A count of review articles on genetic disease listed in Medline reveals a more than sevenfold increase over the years 1986 to 1989 alone. Fifty-one articles are listed for 1986, 152 for 1987, 288 for 1988, and 366 in 1989.

promise that the full sequence of the human genome will teach us, finally, "what it means to be human"; it will enable us to "decipher the mysteries" of our own existence. In spite of the fact that the actual genomes of any two individuals will differ by as much as three million bases, from a molecular biological point of view, the "essential underlying definition" of the human being is a single entity.[13] Advocates for the human genome project continue by arguing that the characterization of this entity (namely, its genetic sequence) therefore constitutes a critical question for medicine. But what is sometimes presented as a sequitur is more commonly presented as an independent appeal to the "major [or 'revolutionary'] impact" such a data base will have "on health care and disease prevention." In the official report issued in 1988 by the National Research Council Committee on Mapping and Sequencing the Human Genome, the value of this information for the "diagnosis, treatment, and prevention" of human disease is repeatedly emphasized. It is argued:

> Encoded in the DNA sequence are fundamental determinants of those mental capacities—learning, language, memory—essential to human culture. Encoded there as well are the mutations and variations that cause or increase susceptibility to many diseases responsible for much human suffering.[14]

The committee concludes "that a project to map and sequence the human genome should be undertaken" in order to "allow rapid progress to occur in the diagnosis and ultimate control of many human diseases."[15] James Watson makes the point even more strongly. For him, the human genome project is "our best go at diseases." Indeed, he goes further.

Referring to manic depression as an instance of the kind of disease we seek to control, he argues that we must find the gene because without it "we are lost."[16]

The two central images of the rhetoric employed here—on the one hand the idea of a base-line norm, indicated by "the human genome," and on the other the specter of a panoply of genetic diseases (currently estimated at well over 3,000)—definitively distinguish this discourse from its precursors. The emphasis now is not so much on the "cultural perfection of man" or on the "conscious" and "direct" employment of genetic technology to engineer our "transition to a whole new pitch of evolution,"[17] or even on improving the quality of our genetic pool, but rather on the use of genetics—through diagnosis, treatment, and prevention—to guarantee to all human beings an individual and natural right, the right to health. In its 1988 report on the human genome project, the Office of Technology Assessment concluded that "new technologies for identifying traits and altering genes make it possible for eugenic goals to be achieved through technological as opposed to social control."[18] But even more important, the report sets the project's eugenic implications apart from earlier precedents by distinguishing a "eugenics of normalcy": that is, "the use of genetic information... to ensure that... each individual has at least a modicum of normal genes." The report cites an argument that "individuals have a paramount right to be born with a normal, adequate hereditary endowment."[19]

Just as Sinsheimer predicted twenty years ago, the nineties version of the "new eugenics" (though the word *eugenics* is not now used) is no longer construed as a matter of social policy, the good of the species, or the quality of our collective gene pool; the current concern is the problem (as Watson puts it) of the "disease-causing genes" that "some of us *as individuals* have inherited [my italics]." Accordingly, it is presented in terms of the choices that "they as individuals" will have to make.[20] Genetics merely provides the information enabling the individual to realize an inalienable right to health, where "health" is defined in reference to a tacit norm, signified by "*the* human genome," and in contradistinction to a state of unhealth (or abnormality), indicated by an ever growing list of conditions characterized as "genetic disease."

A number of fairly obvious questions come to mind at this point about the concepts of both "individual" and "choice" that are invoked in this discourse, but first, some basic points stand in need of clarification. The first is that, despite the repeated emphasis on health care, on the diagnosis, treatment, and prevention of genetic disease, it is in fact primarily the possibility of diagnosis that is considered of practical relevance for the near future by even the most enthusiastic proponents of the human genome project; estimates of arrival times for therapeutic benefits run, optimistically, as long as fifty years hence. Thus, "treatment" is at best a long-term goal, and "prevention" means preventing the births of individuals diagnosed as genetically aberrant—in a word, it means abortion. The choices "individuals" are asked to make are therefore choices not on behalf of their own health but on behalf of the health of their offspring and, implicitly, on behalf of the nation's health costs. Pointing to schizophrenia, which he claimed currently accounts for one-half of all hospital beds, Charles Cantor, the former head of the Human Genome Center at the Lawrence Berkeley Laboratory, recently argued in a lecture that the project would more than pay for itself by preventing the occurrence of just this one disease. When asked how such a saving could be effected he could only say: "by preventing the birth" of schizophrenics.[21]

Which brings us to the second point requiring clarification: namely, that these newly available choices, though ostensibly made by individuals, are in fairly obvious ways preconstructed by the categories of disease already presented to the decisionmaker, often on the basis of rather dubious evidence. Psychiatric disorders are a good case in point. In 1987, reports of a genetic locus for manic depression received extensive publicity, as did a similar report for a genetic locus for schizophrenia published in 1988. Less well publicized was the retraction of both these claims in 1989. Three months before Cantor's lecture, *Nature* had reported that the retraction "leaves us with no persuasive evidence linking any psychiatric disease to a single locus." As David Baltimore, then Director of the Whitehead Institute at MIT, said, "Setting myself up as an average reader of *Nature*, what am I to believe?"[22] Even more pressing for my point is the question of what the average reader of *Time* and *Newsweek* is to believe. If the scientific community were in closer agreement on genetic definitions of disease, an individual's choices might be clearer, but they would not be any more "autonomous."

The current disarray surrounding attempts to define "genetic disease" bears in part on a third point that I briefly indicated earlier—namely, the elusiveness of a norm against which the concept of abnormality is implicitly defined. Molecular analysis of human DNA indicates that the genomes of any two individuals will, on average, differ in approximately three million bases. In an attempt to bypass the enormous diversity among even "normal" human beings, a composite genome, with different chromosomes obtained from different individuals, has been adopted as the standard for genomic analysis. This "solution" does nothing, however, to address either the de facto variability in nucleotide sequence within individual chromosomes or the consequent difficulty in deciding what a "normal" sequence would be.

A fourth and final point that needs at least to be mentioned is that many of the categories of genetic disease —especially those referring to mental competence—put into question the very capacity of those individuals who carry the purported "disease-causing genes" to make choices. Such individuals might well be expected, in Watson's own words, to be "genetically incapable of being responsible."[23]

*   *   *

Forty years ago, when the specter of eugenics aroused such intense anxiety, the aims of genetics were made safe by a clear demarcation between biology and culture. The province of genetics, particularly of molecular genetics, was biology—primarily, the biology of lower organisms. To most people in or out of genetics, molecular biology seemed to have little if any bearing on human behavior. At that time, it was culture, not biology, that "made us human"; culture was simultaneously the source and the object of our special, human, freedom to make choices. Today we are being told— and judging from media accounts, we are apparently coming to believe—that what makes us human is our genes. Indeed, the very notion of "culture" as distinct from "biology" seems to have vanished;

in the terms that increasingly dominate contemporary discourse, "culture" has become subsumed under biology.

But if culture is to be subsumed under biology, and if it is our biological or genetic future that we now seek to shape, where are we to locate the domain of freedom by which this future can be charted? The disarming suggestion that is put forth is that this domain of freedom is to be found in the elusive realm of "individual choice"—a suggestion that invokes a democratic and egalitarian ideal somewhere beyond biology. But since there is in this discourse no domain "beyond biology," since it is our genes that "make us what we are," and since they do so with a definitive inequality that compromises even those choices some of us can make, we are obliged to look elsewhere for the implied realm of freedom. I suggest that the locus of freedom on which this discourse tacitly depends is to be found not in the domain of "individual choice," comforting as such a notion might be, but rather in a domain protected by the ambiguous designation of "normality." More generally, I suggest that the distinction that had earlier been made by the demarcation between culture and biology (or between nurture and nature) is now made by a demarcation between the normal and the abnormal; the force of destiny is no longer attached to culture, or even to biology in general, but rather more specifically to the biology (or genetics) of disease. Far from teaching us "what it means to be human," in actual practice, the burden of the new human genetics turns on the elucidation not of human order but of human disorder. Our genes may make us "what we are," but, it would appear, they do so more forcefully for some of us than for others. By general consensus, molecular geneticists do not seek genetic loci for traits that they—and we—accept as normal. Indeed, they, like us, do not even seek to define the meaning of "normal."

It is perhaps inevitable that the appeal to the desire for health translates into a search for the genetic basis of unhealth, but the net effect of this translation is that the nature of normality is allowed silently to elude the gaze of genetic scrutiny—and thereby tacitly to evade its determinist grip. The freedom molecular biology promises to bring is the freedom to rout the domain of destiny inhering in "disease-causing genes" in the name of an unspecified standard of normality—a standard that remains unexamined not simply by oversight but by the internal logic of the endeavor. The "normal" state can be specified in this endeavor only by negation—by the absence of those alleles said to cause disease.

More problematic still is the insistent ambiguity inhering in the very term *normal*, an ambiguity that the philosopher and historian of science Ian Hacking traces to Auguste Comte:

Comte ... expressed and to some extent invented a fundamental tension in the idea of the normal—the normal as existing average, and the normal as figure of perfection to which we may progress. This is an even richer source of hidden power than the fact/value ambiguity that had always been present in the idea of the normal ... On the one hand there is the thought that the normal is what is right, so that talk of the normal is a splendid way of preserving or returning to the status quo ... On the other hand is the idea that the normal is only average, and so is something to be improved upon.[24]

This ambiguity permits all of us a certain latitude in our hopes and expectations for a "eugenics of normalcy." It also clears a large field for the operation of distinctly nongenetic, ideological forces.

Both the definition and the routing of genetic disease express human choices, and even if "individual choice" is an inadequate model for describing the process by which choices actually get made, the very possibility of choice depends on a residual domain of agency that can remain free only to the extent that it remains unexamined. The question, of course, is where, and how, this residual domain of agency gets constructed and articulated, how the authority for prescribing the meaning of "normal" is distributed. The notion of culture (like that of nurture) may have vanished from contemporary biological discourse, but it is here, hidden from view, that the facts of culture continue to exert their undeniable force.

There is no question that eugenics has become a vastly more realizable prospect than it was in the earlier part of the century, and it must be granted that, in many ways, the very notion remains as disturbing as it was in 1945. As Watson has written,

We have only to look at how the Nazis used leading members of the German human genetics and psychiatry communities to justify their genocide programs, first against the mentally ill and then the Jews and the Gypsies. We need no more vivid reminders that science in the wrong hands can do incalculable harm.[25]

It is of course true that, in 1990, we have no Nazi conspiracy to fear. All we have to fear today is our own complacency that there are some "right hands" in which to invest this responsibility—above all, the responsibility for arbitrating normality.

NOTES

1. U.S. Congress, Office of Technology Assessment, *Mapping Our Genes* (Washington, D.C.: Government Printing Office, 1988), p. 85; Daniel Koshland, "Sequences and Consequences of the Human Genome," *Science*, 146 (1989), 189.

2. Office of Technology Assessment, *Mapping Our Genes*, p. 79.

3. Koshland, "Sequences and Consequences," p. 189. In the address on which this editorial was based, delivered at the First Human Genome Conference in October 1989, Koshland was even more explicit. In response to the oft-raised question, "Why not give this money to the homeless?" he said, "What these people don't realize is that the homeless are impaired... Indeed, no group will benefit more from the application of human genetics." Just how the human genome project will aid "the poor, the infirm, and the underprivileged," Koshland did not say.

4. Daniel Koshland, "Nature, Nurture, and Behavior," *Science*, 235 (1987), 1445.

5. Robert Sinsheimer, "The Prospect of Designed Genetic Change," *Engineering and Science*, 32 (1969), 8–13; reprinted in Ruth Chadwick, ed., *Ethics, Reproduction, and Genetic Control* (London: Croom Helm, 1987), p. 145.

6. Ibid.

7. Edward J. Yoxen, "Constructing Genetic Diseases," in Troy Duster and Karen Garett, eds., *Cultural Perspectives on Biological Knowledge* (Norwood, N.J.: Ablex, 1984).

8. Yoxen, "Constructing Genetic Diseases," p. 41.

9. P. A. Baird, "Genetics and Health Care," *Perspectives in Biology and Medicine*, 33 (1990), 203–213.

10. Yoxen, "Constructing Genetic Diseases," p. 49.

11. Ibid., p. 50.

12. Ibid., p. 48.

13. See the chapter by Walter Gilbert in *The Code of Codes: Scientific and Social Issues in the Human Genome Project* (1992), "A Vision of the Grail," pp. 83–97.

14. National Research Council, *Mapping and Sequencing the Human Genome* (Washington, D.C.: National Academy Press, 1988), pp. 1, 12–13, 45.

15. Ibid., p. 11.

16. The quotations are taken from a lecture that Watson gave at the California Institute of Technology, May 9, 1990.

17. Sinsheimer, "Prospect of Designed Genetic Change," p. 146.

18. Office of Technology Assessment, *Mapping Our Genes*, p. 84.

19. Ibid., p. 86.

20. James D. Watson, "The Human Genome Project—Past, Present, and Future," *Science* 248 (April 6, 1990), 44–49.

21. Charles Cantor, informal lecture at the University of California, Berkeley, 1990.

22. Miranda Robertson, "False Start on Manic Depression," *Nature*, 342 (November 18, 1989), 222.

23. Watson lecture, May 9, 1990.

24. Ian Hacking, *The Taming of Chance* (Cambridge: Cambridge University Press, 1990), p. 168.

25. Watson, "The Human Genome Project," p. 46.

NO

Daniel J. Kevles
and Leroy Hood

THE CODE OF CODES

The human genome comprises, in its totality, all the different genes found in the cells of human beings. The Nobel laureate Walter Gilbert has called it the "grail of human genetics," the key to what makes us human, what defines our possibilities and limits as members of the species *Homo sapiens*. What makes us human beings instead of chimpanzees, for example, is a mere 1 percent difference between the ape genome and our own. That distinction amounts to no more than a gross reckoning, however. The substance and versatility of the human genome lie in its details, in specific information about all the genes we possess—the number has been variously estimated at between 50,000 and 100,000—about how they contribute to the vast array of human characteristics, about the role they play (or do not play) in disease, development, and behavior.

The search for the biological grail has been going on since the turn of the century, but it has now entered its culminating phase with the recent creation of the human genome project, the ultimate goal of which is the acquisition of all the details of our genome. That knowledge will undoubtedly revolutionize understanding of human development, including the development of both normal characteristics, such as organ function, and abnormal ones, such as disease. It will transform our capacities to predict what we may become and, ultimately, it may enable us to enhance or prevent our genetic fates, medically or otherwise.

Unquestionably, the connotations of power and fear associated with the holy grail accompany the genome project, its biological counterpart. The project itself has raised professional apprehensions as well as high intellectual expectations. Undoubtedly, it will affect the way that much of biology is pursued in the twenty-first century. Whatever the shape of that effect, the quest for the biological grail will, sooner or later, achieve its end, and we believe that it is not too early to begin thinking about how to control the power so as to diminish—better yet, abolish—the legitimate social and scientific fears. . . .

It is our conviction that the social and ethical issues of human genetics —which the project is not so much raising as intensifying—are analyzed

From Daniel J. Kevles and Leroy Hood, "Preface" and "Reflections," in Daniel J. Kevles and Leroy Hood, eds., *The Code of Codes: Scientific and Social Issues in the Human Genome Project* (Harvard University Press, 1992). Copyright © 1992 by Daniel J. Kevles and Leroy Hood. Reprinted by permission of Harvard University Press.

most usefully when they are tied to the present and prospective realities of the science and its technological capacities. Science-fiction fantasies about the genetic future distract attention from the genuine problems posed by advances in the study of heredity. . . .

* * *

In April 1991, an exposition opened in the hall atop the great arch of La Defense, in Paris, under the title *La Vie en Kit: Éthique et Biologie*. This exhibit concerning "life in a test tube" included displays about molecular genetics and the human genome project. The ethical worries were manifest in a statement by the writer Monette Vaquin that was printed in the catalogue and was also prominently placarded at the genome display:

> Today, astounding paradox, the generation following Nazism is giving the world the tools of eugenics beyond the wildest Hitlerian dreams. It is as if the preposterous ideas of the fathers' generation haunted the discoveries of the sons. scientists of tomorrow will have a power that exceeds all the powers known to mankind: that of manipulating the genome. Who can say for sure that it will be used only to avoid hereditary illnesses?[1]

Vaquin's apprehensions, echoed frequently by scientists and social analysts alike, indicate that the shadow of eugenics continues to hang over the genome project. Commentators have suggested that the project may stimulate state attempts at positive eugenics, the use of genetic engineering to foster or enhance characteristics such as scholastic, scientific, and mathematical intelligence, musical ability, or athletic prowess. The ultimate goal will be the creation of new Einsteins, Mozarts, or Kareem Abdul-

Jabbars (curiously, brilliantly talented women—such as Marie Curie or Nadia Boulanger or Martina Navratilova—are rarely if ever mentioned in the pantheon of superpeople). Other commentators have warned that the project will more likely spark a revival of negative eugenics—state programs of intervention in reproductive behavior so as to discourage the transmission of "bad" genes in the population.

Negative-eugenic programs could well be prompted by economic incentives. Concern for financial costs played a role in the eugenics movement of the early twentieth century, when social pathologies were said to be increasing at a terrible rate. At the Sesquicentennial Exposition in Philadelphia, in 1926, the American Eugenics Society exhibit included a board that, in the manner of the population counters of a later day, revealed with flashing lights that every fifteen seconds a hundred dollars of the observer's money went for the care of persons with "bad heredity" and that every forty-eight seconds a mentally deficient person was born in the United States. The display implied that restricting the reproduction of people with deleterious genes would not only benefit the gene pool but reduce state and local expenditures for "feeblemindedness" in public institutional settings—that is, state institutions and state hospitals for the mentally deficient and physically disabled or diseased. Perhaps indicative of this reasoning is that, in California and several other states, eugenic sterilization rates increased significantly during the 1930s, when state budgets for the mentally handicapped were squeezed.[2]

In our own day, the more that health care becomes a public responsibility, payable through the tax system, and the more expensive this care becomes, the greater the possibility that taxpayers will rebel against paying for the care of those whom genetics dooms to severe disease or disability. Public policy might feel pressure to encourage, or even to compel, people not to bring genetically disadvantaged children into the world— not for the sake of the gene pool but in the interest of keeping public health costs down.

Eugenic promptings might also come from scientists, who, having been lured by ideas of biological imperatives in the past, could find them equally seductive in the future. It is worth bearing in mind that eugenics was not an aberration, the commitment merely of a few oddball scientists and mean-spirited social theorists. It was embraced by leading biologists—not only of the political right but of the progressive left—and it was integral to the research programs of prominent, powerful institutions devoted to the study of human heredity. Indeed, eugenics remained a powerfully attractive idea even after the social prejudice of its early form was recognized and exposed. Objective, socially unprejudiced knowledge is not ipso facto inconsistent with eugenic goals of some type. Indeed, such knowledge may assist in seeking them. The enrichment of human genetics by molecular biology moved Robert Sinsheimer, in 1969, to raise with enthusiasm the possibility of a "new eugenics"—a eugenics that could be free of social bias and, as a result of DNA engineering, scientifically achievable. The more that is learned in the future about human genetics, the more might some biologists be tempted to reunite it with eugenic goals.

In recent years, crude eugenic policies have been promulgated by several governments. In Singapore in 1984, Prime Minister Lee Kwan Yew deplored the relatively low birth rate among educated women, resorting to the fallacy that their intelligence was higher than average and that they were thus allowing the quality of the country's gene pool to diminish. Since then, the government has adopted a variety of incentives—for example, preferential school enrollment for offspring —to increase the fecundity of educated women, and it has offered a similar incentive to their less-educated sisters who would have themselves sterilized after the birth of a first or second child. In 1988, China's Gansu Province adopted a eugenic law that would—so the authorities said—improve "population quality" by banning the marriages of mentally retarded people unless they first submit to sterilization. Since then, similar laws have been adopted in other provinces and have been endorsed by Prime Minister Li Peng. The official newspaper *Peasants Daily* explained, "Idiots give birth to idiots."[3]

Geneticists know that idiots do not necessarily give birth to idiots and that mental retardation may arise from many nongenetic causes. Analysts of civil liberty also know that reproductive freedom is much more easily curtailed in dictatorial governments than in democratic ones. Eugenics profits from authoritarianism—indeed, almost requires it. The institutions of political democracy may not have been robust enough to resist altogether the violations of civil liberties characteristic of the early eugenics movement, but they did contest them effectively in many places. The British government refused to pass eugenic sterilization laws. So did many American states, and where eugenic laws were enacted, they were often unenforced. It is far-fetched to expect a Nazi-like eugenic program to develop in the contemporary United States so long as political democracy and the Bill of Rights continue in force. If a Nazi-like eugenic program becomes a threatening reality, the country will have a good deal more to be worried about politically than just eugenics.

What makes contemporary political democracies unlikely to embrace eugenics is that they contain powerful anti-eugenic constituencies. Awareness of the barbarities and cruelties of state-sponsored eugenics in the past has tended to set most geneticists and the public at large against such programs. Geneticists today know better than their early-twentieth-century predecessors that ideas concerning what is "good for the gene pool" are highly problematic. (We might add, however, that even though they know better, they may not know enough and that, given the human genome project, education in the social and ethical implications of genetic research and genetic claims should probably become a required part of every biologist's professional training.) Then, too, although prejudice continues against persons living with a variety of disabilities and diseases, today such people are politically empowered, as are minority groups, to a degree that they were not in the early twentieth century. For example, in 1990 they obtained passage of the Americans with Disabilities Act, which, among other things, prohibits discrimination against disabled people in employment, public services, and public accommodations. They may not be sufficiently empowered to counter all quasi-eugenic threats to themselves, but they are politically positioned, with allies in the media, the medical profession, and elsewhere, to block or at least to hinder eugenic proposals that might affect them.

The advance of human genetics and biotechnology has created the capacity for a kind of "homemade eugenics," to use the insightful term of the analyst Robert Wright—"individual families deciding what kinds of kids they want to have." At the moment, the kinds they can choose are those without certain disabilities or diseases, such as Down's syndrome or Tay-Sachs. Most parents would probably prefer a healthy baby. In the future, they might have the opportunity —for example, via genetic analysis of embryos—to have improved babies, children who are likely to be more intelligent or more athletic or better looking (whatever that might mean).[4]

Will people exploit such possibilities? Quite possibly, given the interest that some parents have shown in choosing the sex of their child or that others have pursued in the administration of growth hormone to offspring who they think will grow up too short. Benedikt Härlin's report to the European Parliament on the human genome project noted that the increasing availability of genetic tests was generating increasingly widespread pressure from families for "individual eugenic choice in order to give one's own child the best possible start in a society in which hereditary traits become a criterion of social hierarchy." A 1989 editorial in *Trends in Biotechnology* recognized a major source of the pressure: " 'Human improvement' is a fact of life, not because of the state eugenics committee, but because of consumer demand. How can we expect to deal responsibly with human genetic information in such a culture?"[5]

However, genetic enhancement would inevitably involve the manipulation of human embryos, and, for better or for worse, human-embryo research faces governmental prohibitions in the United States and powerful opposition in virtually all the major western democracies, especially from Roman Catholics. The European Parliament did resolve in 1989 to allow for research on human embryos, but only under very restricted circumstances—for example, only if it would be "of direct and otherwise unattainable benefit in terms of the welfare of the child concerned and its mother." The Parliament's action was based on a report from its Committee on Legal Affairs and Citizens' Rights entitled *Ethical and Legal Problems of Genetic Engineering and Human Artificial Insemination*. The rapporteur for the section of the report concerned with genetic engineering was Willi Rothley, who is not only a Green but a Catholic, and the report itself argued against genetic manipulation of the embryo on several philosophical grounds, including the claim that "each generation must be allowed to wrestle with human nature as it is given to them, and not with the irreversible biological results of their forebears' actions."[6]

The idea of human genetic engineering as such offends many non-Catholics, too. A broad spectrum of lay and religious opinion on both sides of the Atlantic agrees with the European Parliament's 1989 declaration that genetic analysis "must on no account be used for the scientifically dubious and politically unacceptable purpose of 'positively improving' the population's gene pool" and its call for "an absolute ban on all experiments designed to reorganize on an arbitrary basis the genetic make-up of humans."[7] In any event, human genetic improvement is not likely to yield to human effort for some time to come. While the human genome project will undoubtedly accelerate the identification of genes

for physical and medically related traits, it is unlikely to reveal with any speed how genes contribute to the formation of those qualities—particularly talent, creativity, behavior, appearance—that the world so much wants and admires. The idea that genetic knowledge will soon permit the engineering of Einsteins or even the enhancement of general intelligence is simply preposterous.[8] Equally important, the engineering of designer human genomes is not possible under current reproductive technologies and is not likely in the near future to become much easier technically.

NOTES

1. *La Vie en Kit: Éthique et Biologie* (Paris: L'Arche de la Defense, 1991), p. 25.

2. Philip R. Reilly, *The Surgical Solution: A History of Involuntary Sterilization in the United States* (Baltimore: The Johns Hopkins University Press, 1991), pp. 91–93. The last state eugenic sterilization law was passed in 1937, in Georgia, partly in response to conditions of overcrowding in the state's institutions for the mentally handicapped. Edward J. Larson, "Breeding Better Georgians," *Georgia Journal of Southern Legal History*, 1 (Spring/Summer 1991), 53–79.

3. Steven Jay Gould, *The Flamingo's Smile: Reflections in Natural History* (New York: W. W. Norton, 1985), pp. 292–295, 301–303; *The New York Times*, August 15, 1991, p. 1.

4. Robert Wright, "Achilles' Helix," p. 27; Joseph Bishop and Michael Waldholz, *Genome: The Story of the Most Astonishing Scientific Adventure of Our Time —The Attempt to Map All the Genes in the Human Body* (New York: Simon and Schuster, 1990), pp. 310–322.

5. Jane E. Brody, "Personal Health," *The New York Times*, November 8, 1990, p. B7; Barry Werth, "How Short Is Too Short?" *The New York Times Magazine*, June 16, 1991, pp. 15, 17, 28–29; European Parliament, Committee on Energy, Research, and Technology, *Report Drawn up on Behalf of the Committee on Energy, Research and Technology on the Proposal from the Commission to the Council (COM/88/424-C2-119/88) for a Decision Adopting a Specific Research Programme in the Field of Health: Predictive Medicine: Human Genome Analysis (1989–1991)*, Rapporteur Benedikt Härlin, European Parliament Session Documents, 1988–89, 30.01.1989, Series A, Doc A2–0370/88 SYN 146,

pp. 25–26; John Hodgson, "Editorial: Geneticism and Freedom of Choice," *Trends in Biotechnology,* September 1989, p. 221.

6. "Resolutions Adopted by the European Parliament on 16 March 1989," in European Parliament, Committee on Legal Affairs and Citizens' Rights, Rapporteurs: Mr. Willi Rothley and Mr. Carlo Casini, *Ethical and Legal Problems of Genetic Engineering and Human Artificial Insemination* (Luxembourg: Office for Publications of the European Communities, 1990), pp. 15, 38–39. Carlo Casini, from Italy, the rapporteur for the section of the report concerned with human artificial insemination, is known in the circles of the Parliament as virtually a papal representative to the legislative body. Embryo research and germ-line engineering are also opposed by many adherents of Islamic religion and by many Protestants, most recently in a 1989 report by the World Council of Churches. Lectures by Azeddine Guessos and Jack Stotts, "II Workshop on International Cooperation for the Human Genome Project: Ethics," Valencia, Spain, November 12, 1990.

7. "Resolutions Adopted by the European Parliament on 16 March 1989," in European Parliament, Committee on Legal Affairs and Citizens' Rights, *Ethical and Legal Problems of Genetic Engineering and Human Artificial Insemination,* p. 12; Daniel J. Kevles, "Unholy Alliance," *The Sciences,* September/October 1986, pp. 25–30.

8. Bishop and Waldholz, *Genome,* pp. 314–316; Sharon Kingman, "Buried Treasure in Human Genes," *New Scientist,* July 8, 1989, p. 37.

POSTSCRIPT

Will the Human Genome Project Lead to Abuses in Genetic Engineering?

The Human Genome Project is currently ahead of schedule and under budget. A significant interim goal—the construction of a genetic linkage map showing the relative positions of genes and DNA sequences on the chromosomes—was not expected until the end of 1995 but was achieved in 1994. Although the discovery of "disease genes" is progressing rapidly, new treatments will take much more time.

In "The Human Genome Project and Eugenic Concerns," *American Journal of Human Genetics* (vol. 54, no. 1, 1994), Kenneth L. Garver and Bettylee Garver analyze German and American eugenics programs in the early twentieth century and conclude that, given present-day social problems and the growing demand for cost-effective genetic services, a resurgence of eugenics is possible. From a different viewpoint, W. French Anderson argues that genetic engineering should not be considered a threat to our humanness, because it can alter only quantitative human characteristics and not our unique, qualitative abilities. See "Genetic Engineering and Our Humanness," *Human Gene Therapy* (vol. 5, 1994). Susan M. Wolf, in "Beyond 'Genetic Discrimination': Toward the Broader Harm of Geneticism," *Journal of Law, Medicine and Ethics* (vol. 23, 1995), argues that the central concern should not be potential discriminatory uses of genetic information but the use of genetic notions to create and reinforce power relationships based on gender and race. Two historical examinations of eugenics are Edward J. Larson, *Sex, Race, and Science: Eugenics in the Deep South* (Johns Hopkins University Press, 1995) and Alan M. Kraut, *Germs, Genes, and the "Immigrant Menace"* (Johns Hopkins University Press, 1994). Also see Dorothy Nelkin and M. Susan Lindee, *The DNA Mystique: The Gene as a Cultural Icon* (W. H. Freeman, 1995) and Diane B. Paul, *Controlling Human Heredity: 1865 to the Present* (Humanities Press, 1995).

In *The Lives to Come: The Genetic Revolution and Human Possibilities* (Simon & Schuster, 1996), Philip Kitcher describes the likely contributions that research will make toward the treatment of disease. Sharon J. Durfy and Amy E. Grotevant have compiled a bibliography, *The Human Genome Project* (Scope Note No. 17, Kennedy Institute of Ethics, 1992), and the U.S. Department of Energy's Office of Energy Research has published *ELSI Bibliography: Ethical, Legal, and Social Implications of the Human Genome Project* edited by Michael S. Yelsey (1993). More information on the ethical implications of genetics and the Human Genome Project can be found at the following Web site of the National Institutes of Health's National Center for Human Genome Research: http://www.nchgr.nih.gov/home.html.

ISSUE 14

Should Health Insurance Companies Have Access to Information from Genetic Testing?

YES: American Council of Life Insurance and Health Insurance Association of America, from *Report of the ACLI-HIAA Task Force on Genetic Testing* (ACLI-HIAA, 1991)

NO: Thomas H. Murray, from "Genetics and the Moral Mission of Health Insurance," *Hastings Center Report* (November/December 1992)

ISSUE SUMMARY

YES: The American Council of Life Insurance and the Health Insurance Association of America assert that while insurers do not currently plan to use genetic information, if they are denied access to genetic test results, the amount paid out in insurance claims could increase, resulting in higher premiums for most policyholders.

NO: Thomas H. Murray, a professor of biomedical ethics, believes that actuarial fairness—the insurance industry's standard—fails to accomplish the social goals of health insurance and that genetic tests should not be used to deny people access to health insurance.

Genetic diseases and predisposition to disease are not uncommon. An estimated 4,000 to 5,000 genetic diseases have already been identified. Some of these diseases are detectable prenatally, such as Down's syndrome, a form of mental retardation, and sickle-cell anemia, a blood disorder. Others are detected at birth, such as PKU, a metabolic disorder. Still others become manifest only in adults, such as Huntington's disease, a lethal neurological disorder.

Approximately 1,100 genes that cause disease have been identified, many of them because of the work of the Human Genome Project and the existence of newer DNA-based technologies. In 1994–1995, for example, two defective genes, labeled BRCA-1 and BRCA-2, were found to be present in Jewish women from Eastern Europe. These genes might explain the high rate of breast cancer in that population. Genetic disorders come in several varieties. Inherited disorders are passed on from parent to child. Acquired disorders appear later in life as a result of genetic alteration, perhaps due to chemical or environmental toxicities. In addition to diseases directly related to a single gene or a pair of genes, a number of common illnesses—such as most breast cancers, Alzheimer's disease, which causes mental and physical deterioration, and coronary artery disease—are most likely caused by a combination of genetics and environment.

Once a disease-causing gene is identified, a test to determine whether or not a particular individual carries that gene is often developed. The ability to test for such genes has benefits and burdens. The most common use is in prenatal screening, in which a fetus can be tested for a number of chromosomal abnormalities. Premarital screening is also used—particularly among ethnic groups predisposed to certain diseases—so that couples can make informed reproductive choices. The knowledge that one is prone to develop a certain disease can lead to preventive measures such as changes in diet, exercise, and early treatment. The knowledge that these tests provide can be reassuring, or it can force difficult choices—such as whether to marry, conceive a child, or abort a pregnancy.

Choices become more problematic in diseases where children may be affected later in life. For example, should a child be tested for Huntington's disease? If the child is tested and found to be carrying the gene, should he or she be told? How would a young person weigh the concern of becoming demented in adult life against the importance of having that information for his or her future mate and potential children?

Whatever the personal decisions made in these cases, nearly everyone concerned about genetic testing worries about its impact on insurance. As the number of genetic tests increases, and as they become routine in medical practice, more and more diseases and predispositions will be identified and entered into a person's medical record. Who will have access to that information? For what purposes? Medical information of all kinds is now transmitted routinely to insurance companies who use it to validate claims, accept or deny applications for insurance, and to set actuarial standards (making estimates of future claims).

The following selections present different points of view about the use of genetic tests for insurance. The American Council of Life Insurance and the Health Insurance Association of America, both large trade associations, assert that while they do not currently use or plan to use genetic test results in their evaluation of individuals, they must remain free to use whatever information is relevant to maintaining fair rates for all their policyholders. Thomas H. Murray sees this use of "fairness" as flawed, particularly because health insurance is a system with social and moral responsibilities to maintain access to medical care for those in need.

YES

**American Council of
Life Insurance and
Health Insurance
Association of America**

REPORT OF THE ACLI-HIAA TASK FORCE ON GENETIC TESTING

THE ADVENT OF GENETIC TESTING

Genetic science has advanced dramatically in recent years. From gene splicing to gene mapping to gene therapy, astounding scientific breakthroughs have occurred frequently with each discovery being more impressive than the last. The federal government's creation in 1988 of the Human Genome Initiative has further accelerated the pace of discovery and captured the public's attention.

Hope abounds that the Human Genome Initiative will find new ways to prevent and cure disease. But there is also real fear that genetic science may unleash undesirable social problems. Some of the deepest concerns that have been raised relate to how insurance companies and employers might someday use genetic test results to infringe on the right to privacy and improperly deny people access to jobs or insurance coverage.

The American Council of life Insurance (ACLI) and the Health Insurance Association of America (HIAA) recognize the public's hopes and fears about genetic testing. The ACLI and the HIAA are acutely aware that the advent of genetic testing will bring with it many questions about the insurance industry's practices in the areas of risk selection, medical expense reimbursement and protection of medical information. Inevitably, insurance issues occupy a central place in the discussions of the legal, ethical and social dimensions of this new-found technology. . . .

PUBLIC CONCERNS ABOUT INSURANCE

The public policy debate already under way in academic circles is raising significant policy issues for the insurance business. At numerous conferences held across the country during the past year, speakers routinely expressed concern for how insurers might use genetic test information. They expressed fears that insurers would begin using genetic information to deny coverage for large segments of the population. And they questioned whether insurers can be trusted to keep sensitive genetic testing records confidential.

The Task Force believes that for insurers, the two most controversial issues to emerge from the debate will be how genetic information might be used in risk classification to determine insurability and how the confidentiality of such information will be protected. Risk classification, at its center, is the ability of the insurer to appraise an applicant's insurability so that coverage may be offered at an appropriate and fair premium. Confidentiality is the protection of personal information obtained in the course of underwriting an application or administering a claim. Genetic testing promises to draw keen public attention to these two aspects of the insurance business.

Public Concerns: Risk Classification and Insurability

The cornerstone of a private voluntary insurance system is risk classification. Insurers must be able to appraise risks in order to group similar risks together, to forecast costs, and to establish fair and adequate premium rates. As fundamental as this may seem to the insurance industry, however, it is a concept seldom comprehended and oftentimes found objectionable by the public at large.

What the public does understand is insurance availability. This is especially true in the area of health insurance, where in recent years accessibility and affordability have been seriously jeopardized by soaring health care costs. Given this orientation towards insurance, the public tends to view genetic testing as yet another threat to insurance accessibility. A concern widely expressed is that genetic testing will create a "genetic underclass" and swell the ranks of uninsured individuals.

At various forums where knowledgeable people have gathered together to discuss genetic testing, some of the strongest concerns have focused on whether genetic testing will foreclose large numbers of people from the health insurance market. Life insurance availability seems not to arouse the same fervent sentiments, presumably because life insurance is not perceived as an entitlement to the same extent as health insurance.

Those who have reflected on genetic testing and insurance have raised a myriad of questions. Would insurers deny coverage to healthy individuals with a genetic predisposition for a particular disease? Will insurers refrain from using genetic tests until they are proven reliable? Would insurers cancel existing coverages based on genetic test results? Would insurers refuse coverage for new-borns if insured parents are asymptomatic carriers of a disease or disorder?

To some extent, it seems that those who ask the questions already have preconceived notions that insurers will use genetic testing to unfairly discriminate against genetically "inferior" individuals. Such questions are often asked in rhetorical fashion as though it were a foregone conclusion that the insurance industry stands ready to fully embrace genetic testing as a means to achieve perfect risk selection.

The truth is that the insurance industry is approaching genetic testing with great caution and a certain degree of trepidation. No one—either inside or outside the insurance industry—knows for sure how genetic testing will affect existing insurance practices. At this point, what is known is that genetic testing has had little or no impact on insurance. And as for the future, there is ample reason to doubt whether genetic testing will ever significantly alter insurance as we know it today.

The Task Force believes that it is important, amidst the rhetoric and anecdotal stories about genetic discrimination, not to lose sight of the important facts we do know about genetic testing and insurance. Those should serve to allay much of the public's uneasiness about genetic testing and ought to serve as a starting point for establishing any public policy with regard to genetic testing and insurance. Here are some of the points which the Task Force finds noteworthy:

- Life insurance is widely available today and likely to stay that way. Statistics show that an overwhelming 97 percent of applications for ordinary life insurance are accepted—92 percent at standard rates and 5 percent substandard. Only 3 percent of those who apply for coverage are declined. The fact is that insurance underwriting is not a barrier to the vast majority of Americans seeking life insurance. It has yet to be shown whether introducing genetic testing into the underwriting process would substantially change the industry's broad acceptance of applicants.

- Most health insurance is not individually underwritten and so genetic testing would have no effect on the vast majority of health insurance consumers. About 85–90 percent of health insurance is currently purchased through group plans which accept all full-time employees and dependents without evidence of insurability. For those individuals who are not members of an employer group and cannot get health insurance today, the issue is more often cost than insurability. Admittedly, there are gaps in our health insurance system for which workable solutions are needed —such as high-risk insurance pools, small-employer market reforms, and increased Medicaid coverage of the poor. However, the fact remains that genetic testing is unlikely to affect the typical American health insurance consumer who gets coverage through an existing employer-based group health plan.

- The difficulty that small employers face in securing health insurance coverage for their employees when one or more of them is high risk has been of tremendous concern to the industry. In response, the HIAA has developed a comprehensive set of legislative reforms aimed at assuring that private insurance coverage is always available to small employers regardless of the health of their employees. Most important for the concerns posed by genetic testing is that these market reforms will assure that high-risk employees are not denied coverage. Furthermore, people with existing health conditions would be required to satisfy pre-existing condition exclusions for a single, specified time only. If the employer were to change insurers or the employee to change jobs, new pre-existing exclusion time periods would not be imposed. Under these reforms, if enacted, genetic conditions would not affect the ability of employees to obtain and maintain affordable health insurance coverage.

- No insurer—life or health—currently requires genetic tests. One simple and practical reason is cost. Most available tests are far too expensive to be routinely used in the underwriting process. The test for Huntington's disease, for example, costs thousands of dollars. Though costs may come down over time (a cystic fibrosis test now exists for about $200) it will be years and perhaps decades before insurers could realistically afford genetic testing on any wide-scale basis.
- Although an estimated 4,000 genetic disorders and diseases have been identified, predispositions to many of these illnesses are already detectable, to some extent. For example, predisposition to heart disease is already detected through high cholesterol and high blood pressure levels. Family history already gives insurers information about an individual's possible predisposition to diseases like Alzheimer's and some cancers.
- Sickle cell anemia can be detected at a very young age without a genetic test. Thus, many of the illnesses potentially predictable through genetic testing are already known and factored into insurers' underwriting decisions.
- Genetic testing is no crystal ball. Genetic tests will not tell when an illness will strike nor will most of them tell for sure whether an illness will strike. Experts agree that environmental and lifestyle factors can have a large influence on inherited diseases. Such factors include diet, smoking, drinking, exercise, stress and occupation. Also, early detection will enable individuals to take precautions or possibly seek treatment to control or eliminate increased risk. Because there are so many variables that influence the onset of a genetic disease, it cannot be assumed insurers would deny coverage based merely on a genetic test result.
- It is estimated that the average person carries six to eight genes that could lead to diseases. Obviously, insurers would soon go out of business if they denied coverage to everyone with a genetically-diagnosed predisposition.

Above all, it cannot be emphasized enough that insurers are not using genetic tests in risk assessment, nor are there any plans to do so. Genetic tests are not of immediate concern for the life and health insurance industry, because health care providers are using them infrequently.

The Task Force believes that genetic research should be allowed to run its course independent of insurance considerations. Premature legal constraints on the use of such technology at this point in time would only serve to preclude the development of balanced guidelines for the responsible use of genetic testing information. In the meantime, however, the insurance industry should be monitoring the progress of genetic testing, periodically re-assessing the potential ramifications of genetic testing on insurance availability, and developing lines of communication with public policymakers on how to harness the positive aspects of genetic testing while mitigating potentially adverse consequences. . . .

INSURERS' CONCERNS ABOUT ADVERSE SELECTION

It is interesting to note that insurers may be more fearful of genetic testing than are consumers. While customers fear how insurers may use genetic testing to deny coverage or invade privacy, insurers fear how consumers could use genetic testing to foresee coverage needs and exploit the insurance system. Insurers are concerned about a phenomenon known as "adverse selection" which ultimately drives up the cost of insurance for most people. Adverse selection (also called, "anti-selection") is the disproportionately heavy purchase of insurance by persons who are higher risks than their insurers are aware.[1] It is notable that a recent survey conducted by the Task Force into the attitudes of insurance underwriting officials reveals that few, if any, insurers see genetic testing as a means to improve risk selection. But those same officials expressed grave concerns about the potential for adverse selection if insurers were ever denied access to the results of genetic tests already known to the applicant.

Based on preliminary actuarial analyses and fundamental principles of anti-selection, these concerns of insurance underwriters are well-founded. Actuarial experts, who took a closer look at the potential for adverse selection in the event insurers were ever denied access to genetic testing information, concluded that the costs of adverse selection would vary widely depending on the particular disease, but that the cumulative cost of adverse selection for the total spectrum of genetic diseases could be quite significant. Simply put, if insurers are denied access to genetic test results, the amount paid out in insurance claims could increase substantially and the result would be higher premiums for most policyholders.

Though it should be self-evident why insurers need all relevant medical information to perform accurate risk assessment and avoid anti-selection, the unfortunate reality is that many policymakers give short shrift to such concerns. Too often there is a failure to appreciate how adverse selection harms the average, well-meaning policyholder. As a result, simplistic proposals to prohibit insurers from obtaining genetic testing information are introduced and advanced in the name of consumer protection.

The Task Force believes legislative initiatives to limit insurer access to genetic test results are forthcoming and will garner considerable political support. Given the ground swell of public awareness and apprehension towards genetic testing, defeating such proposals will be no small task. The challenge facing the insurance industry, as is so often the case with issues involving risk classification, will be to educate lawmakers on the ramifications of adverse selection and to prove the need for full disclosure by the insurance applicants, including the disclosure of genetic test results.

NOTES

1. It is important to distinguish clearly between insurers requiring genetic tests and insurers having access to genetic test information. As discussed above, the prospect of insurers ordering genetic tests in the course of reviewing an insurance application seems highly remote at this time. But genetic testing is slowly seeping into clinical medicine. There will likely be an increasing amount of genetic testing performed by medical specialists. It is the results of those tests—ordered not by the insurers but by the patients and doctors themselves—which may give rise to the problem of adverse selection.

NO

Thomas H. Murray

GENETICS AND THE MORAL MISSION OF HEALTH INSURANCE

All men are created equal. So reads one of the United States of America's founding political documents. This stirring affirmation of equality was not meant as a claim that all people are equivalent in all respects. Surely the drafters of the Declaration of Independence and the Constitution were as aware then as we are now of the wondrous variety of humankind. People differ in their appearance, their talents, and their character, among other things, and those differences matter enormously.

The commitment to equality embodied in our political tradition is not a claim that people, in fact, are indistinguishable from one another. Rather it is an assertion that before this government, this system of laws and courts, all persons are to be given equal standing, and all persons must be treated with equal regard.

Human genetics, in contrast, is a *science of inequality*—a study of human particularity and difference. One of the most difficult challenges facing us in the coming flood tide of genetic information is how to assimilate these evidences of human differences without undermining our commitment to political, legal, and moral equality.

The information about human differences pouring forth from the science of human genetics provides us with a multitude of opportunities to treat people differently according to some aspect of their genetic makeup. Deciding which uses of this information are just and which are unjust will require us to reexamine the ethical significance of a wide variety of human differences and the larger social purposes of a variety of institutions, among them health, life, and other forms of insurance.

Health insurance in the United States has moved from a system based mostly on community rating where, in a given community, all people pay comparable rates, to a system where the cost to the purchasers of insurance is based on the expected claims—a risk- or experienced-based system. This movement has significant ethical as well as economic overtones. Community rating was a system that reflected a notion of community responsibility for providing health care for its members, where the qualifying principle was

From Thomas H. Murray, "Genetics and the Moral Mission of Health Insurance," *Hastings Center Report*, vol. 22, no. 6 (November/December 1992). Copyright © 1992 by The Hastings Center. Reprinted by permission.

community membership. Other differences, such as preexisting risks, did not count as morally relevant distinctions. Risk-and experience-based systems presume that it is fair to charge different prices, or to refuse to insure people entirely, if they will need expensive health care. Such systems treat predicted need for care as a morally relevant difference among persons that justifies differential access to health insurance, and through it, to health care. But this presumes precisely what is in question: what are good moral reasons for treating people differently with respect to access to health insurance and health care? . . .

GENETICS AND DISTRIBUTIVE JUSTICE

Distributive justice, as the term implies, concerns the distribution of social goods or ills: in its simplest formulation it holds that like cases are to be treated alike and unlike cases are to be treated differently. All depends, obviously, on how we fill in the material conditions of this purely formal statement of comparative justice. When we are asking about a particular occasion of just or unjust treatment, the question commonly takes the form, What makes these cases like or unlike in a morally relevant way? Failure to state a morally relevant reason for treating people differently opens one to the charge that one's action was arbitrary, capricious, and unjust.

Human genetics provides a large and rapidly growing set of differences among persons that may be used to try to justify unequal treatment. For many genetic differences and many distributions of social goods, the moral relevance of the difference seems transparently obvious. Height, for example, is largely determined by genetics. Does it make any sense to say that it was unfair to allow Kareem Abdul Jabaar to play center in the National Basketball Association for many years, but not me, just because he is taller than I am, and our differences in height are genetic, rather than anything we can claim credit for accomplishing? Most people would judge that to be absurd. In this instance a genetic difference —height—constitutes a morally relevant difference that justifies treating people differently. That same difference, however, would not justify treating us differently if, for example, we were accused of a crime, or being judged on our literary accomplishments, or in need of health care. . . .

Having health insurance is a way to pay for . . . treatment—the cost of treating a serious illness can easily exceed an average family's ability to pay for it. Health insurance is, for most people, the means to the end of health care. It is not the good of health care itself. But to the extent that it determines who does and who does not have access to care, and who has the peace of mind that comes with knowing that if care is needed it will be available, access to health insurance is a matter of justice.

GENETIC TESTING: THE CHALLENGE FOR HEALTH INSURANCE

Research in human genetics, such as the Genome Project, is likely to increase dramatically our ability to predict whether individuals are at risk for particular diseases. There are tests currently offered for diseases such as Huntington's, where the presence of the gene assures that the individual will develop the disease if he or she lives long enough. There are tests for carrier status such as cystic fibrosis where two copies of the defective gene —one from each parent—must be inherited in order for symptomatic disease to occur. And there will be tests for diseases of complex etiology such as heart disease, cancer, stroke, lung disease, and the like. For certain relatively rare genes there will be a strong connection between having the gene and having the disease. Yet most of the common killing and disabling diseases are more likely to have a complex variety of causes, including perhaps several genes each of which has some predictive relationship with the disease. These risk-oriented genetic predictors potentially are very interesting to employers and insurers.

Genetic information, in fact, is used now by insurers. There may be considerable genetic information in one's medical record. If your policy is being individually underwritten, that entire record can be copied and shipped to the prospective insurer and that information used to justify increasing the price or denying health insurance altogether. But this begs a prior question: should information about genetic differences be used at all in health insurance?

One argument against paying any special attention to genetic predictors of risk is that insurers already use risk predictors that have genetic components. Coronary artery disease is an example. It is well known that people with higher levels of cholesterol, especially the low-density-lipoprotein component, are at higher risk of coronary artery disease and subsequent heart attacks. It also seems clear that an individual's cholesterol level is at least in part determined by genetics. Variations in individual metabolism can have a substantial impact on a person's cholesterol level, such that two people can be equally virtuous (or careless) in diet and exercise and yet have very different cholesterol levels, and, presumably, very different risks for coronary artery disease and heart attack.

In time it is likely that researchers will discover a number of genes that affect cholesterol metabolism and, presumably, cholesterol level, arterial disease, and the risk of a heart attack. We may be able to construct a genetic profile of an individual's risk of heart disease. Does such a predictive index differ in any ethically significant way from today's cholesterol test, which has not evoked similar objections?

Genetic tests differ from a cholesterol test in that the latter, even if significantly influenced by genetics, is still in some measure under the individual's control. The risk of heart attack is affected by a variety of health-related behaviors including diet, exercise, stress, and smoking. To the extent that people can be held responsible for their behavior, their cholesterol level is something for which they have some responsibility. On the other hand, people cannot be said to be responsible for their genes. An old maxim in ethics is "Ought implies can." You should not be held morally accountable for that which you were powerless to influence.

Genetic tests may also have more direct distributional consequences. Alleles occur in different frequencies in different ethnic groups; it would not be surprising to find that an allele associated with an epidemiologically significant disease such as coronary artery disease was more prevalent in some ethnic groups than in others. Alpha-1 antitrypsin deficiency, associated with lung disease, appears to be more common among people of Scandinavian ancestry. If the group in which the allele occurs more often was not historically a target of discrimination, we might not be particularly concerned. If, however, the allele was more common in a group that continues to suffer discrimination, such as sickle-cell trait in people of African descent, we would have good reason for concern. The mere fact that genetic predictors have the potential to affect differentially ethnic groups that experience discrimination does not uniquely distinguish them from other risk predictors. Hypertension, for example, is more prevalent among Americans of African heritage. But the immediate and direct tie between genetics and ethnicity may make genetic testing a more blatant use of a potentially explosive and discriminatory social classification scheme.

A third response to the claim that we need not worry about genetic risk testing because it is essentially similar to things like cholesterol testing is to question the premise that people know about the genetic component of cholesterol. Discussions of cholesterol in the media emphasize the things people can do to lower it. Reminders that cholesterol level is also significantly affected by genetics appear less frequently, and it may well be that most people are unaware that cholesterol level has a substantial genetic component. If people did understand that, perhaps they would be less tolerant of the widespread use of cholesterol testing to determine insurance eligibility, precisely because it was to that extent outside of individuals' control.

There is yet another possibility: that the central notion underlying commercial health insurance underwriting—the greater the likelihood of illness, the more one should pay for coverage—is morally unsound.

ACTUARIAL FAIRNESS

Insurers take a particular view of fairness: actuarial fairness. Actuarial fairness claims that "policyholders with the same expected risk of loss should be treated equally.... An insurance company has the responsibility to treat all its policyholders fairly by establishing premiums at a level consistent with the risk represented by each individual policyholder."[1] This definition of fairness begs the question: Why should we count differences in risk of disease as an ethically relevant justification for treating people differently in their access to health insurance and health care?

Actuarial fairness does have a realm of application in which it seems reasonable. Call it the Lloyds of London model: if two oil tanker companies ask to have their cargoes and vessels insured, one for a trip up the Atlantic to a U.S. port, the other for a voyage through the Arabian Gulf during the height of the war in Kuwait and Iraq, the owner of the first ship would cry foul if she were charged the same extraordinarily high rate as the owner of the second. Most of us, I suspect, would agree that charging the two owners the same rate would be unfair. What makes it so?

For one thing, the two ships are exposed to vastly different risks, and it seems only fair to charge them accordingly. (The process of assessing risks is called underwriting.) Furthermore, the risks were assumed voluntarily. Third, the goal of both owners is profit, and it seems reasonable to ask them to bear the expense of voluntarily assumed risks. We could also ask how commercial insurance divides up the world. In this hypothetical [situation] it divides it into those who prefer prudent business ventures and those willing to take great risks. That does not seem to be an objectionable way to parse the world for the purpose of insuring oil tankers.

In practice, insurers do not behave as if actuarial fairness were an ironclad moral rule. Valid predictors may not be used for a variety of reasons, typically having to do with other notions of fairness —for example, not discriminating on the basis of race, sex, class, or locale, even though these characteristics are related to the likelihood of insurance claims. Deborah Stone, who has studied insurance practices for HIV infection, dismisses the idea of actuarial fairness and argues instead that:

> insurability is the set of policy decisions by insurers about whom to accept. It is not a trait, but a concept of *membership*.... Treated as a scientific fact about individuals, the notion of insurability disguises fundamentally political decisions about membership in a community of mutual responsibility.[2] ...

UNDERWRITING AND THE SOCIAL PURPOSES OF INSURANCE

The threat genetic testing poses to the future of insurance for health-related risks —including health, life, and disability insurance—compels us to reexamine the social purposes served by insurance. Two points are obvious: first, that different types of insurance can have different purposes; and second, that the purpose of a particular form of insurance must be understood within its social context.

Life insurance, for example, is meant to provide financial security for one's dependents in the event that one dies. In the contemporary United States we must evaluate the role of such insurance in the context of a not particularly generous social welfare system that would otherwise leave the surviving dependents of a deceased breadwinner in very poor financial condition. The typical purchaser is an individual with one or more dependents who are unlikely to become financially independent in the immediate future. The benefits from life insurance are intended to tide survivors over until they can become financially self-sufficient, or live out their lives decently; they are not meant to provide windfalls to friends of the deceased. To the extent that life insurance is perceived as serving a need rather than being merely a commodity, we are likely to regard it as something that ought to be available to all. Our public policies toward life insurance suggest we view it otherwise, however. We prohibit certain actuarially valid distinctions such as ethnicity in setting life insurance rates. But we do not require that all persons, whatever their age, employment, or health, be permitted to buy life insurance at identical prices or at all. In consequence, the financial dependents of a person unable to obtain life insurance may suffer devastating changes in their life prospects if the principal earner dies.

Does the Lloyds of London model fit health care? Despite the current enthusiasm for tying voluntary behavior to health, most illness and disability is neither chosen nor in any sense "deserved," distinguishing it from the risks of shipping oil in a war zone. Neither is the goal of health care for those who seek it profit. Daniels argues that "justice requires that we protect *fair equality of opportunity* for individuals in a society." Reasonable access to health care in the contemporary United States is a necessary condition for fair equality of opportunity to pursue other goods that life affords. The social purpose of health insurance, understood in this way, is to provide access to the health care that people need to have a fair opportunity in life.

Lastly, how does underwriting in health insurance divide the world? It sets off the well from the ill and those likely to become ill. For insurers, the concept of actuarial fairness provides a rationale for charging much higher rates or declining to insure persons with a substantial possibility of illness or disability, reasoning that such persons should bear the costs associated with their particular risks. Persons at risk could find it difficult to obtain insurance at affordable rates, or at all. ...

IMPLICATIONS FOR POLICY

The era of predictive genetic testing coincides with a period of grave public concern about health care. ...

There is little doubt that the current ragged system of private and public programs, with its many holes and frayed edges, must be changed. The conviction that health care ought to be available to those who need it seems to be widely shared. That conviction, together with a growing sense that the current patchwork is failing, may be strong enough to overcome the citizenry's hesitations about government inefficiency. Indeed, it seems likely that private health insurance would not have survived this long if not for government intervention. Tax subsidies for employer-sponsored health insurance programs amounted to $39.5 billion in 1991.[3] In addition, we provide direct government coverage for the health needs of people that commercial insurers want to avoid: Medicare, for those much more likely to need health care; and Medicaid, for some of those unable to pay for their own insurance.

Public programs such as Medicare and Medicaid tell us something important about our moral convictions on health care. They suggest that we are not content to allow the old and the poor simply to languish without access to care. Had we not passed such legislation, we well might have overturned or radically restructured the existing system of commercial health insurance decades ago.

There are good reasons to doubt that actuarial fairness is an adequate description of genuine fairness in health insurance. It may be a sufficient principle for commercial insurance against losses of ships at sea, but even a brief inquiry into the social purpose of health insurance suggests that apportioning by risks, as actuarial fairness dictates, fails to accomplish the primary social goals of health insurance. Genetic tests, like other predictors of the need for health care, are not good reasons for treating people differently with respect to access to health insurance.

REFERENCES

Karen A. Clifford and R. P. Iuculano, "AIDS and Insurance: The Rationale for AIDS-Related Testing," *Harvard Law Review* 100 (1987): 1806–24.

Deborah A. Stone, "AIDS and the Moral Economy of Insurance," *American Prospect* 1 (1990): 62–73.

John K. Iglehart, "The American Health Care System: Private Insurance," *NEJM* 326 (1992): 1715–20.

POSTSCRIPT

Should Health Insurance Companies Have Access to Information from Genetic Testing?

The federal Health Insurance Portability and Accountability Act, signed by President Bill Clinton in August 1996, declares that genetic information itself is not a preexisting condition. The law provides that someone who has had a genetic test predicting a high risk of developing a disease later in life but who is not yet ill cannot be denied insurance on the grounds of the test alone. However, insurance rates are not covered by the law. On the state level, in 1996 a comprehensive Genetic Privacy Act intended to protect the rights of people who choose to obtain predictive genetic testing was passed in New Jersey. In 1993 the Human Genome Project's Task Force on Genetic Information and Insurance recommended that "information about past, present or future health status, including genetic information, should not be used to deny health care coverage or services to anyone."

In "Genetic Testing and the Social Responsibility of Private Health Insurance Companies," *Journal of Law, Medicine and Ethics* (Spring 1993), Nancy S. Jecker argues that "socially responsible insurance companies will avoid genetic discrimination." The existence of discrimination as a consequence of genetic testing is documented in an article by Paul R. Billings et al. in the *American Journal of Human Genetics* (vol. 50, 1992). The American Medical Association's position on the use of genetic testing by employers, outlined in the *Journal of the American Medical Association* (October 2, 1991), is that it generally opposes genetic testing by employers, but it recognizes a limited exception in excluding workers who have a genetic susceptibility to occupational illness.

For more general readings on genetic screening, social policy, and the history of modern genetics, see Lori B. Andrews et al., *Assessing Genetic Risks: Implication for Health and Social Policy* (National Academy Press, 1994); Robert F. Weir, Susan C. Lawrence, and Evan Fales, eds., *Genes and Human Self-Knowledge: Historical and Philosophical Reflections on Modern Genetics* (University of Iowa Press, 1994); and Pat Milmoe McCarrick, *Genetic Testing and Genetic Screening* (Scope Note No. 22, Kennedy Institute of Ethics, 1993).

For more resources on this issue, see the following Web site of the University of Pennsylvania's Center for Bioethics: http://www.med.upenn.edu/~bioethic/library/resources/genetics.html. This Web site contains information on ethical issues in genetics and genetic testing as well as links to other helpful sites and centers.

ISSUE 15

Should Parents Always Be Told of Genetic-Testing Availability?

YES: Mary Z. Pelias, from "Duty to Disclose in Medical Genetics: A Legal Perspective," *American Journal of Medical Genetics* (vol. 39, 1991)

NO: Diane E. Hoffmann and Eric A. Wulfsberg, from "Testing Children for Genetic Predispositions: Is It in Their Best Interest?" *Journal of Law, Medicine and Ethics* (vol. 23, no. 4, 1995)

ISSUE SUMMARY

YES: Mary Z. Pelias, attorney and professor of genetics, argues that parental autonomy and family privacy should govern decisions about whether or not to test children for genetic predispositions to disease and that physicians and genetic counselors have an obligation to disclose full information.

NO: Law professor Diane E. Hoffmann and pediatrician Eric A. Wulfsberg assert that caution and restraint should govern decisions on testing for genetic predispositions in children and that safeguards should be adopted to diminish the potentially negative effects of testing and to protect children's best interests.

Among the most dramatic results of the Human Genome Project, which is designed to determine the complete chemical sequence of human DNA, is the identification of an ever-increasing number of genetically linked conditions. To date, more than 900 genes associated with disease have been found. One example is Huntington's disease, a disorder that leads to mental and neurological deterioration and eventually death. About 100,000 people in the United States are at risk for this disease, which typically begins to be noticed in the patient's late 30s or early 40s. Another genetically linked condition is adult polycystic kidney disease, which accounts for about 10 percent of all end-stage renal disease in the United States. Still another condition is alpha1-antitrypsin deficiency, an enzyme deficiency that leads to a high risk of early-onset emphysema in at-risk individuals of Scandinavian ancestry. Genes linked to particular forms of breast cancer and colon cancer have also been identified, and genes that predict a high risk of other forms of cancer, heart disease, and Alzheimer's disease are likely to be found before long.

Tests for detecting predisposition to a number of genetic disorders are already available, and others are likely to enter the marketplace in coming years. Screening of newborns for some genetically linked or maternally transmitted diseases, especially those that are treatable and likely to manifest symptoms in childhood, is well established, although in some cases it remains controversial. In many states, newborns are routinely screened for sickle-cell disease, a blood condition that targets African Americans in particular, and for phenylketonuria (PKU), a rare but treatable enzyme deficiency that affects a child's ability to absorb certain types of nutrition. Some forms of screening are used primarily to aid reproductive decision making—the goal is to determine if one or both partners carry a disease-linked gene that may put their offspring at risk. Tay-Sachs disease, which primarily affects Jewish families from Eastern Europe and kills affected infants within a few years, is one example. As a result of prenatal screening, fewer babies have been born with Tay-Sachs disease since 1989. A DNA test was also initiated for cystic fibrosis; it has been used primarily by couples with a family history that puts them at risk. Cystic fibrosis is the most common life-threatening genetic disorder to affect people of European descent, but other population groups may be affected as well. About 8 million Americans are believed to carry the cystic fibrosis gene.

For adults, the decision to be tested for genetic conditions is difficult and troubling, carrying as it does the risks of learning negative information, the potential for insurance and employment discrimination, and the sense that life choices have become restricted. Decisions about whether or not to test one's children are even weightier. While testing for a genetic condition for which treatment exists (as is now the case with sickle-cell disease) involves one set of considerations, testing for a condition that cannot be treated or may not show up until the individual is well into adulthood, if at all, involves markedly different and more complex decision making.

The authors of the following selections take opposing views as to whether or not children should be tested for genes that may predict illness and as to who should decide. Mary Z. Pelias invokes the long history of patient and parental autonomy, full disclosure, and informed consent in claiming that physicians' withholding of genetic testing for children is a form of medical paternalism. Diane E. Hoffmann and Eric A. Wulfsberg call on another long-standing tradition—protecting the best interests of children—in urging restraint and caution in utilizing testing that may have serious negative effects with no balancing benefits.

YES
Mary Z. Pelias

DUTY TO DISCLOSE IN MEDICAL GENETICS: A LEGAL PERSPECTIVE

IMPLICATIONS IN MEDICAL GENETICS: TESTING AND COUNSELING FOR DELETERIOUS GENES

The power of geneticists to detect the presence of deleterious genes has increased rapidly with progressive refinements in the use of DNA markers. As technical knowledge expands, so does the power of the geneticist to influence the lives of clients who seek counseling about their own genetic status or the status of their children. In this developing context, the geneticist may experience most vividly the contrast between the beneficent care-giver and the client whose autonomy must be respected. Here, depending on the law of the state where a lawsuit arises, the geneticist may appreciate the full impact of the judicial mandate to impart all information that is material to a patient's decision-making process (Canterbury v. Spence, 1972).

Nowhere has the power of the medical geneticist been expressed more clearly than in recent suggestions about predictive testing for the gene that causes Huntington disease. Several authors have recommended that predictive testing should be unavailable both for minor children and for couples who seek prenatal testing but equivocate about terminating a high risk pregnancy (Bloch and Hayden, 1990; Committee of IHA and WFN, 1990). Parents of minor children would be classified as third parties, whose interests in their own minor children are equated with interests of "adoption agencies, educational institutions, insurance companies, and other third parties." Limiting the interests of parents by classifying them as third parties is proposed as a means of protecting the privacy and autonomy of the minor child. Genetic counseling would be directed toward discouraging parents and at-risk couples from seeking information. Since no immediate advantage can be predicted for minor children whose genetic status is investigated, the refusal by professionals to test children or at-risk couples is viewed as a policy that supports the best interests of family life and the emotional and psychological security of children who may harbor the gene. These arguments against disclosure rest on the facts that Huntington disease is a late-onset disorder and that no treatment is presently available.

These suggestions must have resulted from considerable deliberation, and they are unquestionably sincere. However, they raise serious questions about paternalism in genetic counseling and about the duty of a counselor to his client. They also challenge the principles of parental autonomy and of the privacy of the family unit in our culture. The fundamental issue is neither the nature of the specific genetic disease nor the availability of any treatment but, rather, a renewed tension between the beneficence model of patient care and the rights of parents to their own autonomy and to the protection of their family units.

Although references to constitutional history may have only peripheral interest in suits of professional negligence, the holdings of the Supreme Court are nonetheless regarded as reflections of the values of our society. On several occasions the Supreme Court has affirmed the sanctity of the family unit, so that courts and legislatures are now loathe to interfere with this most basic social group. The scope of "liberty" guaranteed to every American by the fourteenth amendment was addressed in a frequently quoted case involving the role of parents in making educational decisions for their children:

Without doubt, [liberty] denotes not merely freedom from bodily restraint but also the right of the individual to contract, to engage in any of the common occupations of life, to acquire useful knowledge, to marry, establish a home and bring up children, to worship God according to the dictates of his own conscience, and generally to enjoy those privileges long recognized at common law as essential to the orderly pursuit of happiness by free men (Meyer v. Nebraska, 1923).

This holding was reinforced when the Court later affirmed "the liberty of parents and guardians to direct the upbringing and education of children under their control" (Pierce v. Society of Sisters, 1925). More recently, in the context of making medical decisions for minor children, the Court noted that "[s]tate law vests decisional responsibility in the parents, in the first instance" (Bowen v. American Hosp. Ass'n, 1986). This judicial thrust was supported by the President's Commission for the Study of Ethical problems in Medicine and Biomedical and Behavioral Research when it noted that

[T]here is a presumption, strong but rebuttable, that parents are the appropriate decisionmakers for their infants. Traditional law concerning the family, buttressed by the emerging right of privacy, protects a substantial range of discretion for parents (President's Commission, 1983).

Considerations by both the judicial and administrative branches of federal government have thus affirmed the role of parents as the primary decision makers in the lives of their children. Any attempt to usurp the parental role contradicts this clearly expressed public policy, and justification of such an effort would indeed have to be compelling in order to survive a constitutional challenge. The geneticist who defines parents as "third parties" in relation to their own children and assumes the right to make parental decisions acts without regard to our history of protecting the parental prerogative.

A more realistic hazard for the medical geneticist lies in the possibility of being sued in tort for failure to disclose all information material to the plaintiff's decision-making process. When a practicing geneticist assumes the role of guardian of the privacy and autonomy of children who may have deleterious genes, he assumes the role of the parents of these children. If the geneticist then fails to disclose complete information to the parents of these children, he risks allegations of injury to both the parents and the child. Parents deprived of complete information about the genetic status of their children will assert that their parental autonomy was compromised when they were deprived of the chance to explore every available opportunity for their child with a deleterious gene. Children will also claim injury resulting from these diminished opportunities. Parents denied prenatal testing when they refuse to commit to aborting an affected, or high risk, fetus, will have actions in wrongful birth, and children born to these parents may have actions in wrongful life.[1] The plaintiffs may demonstrate that these lost opportunities should be compensable and may well recover substantial damages.

Beyond the practical aspects of litigation may lie a far greater hazard to the profession of medical genetics. Most medical geneticists have adopted a policy of non-directive counseling aimed at communicating information and helping clients understand and cope with their situations (Fraser, 1974; Ad Hoc Committee on Genetic Counseling, 1975). If medical geneticists now adopt a policy of limiting the information available for disclosure, or if counseling becomes so directive as to solicit an agreement to terminate an affected pregnancy in return for prenatal testing, it can only be a matter of time before these situations are exposed in court and exploited in the media. Such exposure and exploitation could severely damage the credibility of the profession. This risk can be avoided, however, by respecting the autonomy of clients and adopting a policy and a practice of full, unconditional disclosure.

Another question of disclosure that arises in the context of testing for deleterious genes is whether the geneticist has any obligation, or right, to disclose genetic information to third parties, including collateral relatives who participate in a study, or schools, employers, or insurance companies. With respect to disclosure to participating collateral relatives, 3 facts must be considered. First, both the client and the relative are protected by their rights to privacy and to personal autonomy. Second, any exchange between a physician and his patient is confidential. The only legal precedent for breaking this confident is knowledge by the physician that the patient poses a foreseeable danger to an identifiable third party, in particular, a psychiatrist's knowledge of a patient's threats of bodily harm to his former girlfriend (Tarasoff v. Regents of the Univ. of Cal., 1976; Davis v. Lhim, 1983). Third, while the geneticist may not discover information that is immediately life-threatening, as in *Tarasoff* or *Davis*, the information may well have a significant influence on a relative's family planning decisions and on the children who are born to that relative. With these facts in mind, then, the geneticist should have the consent of both his client and the participating collateral relative before revealing any information to the relative. Any fortuitous information about non-participating relatives should ideally be kept in confidence until an inquiry is initiated by that relative himself. Certainly the geneticist is in a position to encourage communication among family members, but he is obliged to respect the privacy, autonomy, and confidentiality of those with whom he has direct contact....

SUMMARY AND CONCLUSIONS

During the past century the physician-patient relationship has evolved from the beneficent approach to providing health care to an approach that gives great deference to the patient's moral and legal right to personal autonomy. Decisions formerly made by health care providers for the benefit of their patients are now made by patients themselves. This shift in decision-making prerogative has been accompanied by the evolution of the legal doctrine of informed consent. Caregivers are now required to impart information that meets either the standard of care practiced among professionals or the standard of care determined to include all information material to a patient's decision. Professional conduct that fails to meet the applicable standard of care constitutes a breach of duty owed to the patient. If the patient is injured as a result of this breach, he may sue in tort for medical negligence to recover his damages.

Full disclosure and communication of genetic information often involves information that is unpleasant, even devastating, to counseling clients. The hard reality of genetic counseling is that clients must often learn of poor prognoses, limited if any treatment options, and diminished life expectancy of loved ones. This reality applies equally to chromosomal problems and to single gene disorders, whether dominant or recessive, across the full range of hereditary problems that affect human beings. Geneticists who intentionally restrict information that is sought by clients place themselves at risk of being sued for inadequate disclosure

under the doctrine of informed consent. Geneticists who make decisions on behalf of minor children also disregard the constitutional status of parents as the primary decision-makers for their own children. Beyond the detriment to the immediate parties in genetic counseling, however, lies a grave risk to the profession of medical genetics of allegations of directive counseling aimed at controlling the lives and the reproductive decisions of genetic counseling clients. These dangers must be avoided. They will be best avoided by recognizing a policy of full disclosure to clients who seek information about any hereditary problem.

Respect for patient autonomy and the need for full disclosure in the treatment of genetic disease has also acquired new facets as medical and surgical therapies have become more refined. While parents are usually regarded as the sole decision-makers for their children in questions about treatment, there has recently been a growing recognition in the legislatures and courts of the ability of mature minors to understand and to participate in these decisions. This ability is recognized both in accepting and in refusing a proposed course of treatment. Full disclosure is also mandated when experimental treatment regimes are proposed, with the additional caveat that this is a controversial area, with no professional consensus about ethical standards. Such tenuous treatment situations demand utmost sensitivity to the needs and expectations of all persons involved. Failure of the geneticist to disclose all available information to clients, or patients, who must make critical decisions will be an invitation for allegations of malpractice.

The doctrine of informed consent may eventually be extended to include a duty of the medical geneticist to re-contact counseling clients when new information is amassed that could be material in decisions made by these persons. Based on relevant case law, the geneticist, as the knowledgeable professional, may be required to disclose new information, but he can mitigate the chances of litigation by including his clients in the counseling process, by stressing the importance of communicating changes of address and status, and by making good faith efforts to re-contact patients who seem to have disappeared.

The history of medical genetics acknowledges the difficult aspects of genetic counseling, but it also supports the need for candid and complete disclosure of information to counseling clients. For many years one thrust of counseling has been to help families "make the best possible adjustment to the disorder in an affected family member" (Committee on Genetic Counseling, 1975). How one family deals with genetic information may differ greatly from the way another family deals with the same information, and these decisions are appropriately made within the privacy of each family. The geneticist should continue to serve as the trustee of genetic information. Counseling clients and patients, as the beneficiaries of this trust, are morally and legally entitled to full disclosure and to the right to give truly informed consent.

NOTES

1. Wrongful life actions are brought by children who are born with defects that could have been predicted or detected prenatally. These children claim that it would be better not to be born at all than to be born to a life of suffering and pain. The success of wrongful life actions is considerably more dubious than the success of wrongful birth actions because the courts have demonstrated a reluctance to make judgments about the value of a diminished life in relation to not being born at all (Pelias, 1986).

REFERENCES

Bloch M., Hayden MR (1990): Opinion: Predictive testing for Huntington disease in childhood: Challenges and implications. Am J Hum Genet 46:1–4.
Bowen v. American Hospital Association, 476 U.S. 610 (1986).
Canterbury v. Spence, 464 F.2d 772 (D.C. Cir. 1972).
Committee of the International Huntington Association and the World Federation of Neurology (1990): Ethical issues policy statement on Huntington's disease molecular genetics predictive test. J. Med Genet 27:34–38.
Committee on Genetic counseling (1975): Genetic counseling. Am J Hum Genet 27:240–242.
Davis v. Lhim, 124 Mich. App. 291, 335 N.W.2d 481 (1983).
Fraser FC (1974): Genetic counseling. Am J Hum Genet 26:636–659.
Meyer v. Nebraska, 262 U.S. 390 (1923).
Pelias MZ (1986): Torts of wrongful birth and wrongful life: A review. Am J Med Genet 25: 71–80.
Pierce v. Society of Sisters, 268 U.S. 510 (1925).
President's Commission (1983): Report of the President's Commission for the Study of Ethical Problems in Medicine and Biomedical and Behavioral Research. Washington, D.C.: Government Printing Office.
Tarasoff v. Regents of Univ. of Cal., 17 Cal. 3d 425, 131 Cal. Rptr. 14, 551 P.2d 334 (1976).

NO

Diane E. Hoffmann and Eric A. Wulfsberg

TESTING CHILDREN FOR GENETIC PREDISPOSITIONS: IS IT IN THEIR BEST INTEREST?

Researchers summoned a Baltimore County woman to an office at the Johns Hopkins School of Public Health last spring to tell her the bad news. They had found a genetic threat lurking in her 7-year-old son's DNA—a mutant gene that almost always triggers a rare form of colon cancer. It was the same illness that led surgeons to remove her colon in 1979. While the boy, Michael, now 8, is still perfectly healthy, without surgery he is almost certain to develop cancer by age 40.

This genetic fortune-telling was no parlor trick. It was the product of astonishing advances in recent decades in understanding how genes build and regulate our bodies. And as scientists pinpoint new genes and learn to forecast the onset of more inherited disorders, millions of people are likely to demand their medical prognosis.[1]

Testing healthy newborns and children for genetic DNA abnormalities that will not manifest disease symptoms for many years, if ever, is now rarely done. However, the entry of such tests into the marketplace is raising the specter of their widespread use. Tests that predict the likelihood of cancer are attracting the greatest attention, and they may be the first such tests to be administered on a large-scale basis.[2] Currently, tests are available for predisposition to breast cancer, colon cancer, melanoma, and thyroid cancer.[3]

Marketing these tests to the general population is highly controversial, with proponents arguing that people have a right to know if they or their children are at increased risk and that it would be unethical to deny them that information. Much of the advocacy for widespread use of the tests comes from the biotechnology companies offering them.[4] For example, a recent news article about marketing these genetic tests described the question of testing children as "delicate." Yet it also reported, in a letter to dermatologists on testing for melanoma predisposition, that the manufacturer of the tests

From Diane E. Hoffmann and Eric A. Wulfsberg, "Testing Children for Genetic Predispositions: Is It in Their Best Interest?" *Journal of Law, Medicine and Ethics*, vol. 23, no. 4 (1995), pp. 331–344. Copyright © 1995 by The American Society of Law, Medicine and Ethics. Reprinted by permission.

believed "[e]arly screening with this easy and painless test is particularly useful when testing children."[5]

Some advocates of testing children go so far as to state that a geneticist has a medical and legal duty to advise parents about presymptomatic testing procedures for some (even late-onset) diseases and either to administer the procedure or to refer the child to a colleague for administration (presuming the child meets certain pre-administration criteria).[6] Others describe the effort to keep the tests from patients as medical paternalism.[7] Opponents have characterized the initiative to market the genetic tests as "alarming," arguing that this area of genetic testing is still in the research phase and that the tests should not be marketed now.[8] Others argue that, due to the uncertain psychological consequences for children of predictive testing, such testing should not generally be done at this time or should be restricted.[9]

We support those who express caution and urge restraint[10] in conducting predictive genetic tests on children, and we suggest policy recommendations to safeguard children's interests from possible negative effects of such testing. Many of our suggestions are consistent with the recently published joint statement of the American Society of Human Genetics (ASHG) and the American College of Medical Genetics (ACMG) on genetic testing of children and adolescents.[11] ...

Throughout, we use the term *genetic disease* to refer to that rare group of disorders in which an abnormality (or abnormalities) in the genetic code (DNA) of an individual is associated with a near certainty of developing disease. In contrast, we use *genetic predisposition* to refer to an abnormality in the genetic code of an individual that results in an increased risk of developing a disease.

Current Testing of Newborns and Children

Little genetic testing of children is currently performed, other than newborn screening for a small number of treatable genetic diseases that are expected to cause symptoms if not treated during infancy. When testing is performed on older children, it is generally limited to those few individuals who either are suspected of having a genetic disease or are in families at high risk for having a genetic disease. Several attempts have been made to categorize reasons to do genetic testing on infants and children.[12] Using the work of Wertz et al. and Fost as a starting point, we employ a comprehensive list of seven categories: (1) testing of immediate benefit to the infant or minor, including newborn screening, disease testing for a symptomatic condition in the child, or presymptomatic testing for which treatment during childhood is available and beneficial; (2) reproductive-associated testing and counseling for older adolescents that is mainly genetic carrier rather than genetic disease testing; (3) testing for the benefit of other family members' reproductive decision making, where it may be necessary to test both affected and unaffected family members to understand the inheritance of a genetic disease; (4) research-related testing that is generally conducted under informed consent protocols approved by institutional review boards; (5) testing by insurance companies for the purpose of excluding individuals from coverage; (6) presymptomatic testing to predict a child's future risk of developing a genetic disease or of having a genetic predisposition for which no current treatment or effective prevention exists; and (7) testing for carrier status at an age when the child cannot procreate.

Predictive Testing

Our primary focus is category (6)—testing for presymptomatic genetic diseases or predispositions. While a relatively recent survey indicates that many British geneticists and pediatricians would presymptomatically test children for a genetic condition at the request of the parents and with little immediate benefit to the child,[13] many ethicists and professional genetics societies agree that testing children for genetic diseases, predispositions, or carrier status is only appropriate when a clear and timely benefit to the minor exists.[14] And the debate, in large part, has focused on determining what constitutes a clear and timely benefit and who would benefit from the information. While many professionals argue that there is insufficient benefit to the child to warrant widespread screening or even high-risk family testing for most genetic diseases during childhood,[15] some argue that the information may be beneficial to the child's family. Whether this benefit would outweigh the negative aspects of being identified as having a disease, such as being treated differently by one's parents (no college fund or other long-term plans), has significant ramifications for the appropriateness of predictive testing....

Psychological Impact

Concerns about testing children solely for predictive purposes have focused largely on the potential psychological implications to the child, especially in cases of predisposition to an incurable disease.[16] Wertz et al. have summarized some of the psychological and emotional consequences of such testing. They argue that in requesting testing, parents typically think only of the benefits of a negative test result and not of the potentially damaging effects of a positive result:

> "Planning for the future," perhaps the most frequently given reason for testing, may become "restricting the future" (and also the present) by shifting family resources away from a child with a positive diagnosis.... In families with a chronically ill child, there is less socialization to future roles for all the children, including those who are "healthy." Parents are less likely to say "When you grow up..." or "When you have children of your own..." to any of their children, because they cannot say these words to the ill child.... "Alleviation of anxiety," another reason commonly given by parents for predictive genetic testing, does not necessarily benefit the children. A positive diagnosis may create serious risks of stigmatization, loss of self-esteem, and discrimination [by] family or by institutional third parties such as employers or insurers. Testing may disrupt parent-child or sibling-sibling bonds, may lead to scapegoating a child with a positive result or to continued anxiety over a child despite a negative result....[17]

Identifying a child with a genetic predisposition may lead to the "vulnerable child syndrome" in which parents become overprotective and unnecessarily restrict a child's activities.[18] Also, those who test negative have been shown to experience "survivor guilt."[19] Given these concerns, the International Huntington's Disease Association and the World Federation of Neurology have issued policy statements recommending that minors not be tested for Huntington's disease,[20] and the National Kidney Foundation has recommended that minors not be tested for the gene for adult polycystic kidney disease except in specific circumstances where preventive measures are applicable for stroke.[21] . . .

Should Physicians Disclose the Availability of Presymptomatic Genetic Tests for Children?

The controversy surrounding presymptomatically testing children for genetic disease may soon cause anxiety for some physicians as to whether they must or should disclose the availability of genetic tests to parents of healthy children. Physicians may be concerned about potential liability for failure to inform parents about such tests. Some have contributed to this concern by arguing that physicians may have a legal duty to disclose the availability of these tests.[22] They rely erroneously on case law on prenatal testing and wrongful birth. In these cases, parents have successfully claimed that had they known about the test, they would have consented to it; and, if it had indicated that their fetus had a serious genetic condition, they would have terminated the pregnancy. Instead, the physician's failure to inform them of the test resulted in their having a child with a severe genetic abnormality that could have been detected.[23]

The problem with this analogy is that, in the prenatal context, parents could use the information to make a decision to terminate the pregnancy. In the context of testing children for a genetic predisposition for which the parent can do nothing to alter the likely manifestation of the disease, the physician would be not be legally liable. Liability would only attach when a beneficial intervention exists and failure to test or to test in a timely manner would result in harm to the child.

Thus, for a genetic disease for which we have no effective preventive intervention or treatment, a physician would have no legal duty and should not fear liability for failure to inform parents of a genetic test. We argue that this is the case both when there is no family history or probable cause for believing the child has a genetic predisposition and when there is a family history of the disease. While courts have made a distinction between informing parents about a test for a genetic disease when there is and is not a family history of the disease,[24] these cases are based on the prenatal testing paradigm, in which parents have the option of terminating the pregnancy.

We argue further that, as a policy matter, a physician should not be obligated to disclose the availability of the tests under these circumstances. Where no family history of a genetic condition exists, requiring disclosure of all available tests would take considerable time on the part of a physician or other health professional for no likely benefit to the child or parents. Disclosure in this circumstance arguably wastes resources, and it has the potential for psychological harm. . . .

Should Physicians Perform Predictive Genetic Testing on Children?

With the increased availability of tests for genetic predispositions, physicians will undoubtedly encounter parents who have read about the tests and request one or more of them for their child. Do physicians have a legal duty to perform such tests? More importantly, *should* physicians perform such tests?

As to the first question, physicians are under no legal obligation to provide the test. They are free not to provide a treatment or diagnostic test to a patient under most circumstances. In some cases, if the treatment or diagnostic test is considered part of standard medical care, a physician would need to inform a patient of it but would not be required to provide it. In some jurisdictions, under certain circumstances, they may have a legal obligation to refer the patient to another provider who would provide the test or treatment.[25] In a recent article, Clayton ably dispels the myth that parents have a constitutional right to demand medical treatment or testing for their child, as well as the belief held by some physicians that they will be liable under tort law for failure to provide the tests.[26] Her persuasive analysis should provide comfort to physicians who refuse to test children for genetic predispositions.

As to whether a physician *should* provide such tests for genetic dispositions, we argue generally that such tests should not be provided but that a distinction may be made between cases in which there is and is not a family history of a genetic disease. If there is no family history or other risk factors, to test a healthy child for predisposition to genetic diseases is simply a fishing expedition with no foundation. If there is a family history, we concur with the ASHG-ACMG position that the decision to test should be made by a physician in discussion with the child and the child's parents.

In very young children, testing should be delayed in most cases until the child can understand the implications of the test. For example, where a mother and her three-year-old daughter visit a pediatrician for the first time and a medical history of the child reveals that the mother's mother and sister both had breast cancer, the physician should inform the mother about the availability of the test for herself, and might suggest that, if interested in it, she talk to her internist who can refer her to a geneticist. With respect to her three year old, the physician should simply state that, at some time in the future (when the child is sufficiently mature to understand the information), the child's mother might want to talk to her daughter about the family history and the test and to let the daughter decide if she would like to have the test done and, if so, when.

In some cases, however, parents may persistently demand a test for their child. Some have argued that to deny the parents the test is medical paternalism and flies in the face of our general deference to parents regarding medical decision making for their children.[27] The law clearly gives parents this authority and assumes that parents will act in their child's best interests when making such decisions. Very seldom, in fact, are parents denied the right to make medical decisions for their children, and, when denied, the cases usually involve questions of parental abuse or neglect. But cases deferring to parental decision making are not analogous to the case of genetic testing. Virtually all cases of deference to parental decision making involve circumstances in which a medical professional is recommending a course of treatment for a child, for example, surgery or chemotherapy, and the parents refuse it. Although parental decision making can be taken away when failure to provide the treatment would threaten the child's life, in virtually all other cases the parents have the right to decide not to consent to a proposed treatment.

This stands in stark contrast to cases in which the parent wants a treatment or procedure for the child that is not recommended by the physician. An example might be a common parental request to have the child's blood type determined. Pediatricians generally will not draw a child's blood simply to satisfy the parents' curiosity—he/she must have a medical reason to perform the test. Genetic tests may be somewhat more complex, and physicians may need guidance in determining where or under what circumstances a test should or might be provided.... We recommend that ... guidelines not be rigid, however, so that physicians have some latitude in deciding whether testing is warranted in a particular case. This flexibility should also allow a physician to converse with a child's parents or a child (if sufficiently mature) regarding the desire for the testing.

Although parents generally know their child best and care most about the child's welfare, we believe that physicians and health care providers have an obligation to provide them with sufficient information to make a true informed decision about the benefits and risks associated with testing for a genetic predisposition. If parents, despite a statement from their child's physician that the physician does not generally perform predictive genetic testing, want the test performed, we recommend that the physician refer them to an appropriately trained genetic counselor or another physician who can objectively explain the risks and benefits of such testing. If they still desire the testing, the health care provider must obtain their informed consent....

Safeguards Protecting Children— A Recommendation

Given concerns about testing children for genetic predispositions, we urge adoption of safeguards to ensure that the tests are administered consistent with the child's best interests. While an argument can be made that safeguards should be in place for all tested, children are particularly vulnerable to the potential negative effects of predisposition testing. The most compelling argument for this is the impact a positive test result may have on how a child will be treated by his parents, family, and, potentially, society. Few empirical studies have been done on this issue..., but caution in this type of testing is now warranted, and professional societies must play a role in encouraging physicians to exercise restraint in this area....

Where the guidelines indicate that testing might be appropriate and the parents want that genetic testing performed, we recommend that the child's physician, if not qualified himself, refer the child and his/her parents to a genetic counselor or knowledgeable physician to discuss the test risks (including the psychological risks and the potential impact on family dynamics). We urge that counselors discuss with parents the risk of overvaluing information that can be obtained from genetic tests and not discount the subtle ways in which this information might psychologically harm a child by virtue of treatment by family, friends, and school systems. Finally, counselors should help parents to think through how they will use the information and at what point and under what conditions they will tell their child about a positive test result. The family, after meeting with the counselor, may still desire the test, but the additional counseling and discussion should clarify the issues and make parents more knowledgeable about the risks of the tests.

In addition, all parents seeking genetic testing of a child should give written consent to the procedure. State departments of public health (or comparable agencies) should consider designing model consent forms that list the potential risks and benefits of the proposed test, including the psychological risks and the impact on family dynamics. Forms prepared by some state health departments for HIV testing may serve as models. We also recommend, in all cases where a child tests positive for a genetic predisposition, that the child (if sufficiently mature) and his parents be provided the opportunity to meet with a genetic counselor or knowledgeable physician to explain the results. If necessary, psychological counseling should also be made available to the family.

As regards follow-up, physicians who offer or perform a predictive genetic test on a child have an obligation to tell the family that they should check back periodically with the physician to determine whether any new developments might benefit the child. Physicians should also know about possible resources for the family, including toll-free numbers, family support groups, or disease registries, that could assist them in keeping up-to-date regarding their child's condition. Finally, for certain life-threatening conditions or conditions that have the potential to affect the quality of a child's life significantly, registries should be established by national public health agencies or private disease associations. These registries would be voluntary, would track cases of genetic predispositions, and would inform registrants of new developments that could benefit them.

Conclusion
The availability of more and more genetic tests will create unique dilemmas for parents, their children, and their health care providers. We advise caution in the administration of these tests to children when such testing is solely for predictive purposes. Professional associations must take a strong stand on this issue and should provide physicians with guidance

as to when they should disclose the availability of tests to families as well as to when it would be appropriate to perform such tests. If a predictive test is appropriate for a child, based on established guidelines, safeguards must be in place to ensure accurate and informed decision making by parents and child (if sufficiently mature). Finally, if predictive testing is done on a young child, resources should be made available, through government funding or private agencies, to assist parents in keeping informed about their child's condition and any beneficial interventions. In addition to the establishment of registries for some conditions, public health education and information dissemination strategies should be implemented to ensure that when new information is available, it reaches a large segment of the population. This way, parents of children like Michael, with the predisposing gene for colon cancer, will bring their children in to see a physician when a treatment or cure for colon cancer is available.

ACKNOWLEDGMENTS

Research for this paper was supported by a grant (RO1HG00419) from the National Institutes of Health Center for Human Genome Research. The authors are grateful for the comments of Robert Wachbroit and Karen Rothenberg on an earlier draft.

NOTES

1. D. Birch, "Genetic Fortune-Telling," *Baltimore Sun*, May 9, 1995, at A1.

2. Tests are also predicted to be available for predispositions to "complex conditions and behaviors," such as "mental illness, Alzheimer's disease, hyperactivity, heart disease,... and susceptibility to alcoholism, addiction, and even violence." Some

have described those persons who test positive for these conditions as the "pre-symptomatically ill" or the "person 'at-risk'." R. C. Dreyfuss and D. Nelkin, "The Jurisprudence of Genetics," *Vanderbilt Law Review*, 45 (1992): at 318.

3. According to newspaper reports, the tests cost approximately $800 for the first family member and $250 for each additional member. They are being offered under research protocols to cancer families by at least one biotechnology company. See G. Kolata, "Tests to Assess Risks for Cancer Raising Questions," *New York Times*, Mar. 27, 1995, at A1.

4. See M. R. Natowicz and J. S. Alper, "Genetic Screening: Triumphs, Problems, and Controversies," *Journal of Public Health Policy*, 12 (1991): at 485.

5. Kolata, *supra* note 3, at A9.

6. See, for example, N. F. Sharpe, letter, "Pre-Symptomatic Testing for Huntington Disease: Is There a Duty to Test Those Under the Age of Eighteen Years?," *American Journal of Medical Genetics*, 46 (1993): 250–53.

7. M. Z. Pelias, "Duty to Disclose in Medical Genetics: A Legal Perspective," *American Journal of Medical Genetics*, 39 (1991): at 350.

8. Kolata, *supra* note 3.

9. See, for example, N. Fost, "Genetic Diagnosis and Treatment: Ethical Considerations," *American Journal of Diseases of Children*, 147 (1993): 1190–95; D. C. Wertz et al., "Genetic Testing for Children and Adolescents: Who Decides?," *JAMA*, 272 (1994): 875–82; and P. S. Harper and A. Clarke, "Viewpoint: Should We Test Children for 'Adult' Genetic Disease?," *Lancet*, 335 (1990): 1205–06.

10. *Id.*

11. American Society of Human Genetics and American College of Medical Genetics, "Points to Consider: Ethical, Legal, and Psychosocial Implications of Genetic Testing in Children and Adolescents," *American Journal of Human Genetics*, 57 (1995): 1233–41.

12. Wertz et al., *supra* note 9; and Fost, *supra* note 9.

13. *Id.*

14. The Committee on Assessing Genetic Risks, which was appointed by the Institute of Medicine, recommends that "[c]hildren should generally be tested only for genetic disorders for which there exists an effective curative or preventive treatment that must be instituted early in life to achieve maximum benefit." See Institute of Medicine, L. B. Andrews et al., eds., *Assessing Genetic Risks: Implications for Health and Social Policy* (Washington, D.C.: National Academy Press, 1994): at 10. Detailed statements on the testing of children have been prepared by the Working Party of the Clinical Genetics Society in the United Kingdom and, more recently, by ASHG and ACMG, see

supra note 11. The Working Party makes several recommendations, including the following:

(1) The predictive genetic testing of children is clearly appropriate where onset of the condition regularly occurs in childhood or there are useful medical interventions that can be offered (for example, diet, medication, surveillance for complications). (2) In contrast, the working party believes that predictive testing for an adult onset disorder should generally not be undertaken if the child is healthy and there are no medical interventions established as useful that can be offered in the event of a positive test result.

A. Clarke, Working Party of the Clinical Genetics Society, "The Genetic Testing of Children," *Journal of Medical Genetics*, 31 (1994): at 785.

15. Clarke, *supra* note 14; but see Harper and Clarke, *supra* note 9.

16. Wertz et al., *supra* note 9; and Clarke, *supra* note 14.

17. Wertz et al., *supra* note 9, at 878, citing J. H. Fanos, *Developmental Consequences for Adulthood of Early Sibling Loss* (Ann Arbor: University of Michigan Microfilms, 1987), and J. Dunn, *Sisters and Brothers* (Cambridge: Harvard University Press, 1985).

18. Fost, *supra* note 9, at 1193. citing A. Tluczek et al., "Parents' Knowledge of Neonatal Screening and Response to False-Positive Cystic Fibrosis Screening," *Journal of Developmental and Behavioral Pediatrics*, 13 (1992): 181–86.

19. D. Ball et al., "Predictive Testing of Adults and Children," in A. Clarke, ed., *Genetic Counselling: Practice and Principles* (London: Routledge, 1994): at 70.

20. *Id. at* 74.

21. Wertz et al., *supra* note 9, at 876, citing A. Gabow et al., "Gene Testing in Autosomal Dominant Adult Polycystic Kidney Disease: Results of a National Kidney Foundation Workshop," *American Journal of Kidney Diseases*, 13 (1989): 85–87. Also, according to Biesecker et al., the long-term outcome of polycystic kidney disease is not altered by early identification. The impetus for testing individuals for the disease comes primarily from "efforts to identify unaffected living related renal transplant donors at an age where renal ultrasound will not accurately identify all pre-symptomatic carriers; this can result in the identification of carriers for a disease in which early clinical intervention does not alter the course." The National Kidney Foundation only endorses testing presymptomatically for the disease as part of evaluation for renal transplant donation. B. B. Biesecker et al., "Genetic Counseling for Families with Inherited Susceptibility to Breast and Ovarian Cancer," *JAMA*, 269 (1993): at 1971.

22. See, for example, Pelias, *supra* note 7; and Sharpe, *supra* note 6.

23. See, for example, *Berman v. Allan*, 404 A.2d 8, 15 (N.J. 1979) (court held that parents of a congenitally defective child had a valid claim for compensation for their mental and emotional suffering over the birth of the child when the claim was based on the failure of the expectant mother's doctors to inform the parents of the availability of the diagnostic procedure known as amniocentesis); see also *Phillips v. United States*, 566 F. Supp. 1 (D.S.C. 1981); and *Becker V. Schwartz*, 386 N.E.2d 807 (N.Y. 1978). These cases are often referred to as wrongful birth cases.

24. See, for example, *Munro v. Regents of the University of Cal.*, 263 Cal. Rptr. 878, 882 (Cal. Ct. App. 1989) (doctor did not commit medical malpractice in failing to check whether pregnant woman and her husband were carriers of Tay-Sachs disease, even though the couple's child was later born with Tay-Sachs, when defendants submitted expert evidence that the couple did not meet the profile characteristics necessary to warrant performing a Tay-Sachs carrier screening test); see also *Roth v. Group Health Ass'n, Inc.*, Dkt. No. 88-1005 (D.D.C., settled June 12, 1989) (woman who knew she had a genetic defect in her family sued her doctor and HMO for failing to perform amniocentesis because she was under the age of thirty-five; when her child was born with the defect, she filed a malpractice suit and received a $925,000 settlement).

25. See, for example, Md. Code Ann., Health-Gen. §5-613(a) (1994) (if a patient or his agent or surrogate requests that everything be done for a seriously ill patient, including CPR, and the treating physician believes that CPR would be medically ineffective, the physician must inform the patient of the option to transfer the patient to another provider and must assist in that process).

26. E. W. Clayton, "Removing the Shadow of the Law from the Debate about Genetic Testing of Children," *American Journal of Medical Genetics*, 57 (1995): at 630–32.

27. Pelias, *supra* note 7.

POSTSCRIPT

Should Parents Always Be Told of Genetic-Testing Availability?

Most of the major organizations that have analyzed the issues raised by genetic testing of children for adult-onset diseases have urged caution. In June 1995 the American Medical Association's Council on Ethical and Judicial Affairs said, "If parents have complete freedom to consent to genetic testing for their children, the testing may disclose information that precipitates discrimination against the children. Even if no discrimination results, the parents have preempted their children's right to decide, upon maturity, that they would prefer not to know their genetic status. Accordingly, unless there are important benefits for a child from diagnostic testing, the risks of testing suggest that parents should not be able to require genetic testing of their child." In a 1995 resolution the National Society of Genetic Counselors emphasized the need to explore the psychological and social risks and benefits for both the children and the parents that are inherent in early genetic identification. The society concluded, "Until more data is gathered on the impact of this type of testing, extreme caution should be taken regarding the use of such tests."

Nonetheless, the scientific field of genetics is advancing rapidly, as Philip Kitcher indicates in *The Lives to Come: The Genetic Revolution and Human Possibilities* (Simon & Schuster, 1996). For a historical perspective, see *Controlling Human Heredity: 1865 to the Present* by Diane B. Paul (Humanities Press, 1995). Peter S. Harper and Angus Clarke, in "Should We Test Children for 'Adult' Genetic Diseases," *The Lancet* (May 19, 1990), urge a fuller debate of the ethical and professional issues involved with widespread testing of a significant number of disorders and careful consideration of individual circumstances. The issues raised by testing are also explored at both the professional and societal level in Eric T. Juengst, "The Ethics of Prediction: Genetic Risk and the Physician-Patient Relationship," *Genome Science and Technology* (vol. 1, no. 1, 1995). In "Genetic Testing for Children and Adolescents: Who Decides?" *Journal of the American Medical Association* (September 21, 1994), Dorothy C. Wertz, Joanna H. Fanos, and Philip R. Reilly propose guidelines for predictive genetic testing and counseling. Lisa Geller provides an update of genetic testing issues in "Individual, Family, and Society Dimensions of Genetic Discrimination," *Science and Engineering Ethics* (vol. 2, 1996). In their book *Morality and the New Genetics* (Jones & Barlett, 1996), Bernard Gert et al. show how a philosophical analysis can be used to contend with the moral issues that arise from the new genetics.

Articles on testing for specific genetic diseases include "Consensus Statement on Predictive Testing for Alzheimer Disease," *Alzheimer Disease and Associated Disorders* (vol. 9, no. 4, 1995); Barbara B. Biesecker et al., "Genetic Counseling for Families With Inherited Susceptibility to Breast and Ovarian Cancer," *Journal of the American Medical Association* (April 21, 1993); Benjamin S. Wilfond and Kathleen Nolan, "National Policy Development for the Clinical Application of Genetic Diagnostic Technologies: Lessons from Cystic Fibrosis," *Journal of the American Medical Association* (December 22/29, 1993); Riyana Babul et al., "Attitudes Toward Direct Predictive Testing for the Huntington Disease Gene: Relevance for Other Adult-Onset Diseases," *Journal of the American Medical Association* (November 17, 1993); and Sandi Wiggins et al., "The Psychological Consequences of Predictive Testing for Huntington's Disease," *The New England Journal of Medicine* (November 12, 1992). A personal account of the decision to be tested for Huntington's disease, Catherine V. Hayes's "Genetic Testing for Huntington's Disease—A Family Issue," also appears in the November 12, 1992, issue of *The New England Journal of Medicine*. An article that demonstrates how screening for sickle-cell disease can decrease patient mortality is Elliott Vichinsky et al., "Newborn Screening for Sickle Cell Disease: Effect on Mortality," *Pediatrics* (June 1988). The issue of prenatal testing is explored in *Women and Prenatal Testing: Facing the Challenges of Genetic Technology* edited by Karen H. Rothenberg and Elizabeth J. Thomson (Ohio State University Press, 1994).

PART 6

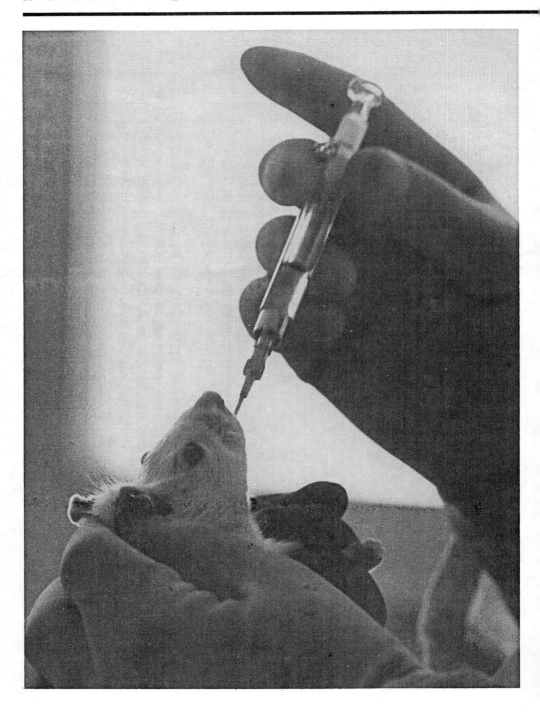

Human and Animal Experimentation

The goal of scientific research is knowledge that will benefit society. But achieving that goal may subject humans and animals to some risks. Questions arise about not only how research should be conducted but whether or not it should be conducted at all, such as in the use of animals or fetal tissue. These questions transcend national boundaries and raise questions of whether or not research can be "ethical" in one country and not in another. This section contends with issues that will shape the future of experimental science.

- Should Animal Experimentation Be Permitted?

- Will Fetal Tissue Research Encourage Abortions?

ISSUE 16

Should Animal Experimentation Be Permitted?

YES: Jerod M. Loeb et al., from "Human vs. Animal Rights: In Defense of Animal Research," *Journal of the American Medical Association* (November 17, 1989)

NO: Tom Regan, from "Ill-Gotten Gains," in Donald Van DeVeer and Tom Regan, eds., *Health Care Ethics: An Introduction* (Temple University Press, 1987)

ISSUE SUMMARY

YES: Jerod M. Loeb and his colleagues, representing the American Medical Society's Group on Science and Technology, assert that concern for animals, admirable in itself, cannot impede the development of methods to improve the welfare of humans.

NO: Philosopher Tom Regan argues that conducting research on animals exacts the grave moral price of failing to show proper respect for animals' inherent value, whatever the benefits of the research.

In 1865 the great French physiologist Claude Bernard wrote, "Physicians already make too many dangerous experiments on man before carefully studying them in animals." In his insistence on adequate animal research before trying a new therapy on human beings, Bernard established a principle of research ethics that is still considered valid. But in the past few decades this principle has been challenged by another view—one that sees animals not as tools for human use and consumption but as moral agents in their own right. Animal experimentation, according to this theory, cannot be taken for granted but must be justified by ethical criteria at least as stringent as those that apply to research involving humans.

Philosophers traditionally have not ascribed any moral status to animals. Like St. Thomas Aquinas before him, René Descartes, a seventeenth-century French physiologist and philosopher, saw no ethical problem in experimentation on animals. Descartes approved of cutting open a fully conscious animal because it was, he said, a machine more complex than a clock but no more capable of feeling pain. Immanuel Kant argued that animals need not be treated as ends in themselves because they lacked rationality.

Beginning in England in the nineteenth century, antivivisectionists (people who advocate the abolition of animal experimentation) campaigned, with varying success, for laws to control scientific research. But the internal dissensions in the movement and its frequent lapses into sentimentality made it only partially effective. At best the antivivisectionists achieved some legislation that mandated more humane treatment of animals used for research, but they never succeeded in abolishing animal research or even in establishing the need for justification of particular research projects.

The more recent movement to ban animal research, however, is both better organized politically and more rigorously philosophical. The movement, often called animal liberation or animal rights, is similar in principle to the civil rights movement of the 1960s. Just as blacks, women, and other minorities sought recognition of their equal status, animal advocates have built a case for the equal status of animals.

Peter Singer, one of the leaders of this movement, has presented an eloquent case that we practice not only racism and sexism in our society but also "speciesism." That is, we assume that human beings are superior to other animals; we are prejudiced in favor of our own kind. Experimenting on animals and eating their flesh are the two major forms of speciesism in our society. Singer points out that some categories of human beings—infants and mentally retarded people—rate lower on a scale of intelligence, awareness, and self-consciousness than some animals. Yet we would not treat these individuals in the way we do animals. He argues that "all animals are equal" and that the suffering of an animal is morally equal to the suffering of a human being.

Proponents of animal research counter that such views are fundamentally misguided, that human beings, with the capacity for rational thought and action, are indeed a superior species. They contend that, while animals deserve humane treatment, the good consequences of animal research (i.e., knowledge that will benefit human beings) outweigh the suffering of individual animals. No other research techniques can substitute for the reactions of live animals, they declare.

In the selections that follow, Jerod M. Loeb and his colleagues reaffirm the American Medical Association's defense of animal research because it is essential for medical progress and it would be unethical to deprive humans and animals of advances in medicine that result from this research. Tom Regan disputes the view that benefit to humans justifies research on animals. Pointing to their inherent value, he says that "whatever our gains, they are ill-gotten," and he calls for an end to such research.

YES

Jerod M. Loeb et al.

HUMAN VS. ANIMAL RIGHTS: IN DEFENSE OF ANIMAL RESEARCH

Research with animals is a highly controversial topic in our society. Animal rights groups that intend to stop all experimentation with animals are in the vanguard of this controversy. Their methods range from educational efforts directed in large measure to the young and uninformed, to promotion of restrictive legislation, filing lawsuits, and violence that includes raids on laboratories and death threats to investigators. Their rhetoric is emotionally charged and their information is frequently distorted and pejorative. Their tactics vary but have a single objective—to stop scientific research with animals.

The resources of the animal rights groups are extensive, in part because less militant organizations of animal activists, including some humane societies, have been infiltrated or taken over by animal rights groups to gain access to their fiscal and physical holdings. Through bizarre tactics, extravagant claims, and gruesome myths, animal rights groups have captured the attention of the media and a sizable segment of the public. Nevertheless, people invariably support the use of animals in research when they understand both sides of the issue and the contributions of animal research to relief of human suffering. However, all too often they do not understand both sides because information about the need for animal research is not presented. When this need is explained, the presentation often reveals an arrogance of the scientific community and an unwillingness to be accountable to public opinion.

The use of animals in research is fundamentally an ethical question: is it more ethical to ban all research with animals or to use a limited number of animals in research under humane conditions when no alternatives exist to achieve medical advances that reduce substantial human suffering and misery? . . .

ANIMALS IN SCIENTIFIC RESEARCH

Animals have been used in research for more than 2000 years. In the third century BC, the natural philosopher Erisistratus of Alexandria used animals

From Jerod M. Loeb, William R. Hendee, Steven J. Smith, and M. Roy Schwarz, "Human vs. Animal Rights: In Defense of Animal Research," *Journal of the American Medical Association*, vol. 262, no. 19 (November 17, 1989), pp. 2716–2720. Copyright © 1989 by The American Medical Association. Reprinted by permission.

to study bodily function. In all likelihood, Aristotle performed vivisection on animals. The Roman physician Galen used apes and pigs to prove his theory that veins carry blood rather than air. In succeeding centuries, animals were employed to confirm theories about physiology developed through observation. Advances in knowledge from these experiments include demonstration of the circulation of blood by Harvey in 1622, documentation of the effects of anesthesia on the body in 1846, and elucidation of the relationship between bacteria and disease in 1878.[1] In his book *An Introduction to the Study of Experimental Medicine* published in 1865, Bernard[2] described the importance of animal research to advances in knowledge about the human body and justified the continued use of animals for this purpose.

In this century, many medical advances have been achieved through research with animals.[3] Infectious diseases such as pertusis, rubella, measles, and poliomyelitis have been brought under control with vaccines developed in animals. The development of immunization techniques against today's infectious diseases, including human immunodeficiency virus disease, depends entirely on experiments in animals. Antibiotics that control infection are always tested in animals before use in humans. Physiological disorders such as diabetes and epilepsy are treatable today through knowledge and products gained by animal research. Surgical procedures such as coronary artery bypass grafts, cerebrospinal fluid shunts, and retinal reattachments have evolved from experiments with animals. Transplantation procedures for persons with failed liver, heart, lung, and kidney function are products of animal research.

Animals have been essential to the evolution of modern medicine and the conquest of many illnesses. However, many medical challenges remain to be solved. Cancer, heart disease, cerebrovascular disease, dementia, depression, arthritis, and a variety of inherited disorders are yet to be understood and controlled. Until they are, human pain and suffering will endure, and society will continue to expend its emotional and fiscal resources in efforts to alleviate or at least reduce them.

Animal research has not only benefited humans. Procedures and products developed through this process have also helped animals.[4,5] Vaccines against rabies, distemper, and parvovirus in dogs are a spin-off of animal research, as are immunization techniques against cholera in hogs, encephalitis in horses, and brucellosis in cattle. Drugs to combat heartworm, intestinal parasites, and mastitis were developed in animals used for experimental purposes. Surgical procedures developed in animals help animals as well as humans.

Research with animals has yielded immeasurable benefits to both humans and animals. However, this research raises fundamental philosophical issues concerning the rights of humans to use animals to benefit humans and other animals. If these rights are granted (and many people are loath to do so), additional questions arise concerning the way that research should be performed, the accountability of researchers to public sentiment, the nature of an ethical code for animal research, and who should compose and approve the code. Today, some animal activists are asking whether humans have the right to exercise dominion over animals for any purpose, including research. Others suggest that because humans have dominion over other forms of life, they are obligated to protect and preserve animals and ensure that they are not exploited. Still others agree that animals can be used to help people, but only under circumstances that are so structured as to be unattainable by most researchers. These attitudes may all differ, but their consequences are similar. They all threaten to diminish or stop animal research.

CHALLENGE TO ANIMAL RESEARCH

Challenges to the use of animals to benefit humans are not new—their origins can be traced back several centuries. With respect to animal research, opposition has been vocal in Europe for more than 400 years and in the United States for at least 100 years.[6]

Most of the current arguments against research with animals have historic precedents that must be grasped to understand the current debate. These precedents originated in the controversy between Cartesian and utilitarian philosophers that extended from the 16th to the 18th centuries.

The Cartesian-utilitarian debate was opened by the French philosopher Descartes, who defended the use of animals in experiments by insisting the animals respond to stimuli in only one way —"according to the arrangement of their organs."[7] He stated that animals lack the ability to reason and think and are, therefore, similar to a machine. Humans, on the other hand, can think, talk, and respond to stimuli in various ways. These differences, Descartes argued, make animals inferior to humans and justify their use as a machine, including as experimental subjects. He proposed that animals learn only by experience, whereas

humans learn by "teaching-learning." Humans do not always have to experience something to know that it is true.

Descartes' arguments were countered by the utilitarian philosopher Bentham of England. "The question," said Bentham, "is not can they reason? nor can they talk? but can they suffer?"[8] In utilitarian terms, humans and animals are linked by their common ability to suffer and their common right not to suffer and die at the hands of others. This utilitarian thesis has rippled through various groups opposed to research with animals for more than a century.

In the 1970s, the antivivisectionist movement was influenced by three books that clarified the issues and introduced the rationale for increased militancy against animal research. In 1971, the anthology *Animals, Men and Morals*, by Godlovitch et al,[9] raised the concept of animal rights and analyzed the relationships between humans and animals. Four years later, *Victims of Science*, by Ryder,[10] introduced the concept of "speciesism" as equivalent to fascism. Also in 1975, Singer[11] published *Animal Liberation: A New Ethic for Our Treatment of Animals*. This book is generally considered the progenitor of the modern animal rights movement. Invoking Ryder's concept of speciesism, Singer deplored the historic attitude of humans toward nonhumans as a "form of prejudice no less objectionable than racism or sexism." He urged that the liberation of animals should become the next great cause after civil rights and the women's movement.

Singer's book not only was a philosophical treatise; it also was a call to action. It provided an intellectual foundation and a moral focus for the animal rights movement. These features attracted many who were indifferent to the emotional appeal based on a love of animals that had characterized anti-vivisectionist efforts for the past century. Singer's book swelled the ranks of the antivivisectionist movement and transformed it into a movement for animal rights. It also has been used to justify illegal activities intended to impede animal research and instill fear and intimidation in those engaged in it....

DEFENSE OF ANIMAL RESEARCH

The issue of animal research is fundamentally an issue of the dominion of humans over animals. This issue is rooted in the Judeo-Christian religion of western culture, including the ancient tradition of animal sacrifice described in the Old Testament and the practice of using animals as surrogates for suffering humans described in the New Testament. The sacredness of human life is a central theme of biblical morality, and the dominion of humans over other forms of life is a natural consequence of this theme.[12] The issue of dominion is not, however, unique to animal research. It is applicable to every situation where animals are subservient to humans. It applies to the use of animals for food and clothing; the application of animals as beasts of burden and transportation; the holding of animals in captivity such as in zoos and as household pets; the use of animals as entertainment, such as in sea parks and circuses; the exploitation of animals in sports that employ animals, including hunting, racing, and animal shows; and the eradication of pests such as rats and mice from homes and farms. Even provision of food and shelter to animals reflects an attitude of dominion of humans over animals. A person who truly does not believe in human dominance over animals would be forced to oppose all of these practices, including keeping animals as household pets or in any form of physical or psychological captivity. Such a posture would defy tradition evolved over the entire course of human existence.

Some animal advocates do not take issue with the right of humans to exercise dominion over animals. They agree that animals are inferior to humans because they do not possess attributes such as a moral sense and concepts of past and future. However, they also claim that it is precisely because of these differences that humans are obligated to protect animals and not exploit them for the selfish betterment of humans.[13] In their view, animals are like infants and the mentally incompetent, who must be nurtured and protected from exploitation. This view shifts the issues of dominion from one of rights claimed by animals to one of responsibilities exercised by humans.

Neither of these philosophical positions addresses the issue of animal research from the perspective of the immorality of not using animals in research. From this perspective, depriving humans (and animals) of advances in medicine that result from research with animals is inhumane and fundamentally unethical. Spokespersons for this perspective suggest that patients with dementia, stroke, disabling injuries, heart disease, and cancer deserve relief from suffering and that depriving them of hope and relief by eliminating animal research is an immoral and unconscionable act. Defenders of animal research claim that animals sometimes must be sacrificed in the development of methods to relieve pain and suffering of humans (and animals) and to affect treatments and cures of a variety of human maladies.

The immeasurable benefits of animal research to humans are undeniable. One example is the development of a vaccine for poliomyelitis, with the result that the number of cases of poliomyelitis in the United States alone declined from 58,000 in 1952 to 4 in 1984. Benefits of this vaccine worldwide are even more impressive.

Every year, hundreds of thousands of humans are spared the braces, wheelchairs, and iron lungs required for the victims of poliomyelitis who survive this infectious disease. The research that led to a poliomyelitis vaccine required the sacrifice of hundreds of primates. Without this sacrifice, development of the vaccine would have been impossible, and in all likelihood the poliomyelitis epidemic would have continued unabated. Depriving humanity of this medical advance is unthinkable to almost all persons. Other diseases that are curable or treatable today as a result of animal research include diphtheria, scarlet fever, tuberculosis, diabetes, and appendicitis.[3] Human suffering would be much more stark today if these diseases, and many others as well, had not been amendable to treatment and cure through advances obtained by animal research.

ISSUES IN ANIMAL RESEARCH

Animal rights groups have several stock arguments against animal research. Some of these issues are described and refuted herein.

The Clinical Value of Basic Research
Persons opposed to research with animals often claim that basic biomedical research has no clinical value and therefore does not justify the use of animals. However, basic research is the foundation for most medical advances and consequently for progress in clinical medicine. Without basic research, including that with animals, chemotherapeutic advances against cancer (including childhood leukemia and breast malignancy), beta-blockers for cardiac patients, and electrolyte infusions for patients with dysfunctional metabolism would never have been achieved.

Duplication of Experiments
Opponents of animal research frequently claim that experiments are needlessly duplicated. However, the duplication of results is an essential part of the confirmation process in science. The generalization of results from one laboratory to another prevents anomalous results in one laboratory from being interpreted as scientific truth. The cost of research animals, the need to publish the results of experiments, and the desire to conduct meaningful research all function to reduce the likelihood of unnecessary experiments. Furthermore, the intense competition of research funds and the peer review process lessen the probability of obtaining funds for unnecessary research. Most scientists are unlikely to waste valuable time and resources conducting unnecessary experiments when opportunities for performing important research are so plentiful....

The Use of Primates in Research
Animal activists often make a special plea on behalf of nonhuman primates, and many of the sit-ins, demonstrations, and break-ins have been directed at primate research centers. Efforts to justify these activities invoke the premise that primates are much like humans because they exhibit suffering and other emotions.

Keeping primates in cages and isolating them from others of their kind is considered by activists as cruel and destructive of their "psychological well-being." However, the opinion that animals that resemble humans most closely and deserve the most protection and care reflects an attitude of speciesism (i.e., a hierarchical scheme of relative importance) that most activists purportedly abhor. This logical fallacy in the drive for special protection of primates apparently escapes most of its adherents.

Some scientific experiments require primates exactly because they simulate human physiology so closely. Primates are susceptible to many of the same diseases as humans and have similar immune systems. They also possess intellectual, cognitive, and social skills above those of other animals. These characteristics make primates invaluable in research related to language, perception, and visual and spatial skills.[14] Although primates constitute only 0.5% of all animals used in research, their contributions have been essential to the continued acquisition of knowledge in the biological and behavioral sciences.[15]

Do Animals Suffer Needless Pain and Abuse?
Animal activists frequently assert that research with animals causes severe pain and that many research animals are abused either deliberately or through indifference. Actually, experiments today involve pain only when relief from pain would interfere with the purpose of the experiments. In any experiment in which an animal might experience pain, federal law requires that a veterinarian must be consulted in planning the experiment, and anesthesia, tranquilizers, and analgesics must be used except when they

would compromise the results of the experiment.[16]

In 1984, the Department of Agriculture reported that 61% of research animals were not subjected to painful procedures, and another 31% received anesthesia or pain-relieving drugs. The remaining 8% did experience pain, often because improved understanding and treatment of pain, including chronic pain, were the purpose of the experiment.[14] Chronic pain is a challenging health problem that costs the United States about $50 billion a year in direct medical expenses, lost productivity, and income.[15]

Alternatives to the Use of Animals
One of the most frequent objections to animal research is the claim that alternative research models obviate the need for research with animals. The concept of alternatives was first raised in 1959 by Russell and Burch[17] in their book, *The Principles of Humane Experimental Technique*. These authors exhorted scientists to reduce the pain of experimental animals, decrease the number of animals used in research, and replace animals with nonanimal models whenever possible.

However, more often than not, alternatives to research animals are not available. In certain research investigations, cell, tissue, and organ cultures and computer models can be used as adjuncts to experiments with animals, and occasionally as substitutes for animals, at least in preliminary phases of the investigations. However, in many experimental situations, culture techniques and computer models are wholly inadequate because they do not encompass the physiological complexity of the whole animal. Examples where animals are essential to research include development of a vaccine against human immunodeficiency virus, refinement of organ transplantation techniques, investigation of mechanical devices as replacements for and adjuncts to physiological organs, identification of target-specific pharmaceuticals for cancer diagnosis and treatment, restoration of infarcted myocardium in patients with cardiac disease, evolution of new diagnostic imaging technologies, improvement of methods to relieve mental stress and anxiety, and evaluation of approaches to define and treat chronic pain. These challenges can only be addressed by research with animals as an essential step in the evolution of knowledge that leads to solutions. Humans are the only alternatives to animals for this step. When faced with this alternative, most people prefer the use of animals as the research model.

COMMENT

Love of animals and concern for their welfare are admirable characteristics that distinguish humans from other species of animals. Most humans, scientists as well as laypersons, share these attributes. However, when the concern for animals impedes the development of methods to improve the welfare of humans through amelioration and elimination of pain and suffering, a fundamental choice must be made. This choice is present today in the conflict between animal rights activism and scientific research. The American Medical Association made this choice more than a century ago and continues to stand squarely in defense of the use of animals for scientific research. In this position, the Association is supported by opinion polls that reveal strong endorsement of the American public for the use of animals in research and testing.[18] . . .

The American Medical Association believes that research involving animals is absolutely essential to maintaining and improving the health of people in America and worldwide.[6] Animal research is required to develop solutions to human tragedies such as human immunodeficiency virus disease, cancer, heart disease, dementia, stroke, and congenital and developmental abnormalities. The American Medical Association recognizes the moral obligation of investigators to use alternatives to animals whenever possible, and to conduct their research with animals as humanely as possible. However, it is convinced that depriving humans of medical advances by preventing research with animals is philosophically and morally a fundamentally indefensible position. Consequently, the American Medical Association is committed to the preservation of animal research and to the conduct of this research under the most humane conditions possible.[19,20]

REFERENCES

1. Rowan AN, Rollin BE. Animal research—for and against: a philosophical, social, and historical perspective. *Perspect Biol Med.* 1983; 27:1–17.
2. Bernard C; Green HC, trans. *An Introduction to the Study of Experimental Medicine.* New York, NY: Dover Publications Inc; 1957.
3. Council on Scientific Affairs. Animals in research. *JAMA*, 1989; 261:3602–3606.
4. Leader RW, Stark D. The importance of animals in biomedical research. *Perspect Biol Med.* 1987; 30:470–485.
5. Kransney JA. Some thoughts on the value of life. *Buffalo Physician,* 1984: 18:6–13.
6. Smith SJ, Evans RM, Sullivan-Fowler M, Hendee WR. Use of animals in biomedical research: historical role of the American Medical Association and the American physician. *Arch Intern Med.* 1988; 148:1849–1853.

7. Descartes R. *'Principles of Philosophy,' Descartes: Philosophical Writings.* Anscombe E. Geach PT, eds. London, England: Nelson & Sons; 1969.

8. Bentham J. *Introduction to the Principles of Morals and Legislation.* London, England: Athlone Press; 1970.

9. Godlovitch S, Godlovitch, Harris J. *Animals, Men and Morals.* New York, NY: Taplinger Publishing Co Inc; 1971.

10. Ryder R. *Victims of Science.* London, England: Davis-Poynter; 1975.

11. Singer P. *Animal Liberation: A New Ethic for Our Treatment of Animals.* New York, NY: Random House Inc; 1975.

12. Morowitz HJ, Jesus, Moses, Aristotle and laboratory animals. *Hosp Pract.* 1988; 23:23–25.

13. Cohen C. The case for the use of animals in biomedical research. *N Engl J Med.* 1986; 315: 865–870.

14. *Alternatives to Animal Use in Research, Testing, and Education.* Washington, DC: Office of Technology Assessment; 1986. Publication OTA-BA-273.

15. Committee on the Use of Laboratory Animals in Biomedical and Behavioral Research. *Use of Laboratory Animals in Biomedical and Behavioral Research.* Washington, DC: National Academy Press; 1988.

16. *Biomedical Investigator's Handbook.* Washington, DC: Foundation for Biomedical Research; 1987.

17. Russell WMS, Burch RL. *The Principles of Humane Experimental Technique.* Springfield, Ill: Charles C Thomas Publisher; 1959.

18. Harvey LK, Shubat SC. *AMA Survey of Physician and Public Opinion on Health Care Issues.* Chicago, Ill: American Medical Association; 1989.

19. Smith SJ, Hendee WR. Animals in research. *JAMA* 1988; 259:2007–2008.

20. Smith SJ, Loeb JM, Evans RM, Hendee WR. Animals in research and testing; who pays the price for medical progress? *Arch Ophthalmol.* 1988; 106:1184–1187.

NO

Tom Regan

ILL-GOTTEN GAINS

THE STORY

Late in 1981 a reporter for a large metropolitan newspaper (we'll call her Karen to protect her interest in remaining anonymous) gained access to some previously classified government files. Using the Freedom of Information Act, Karen was investigating the federal government's funding of research into the short- and long-term effects of exposure to radioactive waste. It was with understandable surprise that, included in these files, she discovered the records of a series of experiments involving the induction and treatment of coronary thrombosis (heart attack). Conducted over a period of fifteen years by a renowned heart specialist (we'll call him Dr. Ventricle) and financed with federal funds, the experiments in all likelihood would have remained unknown to anyone outside Dr. Ventricle's sphere of power and influence had not Karen chanced upon them.

Karen's surprise soon gave way to shock and disbelief. In case after case she read of how Ventricle and his associates took otherwise healthy individuals, with no previous record of heart disease, and intentionally caused their heart to fail. The methods used to occasion the "attack" were a veritable shopping list of experimental techniques, from massive doses of stimulants (adrenaline was a favorite) to electrical damage of the coronary artery, which, in its weakened state, yielded the desired thrombosis. Members of Ventricle's team then set to work testing the efficacy of various drugs developed in the hope that they would help the heart withstand a second "attack." Dosages varied, and there were the usual control groups. In some cases, certain drugs administered to "patients" proved more efficacious than cases in which others received no medication or smaller amounts of the same drugs. The research came to an abrupt end in the fall of 1981, but not because the project was judged unpromising or because someone raised a hue and cry about the ethics involved. Like so much else in the world at that time, Ventricle's project was a casualty of austere economic times. There simply wasn't enough federal money available to renew the grant application.

From Tom Regan, "Ill-Gotten Gains," in Donald Van DeVeer and Tom Regan, eds., *Health Care Ethics: An Introduction* (Temple University Press, 1987). Copyright © 1987 by Temple University. Reprinted by permission.

One would have to forsake all the instincts of a reporter to let the story end there. Karen persevered and, under false pretenses, secured an interview with Ventricle. When she revealed that she had gained access to the file, knew in detail the largely fruitless research conducted over fifteen years, and was incensed about his work, Ventricle was dumbfounded. But not because Karen had unearthed the file. And not even because it was filed where it was (a "clerical error," he assured her). What surprised Ventricle was that anyone would think there was a serious ethical question to be raised about what he had done. Karen's notes of their conversation include the following:

VENTRICLE: But I don't understand what you're getting at. Surely you know that heart disease is the leading cause of death. How can there be any ethical question about developing drugs which *literally* promise to be life-saving?

KAREN: Some people might agree that the goal—to save life—is a good, a noble end, and still question the means used to achieve it. Your "patients," after all, had no previous history of heart disease. *They* were healthy before you got your hands on them.

VENTRICLE: But medical progress simply isn't possible if we wait for people to get sick and then see what works. There are too many variables, too much beyond our control and comprehension, if we try to do our medical research in a clinical setting. The history of medicine shows how hopeless that approach is.

KAREN: And I read, too, that upon completion of the experiment, assuming that the "patient" didn't die in the process—it says that those who survived were "sacrificed." You mean killed?

VENTRICLE: Yes, that's right. But always painlessly, always painlessly. And the body went immediately to the lab, where further tests were done. Nothing was wasted.

KAREN: And it didn't bother you— I mean, you didn't ever ask yourself whether what you were doing was wrong? I mean...

VENTRICLE: (interrupting): My dear young lady, you make it seem as if I'm some kind of moral monster. I work for the benefit of humanity, and I have achieved some small success, I hope you will agree. Those who raise cries of wrongdoing about what I've done are well intentioned but misguided. After all, I use animals in my research— chimpanzees, to be more precise—not human beings.

THE POINT

The story about Karen and Dr. Ventricle is just that—a story, a small piece of fiction. There is no real Dr. Ventricle, no real Karen, and so on. But there *is* widespread use of animals in scientific research, including research like our imaginary Dr. Ventricle's. So the story, while its details are imaginary—while it is, let it be clear, a literary device, not a factual account—is a story with a point. Most people reading it would be morally outraged if there actually were a Dr. Ventricle who did coronary research of the sort described on otherwise healthy human beings. Considerably fewer would raise a morally quizzical eyebrow when informed of such research done on animals, chimpanzees, or whatever. The story has a point, or so I hope, because, catching us off-guard, it brings this difference home to us, gives it life in our experience, and, in doing so, reveals something about ourselves, something about our own constellation of values. If we think what Ventricle did would be wrong if done to human beings but all right if done to chimpanzees, then we must believe that there are different moral standards that apply to how we may treat the two—human beings and chimpanzees. But to acknowledge this difference, if acknowledge it we do, is only the beginning, not the end, of our moral thinking. We can meet the challenge to think well from the moral point of view only if we are able to cite a *morally relevant difference* between humans and chimpanzees, one that illuminates in a clear, coherent, and rationally defensible way why it would be wrong to use humans, but not chimpanzees, in research like Dr. Ventricle's. . . .

THE LAW

Among the difference between chimps and humans, one concerns their legal standing. It is against the law to do to human beings what Ventricle did to his chimpanzees. It is not against the law to do this to chimps. So, here we have a difference. But a morally relevant one?

The difference in the legal status of chimps and humans would be morally relevant if we had good reason to believe that what is legal and what is moral go hand in glove: where we have the former, there we have the latter (and maybe vice versa too). But a moment's reflection shows how bad the fit between legality and morality sometimes is. A century and a half ago, the legal status of black people in the United States was similar to the legal status of a house, corn, a barn: they were property, other people's property, and could legally be bought and sold without regard to their personal interests. But the legality of the slave trade did not make it moral, any more than the law against drinking, during the era of that "great experiment" of Prohibition,

made it immoral to drink. Sometimes, it is true, what the law declares illegal (for example, murder and rape) is immoral, and vice versa. But there is no necessary connection, no pre-established harmony between morality and the law. So, yes, the legal status of chimps and humans differs; but that does not show that their moral status does. Their difference in legal status, in other words, is not a morally relevant difference and will not morally justify using these animals, but not humans, in Ventricle's research.

THE VALUE OF THE INDIVIDUAL

[An] alternative vision [to utilitarian value] consists in viewing certain individuals as themselves having a distinctive kind of value, what we will call "inherent value." This kind of value is not the same as, is not reducible to, and is not commensurate either with such values as preference satisfaction or frustration (that is, mental states) or with such values as artistic or intellectual talents (that is, mental and other kinds of excellences or virtues). We cannot, that is, equate or reduce the inherent value of an individual to his or her mental states or virtues, and neither can we intelligibly compare the two. In this respect, the three kinds of value (mental states, virtues, and the inherent value of the individual) are like proverbial apples and oranges.

They are also like water and oil: they don't mix. It is not only that [a man's] inherent value is not the same as, not reducible to, and not commensurate with *his* satisfaction, pleasures, intellectual and artistic skills, etc. In addition, *his* inherent value is not the same as, is not reducible to, and is not commensurate with the valuable mental states or talents of *other* individuals, whether taken singly or collectively. Moreover, and as a corollary of the preceding, the individual's inherent value is in all ways independent both of his or her usefulness relative to the interest of others and of how others feel about the individual (for example, whether one is liked or admired, despised or merely tolerated). A prince and a pauper, a streetwalker and a nun, those who are loved and those who are forsaken, the genius and the retarded child, the artist and the philistine, the most generous philanthropist and the most unscrupulous used car salesman—all have inherent value, according to the view recommended here, and all have it equally....

WHAT DIFFERENCE DOES IT MAKE?

To view the value of individuals in this way is not an empty abstraction. To the question, "What difference does it make whether we view individuals as having equal inherent value, or as utilitarians do, as lacking such value, or, as perfectionists do, as having such value but to varying degree?"—our response to this question must be, "It makes all the moral difference in the world!" Morally, we are *always* required to treat those who have inherent value in ways that display proper respect for their distinctive kind of value, and though we cannot on this occasion either articulate or defend the full range of obligations tied to this fundamental duty, we can note that we fail to show proper respect for those who have such value whenever we treat them as if they were mere receptacles of value or as if their value was dependent on, or reducible to, their possible utility relative to the interests of others. In particular, therefore, Ventricle would fail to act as duty re-

quires—would, in other words, do what is morally wrong—if he conducted his coronary research on competent human beings, without their informed consent, on the grounds that this research just might lead to the development of drugs or surgical techniques that would benefit others. That would be to treat these human beings as mere receptacles or as mere medical resources for others, and though Ventricle might be able to do this and get away with it, and though others might benefit as a result, that would not alter the nature of the grievous wrong he would have done. And it would be wrong, not because (or only if) there were utilitarian considerations, or contractarian considerations, or perfectionist considerations against his doing his research on these human beings, but because it would mark a failure on his part to treat them with appropriate respect. To ascribe inherent value to competent human beings, then, provides us with the theoretical wherewithal to ground our moral case against using competent human beings, against their will, in research like Ventricle's.

WHO HAS INHERENT VALUE?

If inherent value could nonarbitrarily be limited to competent humans, then we would have to look elsewhere to resolve the ethical issues involved in using other individuals (for example, chimpanzees) in medical research. But inherent value can only be limited to competent human beings by having the recourse to one arbitrary maneuver or another. Once we recognize that we have direct duties to competent and incompetent humans as well as to animals such as chimpanzees; once we recognize the challenge to give a sound theoretical basis for these duties in the case of these humans and animals; once we recognize the failure of indirect duty, contractarian, and utilitarian theories of obligation; once we recognize that the inherent value of competent humans precludes using them as mere resources in such research; once we recognize that perfectionist vision of morality, one that assigns degrees of inherent value on the basis of possession of favored virtues, is unacceptable because of its inegalitarian implications, and once we recognize that morality simply will not tolerate double standards, then we cannot, except arbitrarily, withhold ascribing inherent value, to an equal degree, to incompetent humans and animals such as chimpanzees. All have this value, in short, and all have it equally. All considered, this is an essential part of the most adequate total vision of morality. Morally, none of those having inherent value may be used in Ventricle-like research (research that puts them at risk of significant harm in the name of securing benefits for others, whether those benefits are realized or not). And none may be used in such research because to do so is to treat them as if their value is somehow reducible to their possible utility relative to the interests of others, or as if their value is somehow reducible to their value as "receptacles." What contractarianism, utilitarianism, and the other "isms" discussed earlier will allow is not morally tolerable.

HURTING AND HARMING

The prohibition against research like Ventricle's, when conducted on animals such as chimps, cannot be avoided by the use of anesthetics or other palliatives used to eliminate or reduce suffering. Other things being equal, to cause an animal to suffer is to harm that animal—is, that is, to diminish that individual animal's welfare. But these two notions—harming on the one hand and suffering on the other —differ in important ways. An individual's welfare can be diminished independently of causing her to suffer, as when, for example, a young woman is reduced to a "vegetable" by painlessly administering a debilitating drug to her while she sleeps. We mince words if we deny that harm has been done to her, though she suffers not. More generally, harms, understood as reductions in an individual's welfare, can take the form either of *inflictions* (gross physical suffering is the clearest example of a harm of this type) or *deprivations* (prolonged loss of physical freedom is a clear example of a harm of this kind). Not all harms hurt, in other words, just as not all hurts harm.

Viewed against the background of these ideas, an untimely death is seen to be the ultimate harm for both humans and animals, such as chimpanzees, and it is the ultimate harm for both because it is their ultimate deprivation or loss —their loss of life itself. Let the means used to kill chimpanzees be as "humane" (a cruel word, this) as you like. That will not erase the harm that an untimely death is for these animals. True, the use of anesthetics and other "humane" steps lessens the wrong done to these animals, when they are "sacrificed" in Ventricle-type research. But a lesser wrong is not a right. To do research that culminates in the "sacrifice" of chimpanzees or that puts these and similar animals at risk of losing their life, in the hope that we might learn something that will benefit others, is morally to be condemned, however "humane" that research may be in other respects.

THE CRITERION OF INHERENT VALUE

It remains to be asked, before concluding, what underlies the possession of inherent value. Some are tempted by the idea that life itself is inherently valuable. This view would authorize attributing inherent value to chimpanzees, for example, and so might find favor with some people who oppose using these animals in research. But this view would also authorize attributing inherent value to anything and everything that is alive, including, for example, crabgrass, lice, bacteria, and cancer cells. It is exceedingly unclear, to put the point as mildly as possible, either that we have a duty to treat these things with respect or that any clear sense can be given to the idea that we do.

More plausible by far is the view that those individuals have inherent value who are *the subjects of a life*—who are, that is, the experiencing subjects of a life that fares well or ill for them over time, those who have *an individual experiential welfare*, logically independent of their utility relative to the interests or welfare of others. Competent humans are subjects of a life in this sense. But so, too, are those incompetent humans who have concerned us. And so, too, and not unimportantly, are chimpanzees. Indeed, so too are the members of many species of animals: cats and dogs, monkeys and sheep, cetaceans and wolves, horses and cattle. Where one draws the line between those animals who are, and those who are not, subjects of a life is certain to be controversial. Still there is abundant reason to believe that the members of mammalian species of animals do have a psychophysical identity over time, do have an experiential life, do have an individual welfare. Common sense is on the side of viewing these animals in this way, and ordinary language is not strained in talking of them as individuals who have an experiential welfare. The behavior of these animals, moreover, is consistent with regarding them as subjects of a life, and the implications of evolutionary theory are that there are many species of animals whose members are, like the members of the species *Homo sapiens*, experiencing subjects of a life of their own, with an individual welfare. On these grounds, then, we have very strong reason to believe, even if we lack conclusive proof, that these animals meet the subject-of-a-life criterion.

If, then, those who meet this criterion have inherent value, and have it equally relative to all who meet it, chimpanzees and other animals who are subjects of a life, not just human beings, have this value *and* have neither more nor less of it than we do. (To hold that they have less than we do is to land oneself in the inegalitarian swamp of perfectionism). Moreover, if, as has been argued, having inherent value morally bars others from treating those who have it as mere receptacles or as mere resources for others, then any and all medical research like Ventricle's, done on these animals in the name of possibly benefitting others, stands morally condemned. And it is not only cases in which the benefits for others do not materialize that are condemnable; also to be condemned are cases, such as the research done on chimps regarding hepatitis, for example, in which the benefits for others are genuine. In these cases, as in others like them in the relevant respects, the ends do not justify the means. The *many millions* of mammalian animals used each year for scientific purposes, including medical research, bear mute, tragic testimony to the narrowness of our moral vision.

CONCLUSIONS

This condemnation of such research probably is at odds with the judgment that most people would make about this issue. If we had good reason to assume that the truth always lies with what most people think, then we could look approvingly on Ventricle-like research done on animals like chimps in the name of benefits for others. But we have no good reason to believe that the truth is to be measured plausibly by majority opinion, and what we know of the history of prejudice and bigotry speaks powerfully, if painfully, against this view. Only the cumulative force of informed, fair, rigorous argument can decide where the truth lies, or most likely lies, when we examine a controversial moral question. Although openly acknowledging and, indeed, insisting on the limitations of the arguments . . . , these arguments make the case, in broad outline, against using animals such as chimps in medical research such as Ventricle's. . . .

Those who oppose the use of animals such as chimps in research like Ventricle's and who accept the major themes advanced here, oppose it, then, not because they think that all such research is a waste of time and money, or because they think that it never leads to any benefits for others, or because they view those who do such research as, to use Ventricle's, words, "moral monsters," or even because they love animals. Those of us who condemn such research do so because this research is not possible except at the grave moral price of failing to show proper respect for the value of the animals who are used. Since, whatever our gains, they are ill-gotten, we must bring to an end research like Ventricle's, whatever our losses. A fair measure of our moral integrity will be the extent of our resolve to work against allowing our scientific, economic, health, and other interests to serve as a reason for the wrongful exploitation of members of species of animals other than our own.

POSTSCRIPT

Should Animal Experimentation Be Permitted?

In 1985 Congress passed the Health Research Extension Act, which directed the National Institutes of Health (NIH) to establish guidelines for the proper care of animals to be used in biomedical and behavioral research. The NIH regulations implementing the law require institutions that receive federal grants to establish Animal Care and Use Committees. The Office of Science and Technology Policies' "Principles for the Utilization and Care of Vertebrate Animals Used in Testing, Research and Training," *Federal Register* (May 20, 1985) serves as the basis for the U.S. government's policy. The NIH's *Guide for the Care and Use of Laboratory Animals*, rev. ed. (1985) offers explicit instructions.

In February 1993 a federal judge ruled that the Department of Agriculture's standards on the treatment of laboratory dogs and primates were not stringent enough and that the agency had failed to put into effect the 1985 law. Charles R. McCarthy, in "Improved Standards for Laboratory Animals?" *Kennedy Institute of Ethics* (vol. 3, no. 3, 1993), asserts that this ruling actually lowers the standard for the care of laboratory animals.

Although they do not recommend a complete ban on animal research, some authors have argued that current practices in animal research must be reevaluated and better regulated. See, for example, *Lives in the Balance: The Ethics of Using Animals in Biomedical Research* edited by Jane A. Smith and Kenneth M. Boyd (Oxford University Press, 1991) and *In the Name of Science: Issues in Responsible Animal Experimentation* by F. Barbara Orlans (Oxford University Press, 1993).

For an opposing view, see the Office of Technology Assessment's *Alternatives to Animal Use in Research, Testing, and Education* (Government Printing Office, 1986). Richard P. Vance analyzes what he believes are erroneous myths held by supporters of animal research in "An Introduction to the Philosophical Presuppositions of the Animal Liberation/Rights Movement," *Journal of the American Medical Association* (October 7, 1992). Also see *Current Issues and New Frontiers in Animal Research* edited by Kathryn A. L. Bayne, Molly Greene, and Ernest D. Prentice (Scientists Center for Animal Welfare, 1995); the Hastings Center's "Animals, Science, and Ethics," *Hastings Center Report* (May/June 1990); and the *Hastings Center Report* special supplement "The Brave New World of Animal Biotechnology" (January/February 1994). Also see the *Hastings Center Report* case study "New Creations?" (January–February 1991), which presents opposing views on research on manipulating genes to produce new animal strains.

ISSUE 17

Will Fetal Tissue Research Encourage Abortions?

YES: Douglas K. Martin, from "Abortion and Fetal Tissue Transplantation," *IRB: A Review of Human Subjects Research* (May/June 1993)

NO: Dorothy E. Vawter and Karen G. Gervais, from "Commentary on 'Abortion and Fetal Tissue Transplantation,'" *IRB: A Review of Human Subjects Research* (May/June 1993)

ISSUE SUMMARY

YES: Bioethicist Douglas K. Martin argues that the therapeutic use of fetal tissue cannot be separated from moral concerns over abortion and that the option to donate fetal tissue may influence some women to choose abortion.

NO: Bioethicists Dorothy E. Vawter and Karen G. Gervais contend that knowledge of the option to donate tissue is not an incentive for a woman to abort a fetus she would otherwise carry to term as long as potential recipients remain anonymous and no financial gain is involved.

About 500,000 Americans suffer from Parkinson's disease, a progressively debilitating and incurable nerve disorder that leads to rigidity and tremors. No one knows what causes the disease, and current drug treatments have disturbing side effects. As the disease worsens, patients become incapacitated, unable to carry out even the simplest activities.

In 1987 Mexican surgeon Dr. Ignacio Madrazo Navarro reported success in treating five Parkinson's patients by transplanting fetal tissue into their brains. Previous attempts to transplant adrenal tissue had been disappointing. Transplantation of living tissue is intended to enhance the brain's production of dopamine, a chemical that is important for regulating movement and that is not secreted in normal quantities in Parkinson's patients.

Other potential uses of fetal tissue include the treatment of Alzheimer's disease, brain and spinal cord injuries, some forms of epilepsy, and other serious neurological conditions. It is even possible that fetal tissue might be beneficial in the treatment of diabetes or blood and metabolic disorders. Researchers in Sweden, the United States, China, Canada, and elsewhere are working with animal models and, in a few cases, with human subjects to determine whether or not these techniques will prove beneficial. Before any such use of fetal tissue transplantation can be considered a therapy with proven benefits, research involving human subjects must be conducted. But such studies raise serious ethical questions.

Concern about fetal research arose in the aftermath of the 1973 U.S. Supreme Court decision of *Roe v. Wade*, which legalized abortion. Before *Roe v. Wade*, fetal research had been conducted with little apparent public concern. But reports of research conducted by Scandinavian researchers using live, postabortion fetuses fueled a hot and emotional debate in the United States and led to a moratorium imposed by the National Institutes of Health (NIH) on any research involving a living fetus before or after abortion. In 1975, spurred by public protests, Congress established the National Commission for the Protection of Human Subjects of Biomedical and Behavioral Research to examine the ethical issues surrounding experimentation. The first topic on its agenda was fetal research.

Research that would impose little or no risk to the fetus or that was intended to benefit the fetus posed few ethical difficulties for the commission. However, irreconcilable differences arose when abortion entered the picture. Research using about-to-be-aborted fetuses, for example, might be intended to determine the harmful or beneficial effects on the fetus of drugs given to the pregnant woman during pregnancy or labor. Other types of research might be harmful to the fetus and could not ethically be performed on a fetus that is destined to be delivered at term. The commission (with one dissent) approved minimal-risk research if abortion was anticipated, but they required the approval of a national ethical review body for research that involved more than minimal risk. The commission's recommendations, with some modifications, were incorporated into the federal regulations governing human subject research in 1975. The Reagan and Bush administrations opposed using aborted fetal tissue for research, and during most of the 1980s and early 1990s, there was a federal ban on funding fetal tissue research. In 1988 a National Institutes of Health Fetal Tissue Transplantation Research Panel concluded that funding such research is "acceptable public policy." In May 1992 Congress voted to overturn the ban, but President Bush vetoed it because, he said, it encouraged abortions.

When Bill Clinton became president in 1992, he lifted the ban. Accordingly, the debate has shifted to the question of whether the procedural safeguards recommended by the NIH panel are sufficient to prevent women from aborting fetuses because they want to donate fetal tissue.

The following selections take up this debate. Douglas K. Martin believes that the NIH guidelines are unfeasible and unethical and that the therapeutic uses of aborted tissue cannot be separated from moral concerns about abortion. Dorothy E. Vawter and Karen G. Gervais believe that it is possible to prevent fetal tissue transplantation from leading a woman to abort a fetus she would otherwise carry to term. They argue that procedural safeguards such as timing, restricting the use of tissue to anonymous recipients, and banning payment would address those concerns.

YES

Douglas K. Martin

ABORTION AND FETAL TISSUE TRANSPLANTATION

Government moratoria on public funding for research in fetal tissue transplantation have been based on the concern that knowledge of fetal tissue transplantation, and the option to donate tissue for transplantation, may influence some women to have abortions. In response to this concern, in 1988 the director of the National Institutes of Health, James B. Wyngaarden, convened a research panel to examine the issue. At the conclusion of their deliberations, a majority of the panelists did not consider the concern compelling and recommended procedures they felt would be adequate to morally separate abortion from the use of the fetal tissue. Advocates of fetal tissue transplantation have repeatedly referred to these and similar guidelines as a means of ensuring the ethical acceptability of such therapy.

The NIH panel evaded the fundamental question of whether using tissue from electively aborted fetuses was itself ethically acceptable. The panel report skipped directly to recommending procedures that would enable fetal tissue research to advance. The panel side-stepped the ethical questions by resorting to legal and policy arguments upon which to base its chief recommendation, which was:

> It is of moral relevance that human fetal tissue for research has been obtained from induced abortions. However, in light of the fact that abortion is legal and that the research in question is intended to achieve significant medical goals, the panel concludes that the use of such tissue is acceptable public policy.[1, p. 1]

It is important to emphasize that in asserting that abortion is legal and the research well intended the panel did not comment on the ethical merit of fetal tissue transplantation.

A majority of the panel maintained that permitting research in fetal tissue transplantation was acceptable public policy "either because the source of the tissue posed no moral problem or because the immorality of its source could be ethically isolated from the morality of its use in research."[1, p. 2] To accommodate individuals who believe that abortion is immoral, or at least undesirable, the panel made several recommendations with the express intent of morally

From Douglas K. Martin, "Abortion and Fetal Tissue Transplantation," *IRB: A Review of Human Subjects Research*, vol. 15, no. 3 (May/June 1993). Copyright © 1993 by The Hastings Center. Reprinted by permission.

isolating fetal tissue transplantation from abortion. These recommendations included that:

- the decision to terminate a pregnancy be kept independent from the retrieval and use of fetal tissue;
- informed consent for the research be distinct from and subsequent to consent for the abortion; and
- even preliminary information about tissue donation be withheld from the pregnant woman before she consents to the abortion.

I contend that these and similar proposals, for example the recently considered U.S. federal legislation H.R. 2507, are both unfeasible and unethical, and therefore cannot achieve the stated goal of morally insulating fetal tissue research from abortion. I will address three points of argument: (1) the realities of consent as a process, which makes the recommended constraint on the timing of disclosure unfeasible; (2) the influence that publicized fetal tissue transplantation will have on women confronted with an unwanted pregnancy—an influence that morally and practically cannot be prevented by gag orders on health care professionals; and (3) the autonomy of women considering abortion, and the ethical obligation on professionals to fully inform a woman in the process of making any decision regarding her fetus.

THE CONSENT PROCESS

A simplistic and sometimes callous belief held by many, and implicit in the NIH panel report, is that informed consent is a bureaucratic/legalistic act in which information is disclosed and a consent form is signed at a particular moment in time.[2,3] However, it has been strongly argued that informed consent should be considered an essential part of the professional-patient relationship, a process occurring over a length of time. A metaphor that has been utilized to describe this process is the "conversation model" of informed consent employed by Jay Katz and others.[4,5] During an informed consent process, like a series of conversations, the bidirectional ebb and flow of information is unpredictable. As in conversation, one must go through each process before knowing its outcome.

Despite the fact that in the abortion scenario urgency may curtail the extent of an ongoing physician-patient relationship, a fully explored consent process is still possible and necessary. One could reasonably argue that an extended consent process should be mandatory in an abortion decision because of the emotional distress that often accompanies the circumstances promulgating the decision. Furthermore, as in all medical procedures, a woman contemplating an abortion may sign a consent form and even make an appointment for the procedure before she has fully resolved in her mind what her final decision will be. Her irreversible consent does not occur until she physically submits herself for the procedure. A woman may choose not to go through with the abortion at any time prior to the procedure.

In empirical studies ambivalence and anxiety over the abortion are commonly documented characteristics of women facing this decision;[6] as many as 40 percent of women contemplating abortion reported changing their mind at least once before coming to a final decision, and those who aborted were significantly more likely to rethink their original choice and to regret their decision;[7-9] up to 37 percent of women who abort do not finally decide until just before the procedure.[6-10] Some women who have decided to abort will change their mind at the last minute. One study followed 505 women who went to a clinic and applied to have an abortion: after they filled out the background paperwork, were examined by a gynecologist, and were interviewed by a social worker and psychiatrist, 6 percent changed their minds and decided to continue the pregnancy.[11]

To be prepared to preserve the tissue, researchers must receive consent from the woman for the use of the tissue before the abortion. Therefore, the consent for tissue use will often precede the final consent for the abortion, and always precede the irreversible consent for the abortion. Yet the panel recommended that "the informed consent for the abortion should precede informed consent... for tissue donation.[1, p. 4] This is unfeasible.

THE INFLUENCE OF FETAL TISSUE TRANSPLANTATION ON WOMEN FACING AN UNWANTED PREGNANCY

Regarding the abortion decision, empirical evidence indicates that somewhat less than 10 percent of abortions are chosen for medical reasons. Upwards of 90 percent of abortions are chosen for a multiplicity of reasons (an average of 4) based predominantly on life-style preferences.[12] In one study, up to one-half of women who chose abortion found the decision difficult to make.[7, 8] As previously stated, in another study 40 percent of women who contemplated abortion changed their minds at least once and found the decision difficult to make. For these women, it was reported that the "pros and cons of the decision were somewhat evenly balanced."[9] In other words,

women choose abortion because of a combination of many reasons, most often relating to personal preferences; and the decision is often difficult to make, with a close balance of pros and cons. It is reasonable to suggest that new factors which may be introduced into this decision may well contribute to tipping the balance one way or the other.

It is also reasonable to suggest that the knowledge that aborted fetal tissue might be used to benefit sick people might be an important consideration for some women. Arthur Caplan, an advocate of fetal tissue transplantation, has argued that such an option may provide "solace" to women having abortions.[13] Swedish scientists involved in fetal tissue research have testified that, in their experience, almost all women approached consent to donate the tissue and they do so because they are "glad something positive could come out of it."[14] In research currently underway at the Centre for Bioethics, women aged 18 to 40 were surveyed about their opinions regarding abortion and fetal tissue transplantation. Preliminary results show that 12 percent of these women indicated that, if they were pregnant, they would be more likely to choose abortion if they knew that they could donate tissue for transplantation.[15] Thus the knowledge that a woman may donate the tissue from her aborted fetus for therapeutic transplantation could be an important factor in the decision to abort, and may well be a decisive one.

In addition, it must be stressed that this evidence suggesting that women may be influenced by fetal tissue transplantation was obtained in a social climate where the efficacy of such therapy is not established. Researchers hope that in the near future fetal tissue transplantation might provide significant benefit for patients suffering from Parkinson's disease, Type I diabetes, or any of the more than 20 diseases currently being considered. If it is shown that fetal tissue transplantation would benefit at least some of these millions of patients, it must be presumed that the influence this knowledge will exert on women facing an unwanted pregnancy will be much greater, and that the influence society will exert on these women will be much greater—even in the absence of direct influence or information from a physician.

The NIH panel reported that they "regarded it highly unlikely that a woman would be encouraged to make this decision [the abortion decision] because of the knowledge that fetal remains might be used in research."[1, p. 3] This speculation is not in accord with present evidence and is naive to the future implications of fetal tissue transplantation. Contrary to this presumption, current evidence suggests that the option to donate fetal tissue for transplantation may well influence some women to choose abortion.

THE AUTONOMY OF WOMEN CONSIDERING ABORTION

The Belmont Report, which outlines guidelines for the conduct of biomedical research, states that "to withhold information necessary to make a considered judgment, when there are not compelling reasons to do so" shows lack of respect for autonomous agents. In the matter of clinical practice, consent to treatment is not currently addressed in legislation. However, Canadian case law has determined that, to obtain a valid informed consent, a health professional must explore and disclose all information "material" to the patient's decision.[16, 3] Furthermore, the professional must not withhold information nor present information such that it misleads the patient.[3] As I have argued, for a woman contemplating abortion information regarding the donation of aborted fetal tissue may reasonably constitute important, even decisive, information. Prohibiting disclosure of this information contradicts modern ethical and legal standards of disclosure based on the ethical principle of autonomy.

The NIH advisory committee held that "the decision and consent to abort must precede discussion of the possible use of the fetal tissue."[1, p. 3] and that "informed consent for abortion should precede... the provision of preliminary information for tissue donation."[1, p. 4] The panel also wrote that "in the consent process for termination of pregnancy, we believe there should be no mention at all of the possibility of fetal tissue use in transplantation and research."[1, p. 4] If these guidelines were followed, the consent for the abortion would not be ethically valid, and might not be legally valid, and the autonomy of the woman in question would be violated. Therefore, the guidelines are unfeasible and unethical.

REFERENCES

1. Consultants to the Advisory Committee to the Director, National Institutes of Health, *Report of the Human Fetal Tissue Transplantation Research Panel.* vol. 1. Bethesda, Md.: National Institutes of Health, 1988.
2. For critical discussion, see Faden, RR, and Beauchamp, TL: *A History and Theory of Informed Consent.* New York: Oxford University Press, 1986.
3. Rozovsky, LE, and Rozovsky, FA: *The Canadian Law of Consent to Treatment.* Toronto: Butterworths, 1990.
4. Katz, J: *The Silent World of Doctor and Patient.* New York: Free Press, 1984.
5. Brody, H: Transparency: Informed consent in primary care. *Hastings Center Report.* 1989; 19(5):5–9.

6. Reardon, DC: *Aborted Women*. Westchester, IL: Crossway, 1987; Nadleson, C: Abortion counseling: Focus on adolescent pregnancy. *Pediatrics* 1974; 54:768.

7. Kerenyi, TD, Glascock, EL, and Horowitz, ML: Reasons for delayed abortion: Results of four hundred interviews. *American Journal of Obstetrics and Gynecology* 1973; 117(3):299–311; at 307.

8. Bracken, MB: The stability of the decision to seek induced abortion. In *Report and Recommendations on Research on the Fetus*, National Commission for the Protection of Human Subjects of Biomedical and Behavioral Research, 1975, Appendix 16.

9. Bracken, MB, Klerman, LV, and Bracken, MA: Abortion, adoption, or motherhood: An empirical study of decision-making during pregnancy. *American Journal of Obstetrics and Gynecology* 1978; 130(3):251–62; at 256–57.

10. Diamond, M, et al.: Sexuality, birth control and abortion: A decision-making sequence. *Journal of Biosocial Science* 1973; 5:347.

11. Swigar, ME, Breslin, R, Pouzzner, MG, and Quinlan, D: Interview follow-up of abortion applicant dropouts. *Social Psychiatry* 1976; 11:135–43.

12. Torres, A, Forrest, JD: Why do women have abortions? *Family Planning Perspectives* 1988; 20:170–76.

13. Caplan, AL: Should foetuses or infants be utilized as organ donors? *Bioethics* 1987; 1(2):119–40.

14. Testimony of Lars Olson, 14 September 1988. Reported in J. Bopp and J. Burtchaell: Statement of dissent in consultants to the Advisory Committee to the Director, National Institutes of Health. *Report of the Human Fetal Tissue Transplantation Research Panel*, vol 1; at p. 57.

15. Martin, DK, Lowy, FH, Williams, JI, and Dunn, EV: Women's attitudes toward abortion and fetal tissue transplantation. Unpublished ms.

16. *Reibel v. Hughes*, (1980) 2 S.C.R. 880 (1980), 14 C.C.L.T.1; *Hopp v. Lepp*, (1980) 2 S.C.R. 192, 13 C.C.L.T. 66.

NO

Dorothy E. Vawter
and Karen G. Gervais

COMMENTARY ON "ABORTION AND FETAL TISSUE TRANSPLANTATION"

The former ban on the use of federal funds for fetal tissue transplantation research was based on the belief that it is impossible to prevent women from aborting fetuses for the purpose of donation if such transplants are permitted. One of the few points of agreement in the debate concerning fetal tissue transplantation is that it is wrong to use tissue from fetuses aborted specifically for donation. The major problem with abortion for donation is that it involves grave disrespect for the living fetus; the fetus is valued more for its parts and its usefulness to someone else than for being a potential human person. Whether it is possible to prevent fetal tissue transplants from leading to abortion for donation, and if so, how, remain subjects of contention. Those who believe it is possible to prevent abortion for donation have focused on a set of three policy recommendations to ensure that a woman's decision to abort is made separately from, and prior to, a decision to donate fetal tissue.

The two most important policy recommendations to prevent abortion for donation remove possible incentives, namely, the desire either to save the life of a relative or close friend or to obtain financial benefits. The NIH Human Fetal Tissue Transplantation Research Panel, Congress, and many other groups recommend that women be prohibited from designating the recipient of fetal tissue, and from benefiting financially from donation.[1] Since donating to anonymous recipients is not believed to provide a woman with an incentive to abort, these groups permit women to donate fetal tissue for this purpose. Their third recommendation is directed at preventing abortion clinic personnel from pressuring a pregnant woman to donate tissue before she has consented to an abortion, possibly thereby causing her to abort to donate. They recommend prohibiting abortion clinic personnel from raising the option of fetal tissue donation, and from seeking the woman's consent, until after she has consented to an abortion.

Martin criticizes this third policy recommendation on two grounds. First, restricting the timing of invitations to donate will not prevent women from knowing of the option to abort to donate and ultimately choosing to abort for

From Dorothy E. Vawter and Karen G. Gervais, "Commentary on 'Abortion and Fetal Tissue Transplantation,'" *IRB: A Review of Human Subjects Research*, vol. 15, no. 3 (May/June 1993). Copyright © 1993 by The Hastings Center. Reprinted by permission.

this reason. Second, restricting the timing of invitations to donate is unethical because it requires the withholding of information material to women's abortion decisions. He concludes that it is impossible to prevent fetal tissue transplantation from encouraging women to abort for the purpose of donating tissue to anonymous recipients, and that it is impossible to insulate abortion and fetal tissue transplantation from one another. He stops short, however, of disclosing whether he believes abortion for donation is unethical or whether the transplantation of tissue from electively aborted fetuses should be prohibited.

We believe that it is permissible to transplant tissue from electively aborted fetuses if provisions are in place to adequately respect and protect fetuses as well as women. We support the policy recommendations made by the NIH panel, Congress, and other groups to prevent abortion for donation, including the restriction on when abortion clinic personnel may raise the option to donate. Contrary to Martin, we maintain that:

- It is possible to prevent fetal tissue transplantation from leading a woman to abort a fetus she would otherwise carry to term.
- A woman would not choose abortion in response to knowing there is a chance some of the fetal tissue may be suitable for transplantation in an anonymous recipient.
- If a woman is properly informed of the potential risks to her privacy and well-being from donating tissue for transplantation, she not only has no incentive to donate, but has disincentives as well.
- The primary purpose of restricting the timing of invitations to donate is to

prevent abortion clinic personnel from pressuring women to abort to donate, not to prevent women from knowing of the option to donate.
- Restricting the timing of invitations to donate is ethically required because it is protective and respectful of women as well as fetuses.

There is no basis for assuming that a woman weighs the option to donate fetal tissue to anonymous recipients when considering an abortion. That a woman may be ambivalent about her abortion decision, and may change her mind, does not prove that information about donating to anonymous recipients or an invitation to donate would have any affect on the woman's ambivalence or abortion decision. That 40 to 50 percent of women find the abortion decision difficult does not mean that a woman does not have good reasons for and against it. The option to donate fetal tissue is at least equally irrelevant to a woman's decision to abort as the option to donate hip bone is to a patient considering a hip replacement. Knowledge of the option to donate fetal tissue to anonymous recipients neither generates a dilemma about whether to have an abortion nor assists a woman in resolving such a dilemma.

Believing otherwise rests on confusing the solace a woman may seek from donating fetal tissue with her reasons for having an abortion. A woman may agree to donate fetal tissue out of a desire to relieve some of her pain over her previous and independent decision to abort; she will not, however, choose to have an abortion as a means of obtaining solace. The desire for solace is not a reason to abort; it is a reason for deciding to donate subsequent to a separate decision to abort.

Finally, we have reservations about the preliminary results reported from a study of women's opinions about abortion and fetal tissue transplantation. Martin says that the study supports the claim that women will abort for the purpose of donating tissue (to anonymous others?). Until the details of the study are published it is clearly impossible to fully evaluate this information. However, given how situation-specific women's abortion decisions are, it is unclear what useful information can be obtained from asking women global hypothetical questions about whether they believe the option to donate would affect their decision to terminate a "generic" pregnancy sometime in the future.

It is especially important to know how the questions are framed. For example, might the response to a question about whether the opportunity to donate tissue to anonymous recipients would make the respondent feel better about her abortion be unjustifiably interpreted as evidence that women would abort for the purpose of donating tissue? It is also important to know whether the respondents were provided with the information that a woman should properly receive concerning the donation, procurement, and transplantation of fetal tissue, including the associated risks to her privacy and well-being.[2] Were the respondents informed of the low likelihood that the tissue they donate will be usable or used? Were they informed that they would not be permitted to designate the recipient or to receive financial compensation? The problems inherent in studies involving hypothetical questions are magnified if the respondents lack full understanding of the activity they are asked to imagine participating in.

Martin ends his critique with the startling suggestion that it is unethical not to inform a woman considering abortion of the option to abort to donate. He argues that because some women, in his view, will choose to abort to donate, information about the option to donate must be considered material to a woman's abortion decision and must, therefore, be disclosed to all women considering abortion. This suggests that a woman's decision to abort and her decision to donate should be allowed to be a single decision and that it is wrong for health professionals not to provide a woman the opportunity to abort to donate. By extension this implies that it is wrong for health care providers to fail to inform all patients of the ways they may serve as live donors of tissues and organs, perhaps even of unethical or illegal types of donation.[3]

First, disclosure requirements for therapeutic interventions do not require disclosing options unrelated to the health problem for which the patient is seeking assistance. Inviting a patient to be a live organ or tissue donor, or a human research subject, is never obligatory. Moreover, before making such a request or invitation it is necessary to have special protections in place to assure that the "patient" is respected, is not exposed to unreasonable risks, and is fully informed. Treating all pregnant women considering abortion as persons who must be given the opportunity to undergo an invasive procedure for the purpose of assisting anonymous recipients is disrespectful of, as well as potentially harmful to, the woman seeking medical assistance, the living fetus, and the special relationship between a pregnant woman and her fetus. Second, insofar as it is unethical (and illegal) for a woman to abort to donate, not only is there no obligation to disclose the option to donate, but health providers should be prohibited from inviting the woman to donate before she has consented to abortion.

In our view, the policy recommendation to restrict the timing of invitations to donate is ethically required to protect and respect women as well as fetuses.

- It prevents abortion clinic personnel from pressuring women to abort to donate.
- It protects women considering abortion from being treated merely as potential live tissue donors and from possibly being denied a genuinely therapeutic relationship with their physician.
- It protects living fetuses from being valued for their tissues and being treated as renewable, or optional, tissue specimens of women.
- It prevents any suggestion that it is permissible to abort to donate.

Once the incentives to abort to donate for financial gain or to save the life of a relative or friend are eliminated, there is no reason to be concerned about women knowing of the option to donate tissue. Knowledge of the option to donate tissue to anonymous recipients is not an incentive for a woman to abort a fetus she would otherwise carry to term. However, if clinic personnel are permitted to seek a woman's consent to donate prior to obtaining her consent to an abortion, there is reason to be concerned that women may be pressured to choose abortion. Taken together, the three policy recommendations—prohibiting designated donation, prohibiting the buying and selling of fetal tissue, and prohibiting invitations to donate before a woman has consented to an abortion—prevent abortion for donation, while permitting abortion and donation. Nevertheless, as the fetal tissue bill currently before Congress makes clear, these are only some of the provisions necessary to ensure that the transplantation of fetal tissue is adequately respectful and protective of fetuses and women.

NOTES

1. The National Organ Transplant ACT (NOTA) and most state Uniform Anatomical Gift Acts (UAGAs) already prohibit the buying and selling of fetal tissue.

2. Vawter, DE, Gervais, KG, and Caplan, AL: Risks of fetal tissue donation to women. *Journal of Neural Transplantation and Plasticity* 1992; 3(4), forthcoming.

3. In some jurisdictions abortion providers are legally prohibited from performing an abortion on a woman known to be seeking an abortion for donation.

POSTSCRIPT

Will Fetal Tissue Research Encourage Abortions?

A Swedish study, reported in 1992, demonstrated that impaired brain tissue was repaired by implants of fetal brain tissue. In this study, two American heroin addicts damaged by tainted drugs improved considerably after the transplants, and brain scans revealed that their brains were producing chemicals that had been lacking since their injuries. Two American research groups, at the University of Colorado and at Yale University, also reported small but definite effects in 10 patients with Parkinson's disease who were treated with fetal brain tissue. These research projects were privately funded.

The first grant for fetal tissue research, after the government ban was lifted, was awarded by the National Institute of Neurological Disorders and Stroke in January 1994. The $4.5 million grant went to three institutions to study 40 patients with Parkinson's disease. However, patients will have to pay $40,000 to be in the study because insurance companies will generally not reimburse experimental procedures.

One proposed alternative to the use of fetuses from induced abortions for research is the use of fetal tissue from spontaneous abortions or ectopic pregnancies (nonviable pregnancies that develop outside the uterus). The Human Fetal Tissue Working Group, made up of scientists from around the United States, studied the feasibility of this option. They found that less than 1 percent of 1,250 spontaneous abortions and 247 ectopic pregnancies resulted in tissues that were potentially useful for human transplantation therapy (see D. Ware Branch et al., "Suitability of Fetal Tissues from Spontaneous Abortions and from Ectopic Pregnancies for Transplantation," *Journal of the American Medical Association,* January 4, 1995).

In the United Kingdom, guidelines to protect women undergoing abortions from exploitation have been in place since 1990. Researchers in Edinburgh conducted a survey to explore nearly 700 women's views on research involving fetal tissue. Regardless of whether they were about to have an abortion, had had one in the past, or had never had one, women were overwhelmingly (94 percent) in favor of this kind of research. They also supported the use of fetal tissue for treatment of adult diseases such as Parkinson's. See Fionn Anderson et al., "Attitudes of Women to Fetal Research," *Journal of Medical Ethics* (March 1994). For more analysis about the ethics of using materials from an elective abortion, see Michelle A. Mullen and Frederick H. Lowy, "Physician Attitudes Toward the Regulation of Fetal Tissue Therapies: Empirical Findings and Implications for Public Policy," *Journal of Law, Medicine and Ethics* (Summer 1993).

PART 7

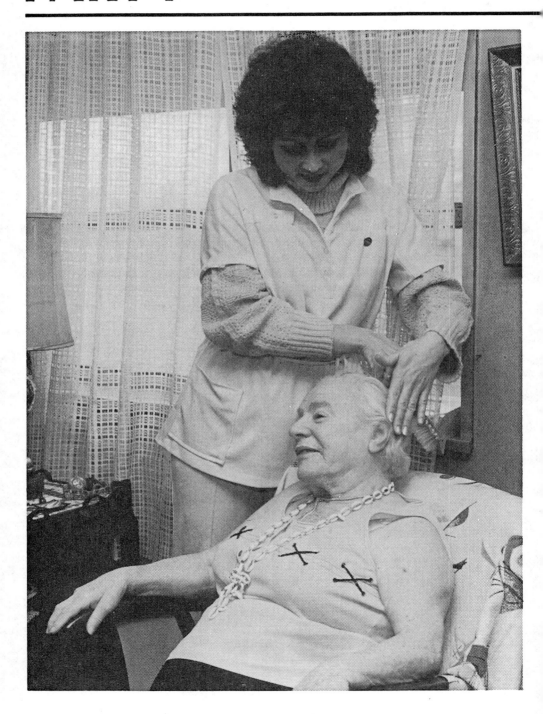

Bioethics and Resource Allocation

In its modern infancy, biomedical ethics was almost exclusively concerned with issues relating to individual doctor-patient relationships. Questions of resource allocation did occur, but mostly within the context of whether or not a patient could pay for certain kinds of care. In the past several decades, as medical care costs have skyrocketed, the issues concerning equitable distribution of scarce resources have become paramount. As medical care became more costly, it became less accessible to the uninsured and to the underinsured (people who have some health insurance but not enough to cover their own illnesses or those of their families). Managed care in many different forms is rapidly replacing the traditional fee-for-service system, and big corporations are rapidly buying up health plans, hospitals, and doctors' groups. In this new world of market-driven health care, some old problems of resource allocation take on new urgency. How can generational equity be obtained? Will physician ethics change under managed care? How far should commercialism extend? This section takes up these issues.

- Should Health Care for the Elderly Be Limited?

- Should Patient-Centered Medical Ethics Govern Managed Care?

- Should There Be a Market in Body Parts?

ISSUE 18

Should Health Care for the Elderly Be Limited?

YES: Daniel Callahan, from "Limiting Health Care for the Old?" *The Nation* (August 15, 1987)

NO: Amitai Etzioni, from "Spare the Old, Save the Young," *The Nation* (June 11, 1988)

ISSUE SUMMARY

YES: Philosopher Daniel Callahan believes that since health care resources are scarce, people who have lived a full natural life span should be offered care that relieves suffering but not expensive life-prolonging technologies.

NO: Sociologist Amitai Etzioni argues that rationing health care for the elderly would encourage conflict between generations and would invite restrictions on health care for other groups.

America is aging. In 1965 the 18.5 million people over the age of 65 accounted for only 9.5 percent of the population. By 1987 the number had climbed to 29 million, or 12 percent of the population. The number of people over 85—the "old old"—is the fastest-growing age group in the United States. By the year 2040 the elderly will represent 21 percent of the population.

Older people are more likely to need health care than the young. In 1980 people over 65 accounted for 29 percent of the total American health care expenditures of $219.4 billion. By 1986 the bill had risen to $450 billion, and the share devoted to the elderly to 31 percent. The costs of Medicare—the federal program that supports the health care of people over 65—are projected to increase from $75 billion in 1986 to $114 billion in the year 2000, measured in current, not inflated, dollars.

Although Medicare coverage of nursing homes and home care remains inadequate to meet the need, organ transplants are now covered. The typical cost of such an operation is $200,000.

Many (but not all) elderly people do not want to have their lives prolonged through the use of expensive technology such as kidney dialysis, respirators, and intensive care. They fear losing control of their medical care and dying "hooked up to tubes."

There are many competing interests vying for the increasingly scarce health care dollar. Groups representing patients suffering from particular diseases —cancer, AIDS, diabetes, and heart disease, to name just a few—advocate increased spending on research and care. Those who speak for the poor, especially poor children, point out that the poor often do not have access to the most basic medical care, such as immunizations. The costs of treating premature, low-birth-weight infants are extremely high; yet programs that provide prenatal care and adequate nutrition to mothers at risk, which might prevent many such births, are inadequately funded.

In such a complex web of competing claims, when not all interests can be met, how should decisions to ration care be determined? Should age be one criterion? In Great Britain, which has a National Health Service and centralized planning, patients over the age of 55 have been routinely denied kidney dialysis ostensibly on "medical" grounds, even though the procedure is performed in the United States on very old patients.

Should this pattern be followed in the United States? The following selections present the contrasting views. Daniel Callahan says that we must confront realities: in the interest of ensuring adequate health care for the younger generation, we must limit the kinds of care that will be available to those who have lived a full natural life span. Amitai Etzioni objects to this call to ration health care to the elderly on the grounds that it will lead to denying care to people of younger ages and other groups deemed less productive to society.

YES

Daniel Callahan

LIMITING HEALTH CARE FOR THE OLD?

Is it sensible, in the face of the rapidly increasing burden of health care costs for the elderly, to press forward with new and expensive ways of extending their lives? Is it possible even to hope to control costs while simultaneously supporting innovative research, which generates new ways to spend money? Those are now unavoidable questions....

Anyone who works closely with the elderly recognizes that the present Medicare and Medicaid programs are grossly inadequate in meeting their real and full needs. The system fails most notably in providing decent long-term care and medical care that does not constitute a heavy out-of-pocket drain. Members of minority groups and single or widowed women are particularly disadvantaged. How will it be possible, then, to provide the growing number of elderly with even present levels of care, much less to rid the system of its inadequacies and inequities, and at the same time add expensive new technologies?

The straight answer is that it will be impossible to do all those things and, worse still, it may be harmful even to try. It may be so because of the economic burdens that would impose on younger age groups, and because of the requisite skewing of national social priorities too heavily toward health care. But that suggests to both young and old that the key to a happy old age is good health care, which may not be true.

In the past few years three additional concerns about health care for the aged have surfaced. First, an increasingly large share of health care is going to the elderly rather than to youth. The Federal government, for instance, spends six times as much providing health benefits and other social services to those over 65 as it does to those under 18. And, as the demographer Samuel Preston observed in a provocative address to the Population Association of America in 1984, "Transfers from the working-age population to the elderly are also transfers away from children, since the working ages bear far more responsibility for childrearing than do the elderly."

Preston's address had an immediate impact. The mainline senior-citizen advocacy groups accused Preston of fomenting a war between the generations. But the speech also stimulated Minnesota Senator David Durenberger

From Daniel Callahan, "Limiting Health Care for the Old?" *The Nation* (August 15, 1987). Adapted from Daniel Callahan, *Setting Limits: Medical Goals in an Aging Society* (Simon & Schuster, 1987). Copyright © 1987 by Daniel Callahan. Reprinted by permission.

and others to found Americans for Generational Equity (AGE) to promote debate about the burden on future generations, particularly the Baby Boom cohort, of "our major social insurance programs." Preston's speech and the founding of AGE signaled the outbreak of a struggle over what has come to be called "intergenerational equity," which is now gaining momentum.

The second concern is that the elderly, in dying, consume a disproportionate share of health care costs. "At present," notes Stanford University economist Victor Fuchs, "the United States spends about 1 percent of the gross national product on health care for elderly persons who are in their last year of life.... One of the biggest challenges facing policy makers for the rest of this century will be how to strike an appropriate balance between care for the [elderly] dying and health services for the rest of the population."

The third issue is summed up in an observation by Dr. Jerome Avorn of the Harvard Medical School, who wrote in *Daedalus*, "With the exception of the birth-control pill, [most] of the medical-technology interventions developed since the 1950s have their most widespread impact on people who are past their fifties—the further past their fifties, the greater the impact." Many of the techniques in question were not intended for use on the elderly. Kidney dialysis, for example, was developed for those between the ages of 15 and 45. Now some 30 percent of its recipients are over 65.

The validity of those concerns has been vigorously challenged, as has the more general assertion that some form of rationing of health care for the elderly might become necessary. To the charge

that old people receive a disproportionate share of resources, the response has been that assistance to them helps every age group: It relieves the young of the burden of care they would otherwise have to bear for elderly parents and, since those young will eventually become old, promises them similar care when they need it. There is no guarantee, moreover, that any cutback in health care for the elderly would result in a transfer of the savings directly to the young. And, some ask, Why should we contemplate restricting care for the elderly when we wastefully spend hundreds of millions on an inflated defense budget?

The assertion that too large a share of funds goes to extending the lives of elderly people who are terminally ill hardly proves that it is an unjust or unreasonable amount. They are, after all, the most in need. As some important studies have shown, it is exceedingly difficult to know that someone is dying; the most expensive patients, it turns out, are those who were expected to live but died. That most new technologies benefit the old more than the young is logical; most of the killer diseases of the young have now been conquered.

There is little incentive for politicians to think about, much less talk about, limits on health care for the aged. As John Rother, director of legislation for the American Association of Retired Persons, has observed, "I think anyone who wasn't a champion of the aged is no longer in Congress." Perhaps also, as Guido Calabresi, dean of the Yale Law School, and his colleague Philip Bobbitt observed in their thoughtful 1978 book *Tragic Choices*, when we are forced to make painful allocation choices, "Evasion, disguise, temporizing... [and]

averting our eyes enables us to save some lives even when we will not save all."

I believe that we must face this highly troubling issue. Rationing of health care under Medicare is already a fact of life, though rarely labeled as such. The requirement that Medicare recipients pay the first $520 of hospital care costs, the cutoff of reimbursement for care after 60 days and the failure to cover long-term care are nothing other than allocation and cost-saving devices. As sensitive as it is to the senior-citizen vote, the Reagan Administration agreed only grudgingly to support catastrophic health care coverage for the elderly (a benefit that will not help very many of them), and it has already expressed its opposition to the recently passed House version of the bill. It is bound to be far more resistant to long-term health care coverage, as will any administration.

But there are reasons other than the economics to think about health care for the elderly. The coming economic crisis provides a much-needed opportunity to ask some deeper questions. Just what is it that we want medicine to do for us as we age? Other cultures have believed that aging should be accepted, and that it should be in part a time of preparation for death. Our culture seems increasingly to dispute that view, preferring instead, it often seems, to think of aging as hardly more than another disease, to be fought and rejected. Which view is correct?

Let me interject my own opinion. The future goal of medical science should be to improve the quality of old people's lives, not to lengthen them. In its longstanding ambition to forestall death, medicine has reached its last frontier in the care of the aged. Of course children and young adults still die of maladies that are open to potential cure; but the highest

proportion of the dying (70 percent) are over 65. If death is ever to be humbled, that is where endless work remains to be done. But however tempting the challenge of that last frontier, medicine should restrain itself. To do otherwise would mean neglecting the needs of other age groups and of the old themselves.

Our culture has worked hard to redefine old age as a time of liberation, not decline, a time of travel, of new ventures in education and self-discovery, of the ever-accessible tennis court or golf course and of delightfully periodic but thankfully brief visits from well-behaved grandchildren. That is, to be sure, an idealized picture, but it arouses hopes that spur medicine to wage an aggressive war against the infirmities of old age. As we have seen, the costs of such a war would be prohibitive. No matter how much is spent the ultimate problem will still remain: people will grow old and die. Worse still, by pretending that old age can be turned into a kind of endless middle age, we rob it of meaning and significance for the elderly.

There is a plausible alternative: a fresh vision of what it means to live a decently long and adequate life, what might be called a "natural life span." Earlier generations accepted the idea that there was a natural life span—the biblical norm of three score and ten captures that notion (even though in fact that was a much longer life span than was typical in ancient times). It is an idea well worth reconsidering and would provide us with a meaningful and realizable goal. Modern medicine and biology have done much, however, to wean us from that kind of thinking. They have insinuated the belief that the average life span is not a natural fact at all, but instead one that is strictly dependent on the state of medical knowledge and skill. And there is much to that belief as a statistical fact: The average life expectancy continues to increase with no end in sight.

But that is not what I think we ought to mean by a natural life span. We need a notion of a full life that is based on some deeper understanding of human needs and possibilities, not on the state of medical technology or its potential. We should think of a natural life span as the achievement of a life that is sufficiently long to take advantage of those opportunities life typically offers and that we ordinarily regard as its prime benefits—loving and "living," raising a family, engaging in work that is satisfying, reading, thinking, cherishing our friends and families. People differ on what might be a full natural life span; my view is that it can be achieved by the late 70s or early 80s.

A longer life does not guarantee a better life. No matter how long medicine enables people to live, death at any time —at age 90 or 100 or 110—would frustrate some possibility, some as-yet-unrealized goal. The easily preventable death of a young child is an outrage. Death from an incurable disease of someone in the prime of young adulthood is a tragedy. But death at an old age, after a long and full life, is simply sad, a part of life itself.

As it confronts aging, medicine should have as its specific goals the averting of premature death, that is, death prior to the completion of a natural life span, and thereafter, the relief of suffering. It should pursue those goals so that the elderly can finish out their years with as little needless pain as possible—and with as much vitality as can be generated in contributing to the welfare of younger age groups and to the community of which they are a part. Above all, the elderly need to have a sense of the meaning and significance of their stage in life, one that is not dependent on economic productivity or physical vigor.

What would medicine oriented toward the relief of suffering rather than the deliberate extension of life be like? We do not have a clear answer to that question, so longstanding, central and persistent has been medicine's preoccupation with the struggle against death. But the hospice movement is providing us with much guidance. It has learned how to distinguish between the relief of suffering and the lengthening of life. Greater control by elderly persons over their own dying—and particularly an enforceable right to refuse aggressive life-extending treatment—is a minimal goal.

What does this have to do with the rising cost of health care for the elderly? Everything. The indefinite extension of life combined with an insatiable ambition to improve the health of the elderly is a recipe for monomania and bottomless spending. It fails to put health in its proper place as only one among many human goods. It fails to accept aging and death as part of the human condition. It fails to present to younger generations a model of wise stewardship.

How might we devise a plan to limit the costs of health care for the aged under public entitlement programs that is fair, humane and sensitive to their special requirements and dignity? Let me suggest three principles to undergird a quest for limits. First, government has a duty, based on our collective social obligations, to help people live out a natural life span but not to help medically extend life beyond that point. Second, government is obliged to develop under its research subsidies, and to pay for under its entitlement programs, only the kind and degree of life-extending technology necessary for medicine to achieve and serve the aim of a natural life span. Third, beyond the point of a natural life span, government should provide only the means necessary for the relief of suffering, not those for life-extending technology.

A system based on those principles would not immediately bring down the cost of care of the elderly; it would add cost. But it would set in place the beginning of a new understanding of old age, one that would admit of eventual stabilization and limits. The elderly will not be served by a belief that only a lack of resources, better financing mechanisms or political power stands between them and the limitations of their bodies. The good of younger age groups will not be served by inspiring in them a desire to live to an old age that maintains the vitality of youth indefinitely, as if old age were nothing but a sign that medicine has failed in its mission. The future of our society will not be served by allowing expenditures on health care for the elderly to escalate endlessly and uncontrollably, fueled by the false altruistic belief that anything less is to deny the elderly their dignity. Nor will it be aided by the pervasive kind of self-serving argument that urges the young to support such a crusade because they will eventually benefit from it also.

We require instead an understanding of the process of aging and death that looks to our obligation to the young and to the future, that recognizes the necessity of limits and the acceptance of decline and death, and that values the old for their age and not for their continuing youthful vitality. In the name of accepting the elderly and repudiating discrimination against them, we have succeeded mainly in pretending that, with enough will and money, the unpleasant part of old age can be abolished. In the name of medical progress we have carried out a relentless war against death and decline, failing to ask in any probing way if that will give us a better society for all.

NO

Amitai Etzioni

SPARE THE OLD, SAVE THE YOUNG

In the coming years, Daniel Callahan's call to ration health care for the elderly, put forth in his book *Setting Limits*, is likely to have a growing appeal. Practically all economic observers expect the United States to go through a difficult time as it attempts to work its way out of its domestic (budgetary) and international (trade) deficits. Practically every serious analyst realizes that such an endeavor will initially entail slower growth, if not an outright cut in our standard of living, in order to release resources to these priorities. When the national economic "pie" grows more slowly, let alone contracts, the fight over how to divide it up intensifies. The elderly make an especially inviting target because they have been taking a growing slice of the resources (at least those dedicated to health care) and are expected to take even more in the future. Old people are widely held to be "nonproductive" and to constitute a growing "burden" on an ever smaller proportion of society that is young and working. Also, the elderly are viewed as politically well-organized and powerful; hence "their" programs, especially Social Security and Medicare, have largely escaped the Reagan attempts to scale back social expenditures, while those aimed at other groups—especially the young, but even more so future generations—have been generally curtailed. There are now some signs that a backlash may be forming.

If a war between the generations, like that between the races and between the genders, does break out, historians may accord former Governor Richard Lamm of Colorado the dubious honor of having fired the opening shot in his statement that the elderly ill have "got a duty to die and get out of the way." Phillip Longman, in his book *Born to Pay*, sounded an early alarm. However, the historians may well say, it was left to Daniel Callahan, a social philosopher and ethicist, to provide a detailed rationale and blueprint for limiting the care to the elderly, explicitly in order to free resources for the young. Callahan's thesis deserves close examination because he attempts to deal with the numerous objections his approach raises. If his thesis does not hold, the champions of limiting funds available to the old may have a long wait before they will find a new set of arguments on their behalf.

In order to free up economic resources for the young, Callahan offers the older generation a deal: Trade quantity for quality; the elderly should not be given life-*extending* services but better years while alive. Instead of the relentless attempt to push death to an older age, Callahan would stop all development of life-extending technologies and prohibit the use of ones at hand for those who outlive their "natural" life span, say, the age of 75. At the same time, the old would be granted more palliative medicine (e.g., pain killers) and more nursing-home and home-health care, to make their natural years more comfortable.

Callahan's call to break an existing ethical taboo and replace it with another raises the problem known among ethicists and sociologists as the "slippery slope." Once the precept that one should do "all one can" to avert death is given up, and attempts are made to fix a specific age for a full life, why stop there? If, for instance, the American economy experiences hard times in the 1990s, should the "maximum" age be reduced to 72, 65 —or lower? And should the care for other so-called unproductive groups be cut off, even if they are even younger? Should countries that are economically worse off than the United States set their limit, say, at 55?

This is not an idle thought, because the idea of limiting the care the elderly receive in itself represents a partial slide down such a slope. Originally, Callahan, the Hastings Center (which he directs) and other think tanks played an important role in redefining the concept of death. Death used to be seen by the public at large as occurring when the lungs stopped functioning and, above all, the heart stopped beating. In numerous old movies and novels, those attending the dying would hold a mirror to their faces to see if it fogged over, or put an ear to their chests to see if the heart had stopped. However, high technology made these criteria obsolete by mechanically ventilating people and keeping their hearts pumping. Hastings et al. led the way to provide a new technological definition of death: brain death. Increasingly this has been accepted, both in the medical community and by the public at large, as the point of demise, the point at which care should stop even if it means turning off life-extending machines, because people who are brain dead do not regain consciousness. At the same time, most doctors and a majority of the public as well continue strongly to oppose terminating care to people who are conscious, even if there is little prospect for recovery, despite considerable debate about certain special cases.

Callahan now suggests turning off life-extending technology for all those above a certain age, even if they could recover their full human capacity if treated. It is instructive to look at the list of technologies he would withhold: mechanical ventilation, artificial resuscitation, antibiotics and artificial nutrition and hydration. Note that while several of these are used to maintain brain-dead bodies, they are also used for individuals who are temporarily incapacitated but able to recover fully; indeed, they are used to save young lives, say, after a car accident. But there is no way to stop the development of such new technologies and the improvement of existing ones without depriving the young of benefit as well. (Antibiotics are on the list because of an imminent "high cost" technological advance—administering them with a pump implanted in the body, which makes their introduction more reliable and better distributes dosages.)

One may say that this is Callahan's particular list; other lists may well be drawn. But any of them would start us down the slope, because the savings that are achieved by turning off the machines that keep brain-dead people alive are minimal compared with those that would result from the measures sought by the people calling for new equity between the generations. And any significant foray into deliberately withholding medical care for those who can recover does raise the question, Once society has embarked on such a slope, where will it stop?

Those opposed to Callahan, Lamm and the other advocates of limiting care to the old, but who also favor extending the frontier of life, must answer the question, Where will the resources come from? One answer is found in the realization that defining people as old at the age of 65 is obsolescent. That age limit was set generations ago, before changes in life styles and medicines much extended not only life but also the number and quality of productive years. One might recognize that many of the "elderly" can contribute to society not merely by providing love, companionship and wisdom to the young but also by continuing to work, in the traditional sense of the term. Indeed, many already work in the underground economy because of the large penalty—a cut in Social Security benefits—exacted from them if they hold a job "on the books."

Allowing elderly people to retain their Social Security benefits while working, typically part-time, would immediately raise significant tax revenues, dramatically change the much-feared dependency-to-dependent ratio, provide a much-needed source of child-care workers and increase contributions to Social Security (under the assumption that anybody who will continue to work will continue to contribute to the program). There is also evidence that people who continue to have meaningful work will live longer and healthier lives, without requiring more health care, because psychic well-being in our society is so deeply associated with meaningful work. Other policy changes, such as deferring retirement, modifying Social Security benefits by a small, gradual stretching out of the age of full-benefit entitlement, plus some other shifts under way, could be used readily to gain more resources. Such changes might be justified prima facie because as we extend life and its quality, the payouts to the old may also be stretched out.

Beyond the question of whether to cut care or stretch out Social Security payouts, policies that seek to promote intergenerational equity must be assessed as to how they deal with another matter of equity: that between the poor and the rich. A policy that would stop Federal support for certain kinds of care, as Callahan and others propose, would halt treatment for the aged, poor, the near-poor and even the less-well-off segment of the middle class (although for the latter at a later point), while the rich would continue to buy all the care they wished to. Callahan's suggestion that a consensus of doctors would stop certain kinds of care for all elderly people is quite impractical; for it to work, most if not all doctors would have to agree to participate. Even if this somehow happened, the rich would buy their services overseas either by going there or by importing the services. There is little enough we can do to significantly enhance economic equality. Do we want to exacerbate the inequalities that already exist by completely eliminating access to major categories of health care services for those who cannot afford to pay for them?

In addition to concern about slipping down the slope of less (and less) care, the *way* the limitations are to be introduced raises a serious question. The advocates of changing the intergenerational allocation of resources favor rationing health care for the elderly but nothing else. This is a major intellectual weakness of their argument. There are other major targets to consider within health care, as well as other areas, which seem, at least by some criteria, much more inviting than terminating care to those above a certain age. Within the medical sector, for example, why not stop all interventions for which there is no hard evidence that they are beneficial? Say, public financing of psychotherapy and coronary bypass operations? Why not take the $2 billion or so from plastic surgery dedicated to face lifts, reducing behinds and the like? Or require that all burials be done by low-cost cremations rather than using high-cost coffins?

Once we extend our reach beyond medical care to health care, if we cannot stop people from blowing $25 billion per year on cigarettes and convince them to use the money to serve the young, shouldn't we at least cut out public subsidies to tobacco growers before we save funds by denying antibiotics to old people? And there is the matter of profits. The high-technology medicine Callahan targets for savings is actually a minor cause of the increase in health care costs for the elderly or for anyone —about 4 percent. A major factor is the very high standard of living American doctors have, compared to those of many other nations. Indeed, many doctors tell interviewers that they love their work and would do it for half their current income as long as the incomes of their fellow practitioners were also cut. Another important area of saving is the exorbitant profits made by the nondoctor owners of dialysis units and nursing homes. If we dare ask how many years of life are enough, should we not also be able to ask how much profit is "enough"? This profit, by the way, is largely set not by the market but by public policy.

Last but not least, as the United States enters a time of economic constraints, should we draw new lines of conflict or should we focus on matters that sustain our societal fabric? During the 1960s numerous groups gained in political consciousness and actively sought to address injustices done to them. The result has been some redress and an increase in the level of societal stress (witness the deeply troubled relationships between the genders). But these conflicts occurred in an affluent society and redressed deeply felt grievances. Are the young like blacks and women, except that they have not yet discovered their oppressors—a group whose consciousness should be raised, so it will rally and gain its due share?

The answer is in the eye of the beholder. There are no objective criteria that can be used here the way they can be used between the races or between the genders. While women and minorities have the same rights to the same jobs at the same pay as white males, the needs of the young and the aged are so different that no simple criteria of equity come to mind. Thus, no one would argue that the teen-agers and those above 75 have the same need for schooling or nursing homes.

At the same time, it is easy to see that those who try to mobilize the young

—led by a new Washington research group, Americans for Generational Equity (AGE), formed to fight for the needs of the younger generation—offer many arguments that do not hold. For instance, they often argue that today's young, age 35 or less, will pay for old people's Social Security, but by the time that they come of age they will not be able to collect, because Social Security will be bankrupt. However, this argument is based on extremely farfetched assumptions about the future. In effect, Social Security is now and for the foreseeable future overprovided, and its surplus is used to reduce deficits caused by other expenditures, such as Star Wars, in what is still an integrated budget. And, if Social Security runs into the red again somewhere after the year 2020, relatively small adjustments in premiums and payouts would restore it to financial health.

Above all, it is a dubious sociological achievement to foment conflict between the generations, because, unlike the minorities and the white majority, or men and women, many millions of Americans are neither young nor old but of intermediate ages. We should not avoid issues just because we face stressing times in an already strained society; but maybe we should declare a moratorium on raising new conflicts until more compelling arguments can be found in their favor, and more evidence that this particular line of divisiveness is called for.

POSTSCRIPT

Should Health Care for the Elderly Be Limited?

Callahan's views are amplified in his book *Setting Limits: Medical Goals in an Aging Society* (Simon & Schuster, 1987). See Paul Homer and Martha Holstein, eds., *A Good Old Age: The Paradox of Setting Limits* (Touchstone, 1990) for responses to Callahan's arguments. Also see Robert L. Barry and Gerard V. Bradley, eds., *Set No Limits: A Rebuttal to Daniel Callahan's Proposal to Limit Health Care for the Elderly* (University of Illinois Press, 1991). In "Elder Choice," *American Journal of Law and Medicine* (vol. 19, no. 3, 1993), Alfred F. Conard argues that artificial prolongation of life is usually undesirable and that health care for the aged should include information about advance directives.

A study of critically ill elderly patients concluded that age alone is not an adequate predictor of long-term survival and quality of life. See L. Chelluri et al., "Long-Term Outcome of Critically Ill Elderly Patients Requiring Intensive Care," *Journal of the American Medical Association* (June 23/30, 1993).

For contrasting views on age as a criterion for medical care, see David C. Thomasma, "Functional Status Care Categories and National Health Policy," *Journal of the American Geriatrics Society* (April 1993); Mark Siegler, "Should Age Be a Criterion for Health Care?" and James F. Childress, "Ensuring Care, Respect, and Fairness for the Elderly," both in the *Hastings Center Report* (October 1984); and Nancy S. Jecker and Robert A. Pearlman, "Ethical Constraints on Rationing Medical Care by Age," *Journal of the American Geriatrics Society* (November 1989). Marshall B. Kapp opposes Callahan's view in "Rationing Health Care: Will It Be Necessary? Can It Be Done Without Age or Disability Discrimination?" *Issues in Law and Medicine* (Winter 1989). Pat Milmoe McCarrick's *The Aged and the Allocation of Health Care Resources* (Scope Note No. 13, Kennedy Institute of Ethics, 1990) offers a good bibliography.

See Edward L. Schneider and Jack M. Guralnik, "The Aging of America: Impact on Health Care Costs," *Journal of the American Medical Association* (May 2, 1990) for a discussion of how the rapid increase in the elderly population will affect health care costs.

An international perspective is taken in Daniel Callahan, Ruud H. T. Ter Meulen, and Eva Topinkova, eds., *A World Growing Old: The Coming Health Care Challenges* (Georgetown University Press, 1995). See also Richard Posner, *Aging and Old Age* (University of Chicago Press, 1995).

ISSUE 19

Should Patient-Centered Medical Ethics Govern Managed Care?

YES: Ezekiel J. Emanuel and Nancy Neveloff Dubler, from "Preserving the Physician-Patient Relationship in the Era of Managed Care," *Journal of the American Medical Association* (January 25, 1995)

NO: Michael J. Malinowski, from "Capitation, Advances in Medical Technology, and the Advent of a New Era in Medical Ethics," *American Journal of Law and Medicine* (vol. 22, nos. 2 and 3, 1996)

ISSUE SUMMARY

YES: Physician Ezekiel J. Emanuel and attorney Nancy Neveloff Dubler argue that the expansion of managed care and the imposition of significant cost controls could undermine critical aspects of the physician-patient relationship, including freedom of choice, careful assessments of physician competence, time available for communication, and continuity of care.

NO: Attorney Michael J. Malinowski contends that medical ethics can no longer be focused on individual patients and physicians but must develop a social conscience, which means recognizing that costs matter, that not everyone can have access to everything, and that resources must be rationed fairly and openly.

Health care in the United States is going through a profound period of economic and structural change. In the past, providers of health care (hospitals, physicians, suppliers of technology and other services) dictated prices and terms. In this system, provider income increased with greater numbers of patients, more procedures, and longer stays. As a result, health care costs grew at a rate that many considered unacceptable, especially since it was not accompanied by significantly broadened access to care. In order to restrain this trend, major purchasers of medical services (large employers and government programs such as the Veterans Administration, Medicare, and Medicaid) began to aggressively seek the best deal at the best price. In this system, fewer patients, fewer procedures, and shorter hospital stays mean lowered costs.

The generic term for this new system is *managed care*, a term that covers a variety of organizational structures and practices, some with long histories and some that are quite new. Some do not even provide health care directly but are "packagers" of a specific group of services. Corporate, for-profit control of health care, in which organizational decisions must consider profit to shareholders as a prime goal, has become an increasingly prominent feature of the system. The presumed benefit is that increased competition, along with tough business practices, will reduce costs without reducing quality.

By the end of 1995 more than 56 million Americans were enrolled in some type of health maintenance organization (HMO). In 1994 publicly traded HMOs completed acquisitions worth more than $4 billion. Hospital mergers are occurring widely, often resulting in the closure of or reduction of services in one of the hospitals. Publicly traded physician practice companies are doing well, as evidenced by a *Wall Street Journal* article predicting that 10 companies would be competing for a potential $200 billion market. In short, health care is a big, profitable business with a growing consolidation of power in a few large corporations.

"Capitation" is a key concept in the new systems. Under the traditional "fee-for-service" approach, patients pay a fee for each visit to the doctor (some or all of which might be reimbursed by insurance) and also for the diagnostic or therapeutic interventions that the doctor recommends. Providers have an economic incentive to do more because each intervention means additional income. Under a capitated system, by contrast, the provider is paid a fixed, or capitated, fee for each person (per head, literally) each year. If the person rarely becomes ill and does not require expensive interventions, the provider realizes a profit at the end of the year. If, however, a great deal of costly medical care is required, the patient is a financial loss to the system. In this framework, the economic incentive is to do less because each intervention reduces profit. Less intervention may mean less unnecessary surgery and fewer expensive and marginally useful procedures, medications, and visits. It may also mean postponing needed care or failing to provide appropriate follow-up.

While most attention has been focused on whether or not managed care actually saves money and whether or not others besides corporate executives and investors are reaping any benefits from the savings, the impact on medical ethics is equally important. The following selections look at managed care from that broad perspective. Ezekiel J. Emanuel and Nancy Neveloff Dubler assert that the physician-patient relationship remains the cornerstone for achieving, maintaining, and improving health. Although they acknowledge that the current system fails many in this regard, they worry that imposing significant cost controls in an environment where financial pressures are intense and omnipresent may restrict patient choice, reduce the time available for communication, and create conflicts of interest between patient and physician. Michael J. Malinowski sees the advent of a new and more realistic era in medical ethics through capitation and advances in medical technology. Physicians must now develop a social conscience, he asserts, and recognize that the prior era's failure to consider costs must give way to an ethic that incorporates the utilitarian principle of doing the most good for the greater number.

YES

Ezekiel J. Emanuel and
Nancy Neveloff Dubler

PRESERVING THE PHYSICIAN-PATIENT RELATIONSHIP IN THE ERA OF MANAGED CARE

THE IDEAL PHYSICIAN-PATIENT RELATIONSHIP

To evaluate the effects of managed care, we need to delineate an ideal conception of the physician-patient relationship. This ideal establishes the normative standard for assessing the effect of the current health care system as well as changes in the system. Although patients receive health care from a diverse number of providers, and the use of nonphysician providers, such as nurse practitioners, physician assistants, and nurse midwives, is likely to increase with more emphasis on primary care and managed care, we chose to concentrate on the physician-patient relationship. The reasons for this focus are many: physicians outnumber nonphysician providers; most Americans continue to receive their health care from physicians rather than nonphysician providers; there have been many more years, indeed, centuries, for reflection on the elements that constitute the ideal physician-patient relationship, while the ethical guidelines and legal rulings on nonphysician provider-patient relationships are more recent and have not been as exhaustively developed; and there is substantially more empirical research on the physician-patient relationship with which to formulate educated projections....

We suggest that the fundamental elements of the ideal physician-patient relationship that are embodied in our intuitions and common to ethical analyses and legal standards can be expressed as six C's: choice, competence, communication, compassion, continuity, and (no) conflict of interest. While many people emphasize the importance of trust in the physician-patient relationship, we believe trust is the culmination of realizing these six C's, not an independent element....

From Ezekiel J. Emanuel and Nancy Neveloff Dubler, "Preserving the Physician-Patient Relationship in the Era of Managed Care," *Journal of the American Medical Association*, vol. 273, no. 4 (January 25, 1995), pp. 323–324, 326–328. Copyright © 1995 by The American Medical Association. Reprinted by permission. Some references omitted.

THE PHYSICIAN-PATIENT RELATIONSHIP IN THE ERA OF MANAGED CARE

Despite the lack of comprehensive health care system reform legislation, significant changes are occurring without legislative and governmental regulation, driven predominantly by the increased efforts of employers to reduce health care costs. These changes include more managed care, increased use of primary care physicians and generalists rather than specialists, increased use of non-physician providers, emphasis on preventive measures, greater commitment to the care of children, and intensive quality assessment.[1,2] Although it is impossible to predict the precise concrete manifestations and effects of all these changes, it is possible to provide some educated reflections on their probable implications for the physician-patient relationship (Table 1). Because the health care system is so complex, the changes may not always tend in a coherent direction; some aspects may enhance a particular element of the physician-patient relationship while others undermine it. It is often difficult to know which tendency will dominate in practice, and so we try to outline the potential trends in both directions.

Admittedly, these predictions are speculative. But they are no more speculative than projections on the cost of certain changes or on the economic consequences of particular managed care programs.[3] And just as economic projections, with uncertainty, are essential in evaluating health care proposals, so too we hope these predictions will provide a basis for planning and promoting those parts of the trend toward managed care that enhance the ideal physician-patient relationship, anticipating threats to the ideal posed by managed care, and acting to mitigate the ill effects.

Potential Improvements

With some expansion of managed care, the range of choice for many insured Americans could also increase. Americans who live in regions without significant managed care penetration, such as the South, will soon have the option of care in a managed care setting. In addition, other Americans could now have several managed care plans as well as fee-for-service options to choose from. However, if managed care expands too much, it may threaten to eliminate fee-for-service practitioners in a region altogether, as it appears to be doing in northern California and Minnesota. Under such circumstances, patients' choice of practice setting, even for well-insured Americans, could be effectively reduced.

Managed care may also provide the insured with a wider range of treatment alternatives. For example, by removing financial barriers, managed care plans should give enrollees more effective choice over utilizing preventive interventions, such as screening tests. Indeed, studies consistently demonstrate greater use of preventive tests and procedures among managed care enrollees.[4-6] In addition, many managed care plans contain benefits packages that include services not currently covered by many insurance programs. Indeed, pediatric patients may significantly benefit from the coverage of vaccinations, small co-payments for well-child visits, and coverage of dental and visual services for children.

Managed care plans are increasingly attempting to develop quality measures; they are trying to use these quality measures for routine assessments of

Table 1
The Effects of Managed Care on the Physician-Patient Relationship

Potential Improvements	Potential Threats
Choice	
• Expanded choice of managed care plans, particularly in areas with low managed care penetration	• "Cherry picking" increasing the number of uninsured Americans
• Expanded choice of preventive and pediatric services	• Employers restricting patients' choice of managed care plans and physicians
	• Price competition forcing patients to choose between continuing with their current physicians or switching to a cheaper plan
	• Financial failures of managed care plans forcing change in managed care plan without choice
	• Restrictions by managed care plans of choice of specialists and particular services
Competence	
• Development and use of measures to assess quality of physicians and managed care plans	• Underutilization of specialists and specialized facilities
• Greater use of preventive medical care	• Unreliable and non–risk-adjusted quality measures providing a distorted view of competence
Communication	
• Increased number of generalists and primary care providers	• Productivity requirements creating shorter office visits, reduced telephone access, and other access barriers to physicians
• Creation of physician–nonphysician provider teams to provide a broader range of providers knowledgeable about the patient's condition	• Advertising creating inflated patient expectations
Compassion	
..	• Less time for interaction with patients during stressful decisions
Continuity	
..	• Price competition forcing patient choice of continuity at a higher price vs the cheapest plan
	• "Deselection" of physicians disrupting existing physician-patient relations
	• Frequent changes by employer of managed care plans forcing changes of physician
(No) Conflict of Interest	
...	• Linking physician salary incentives and bonuses to reduced use of tests and procedures for patients

performance and to provide the public with the performance results based on these quality indicators. While such extensive efforts at quality assessment in medicine have never before been undertaken and there is skepticism that these measures will be reliable and valid, if this effort is successful, many

Americans will have a rigorous and systematic mechanism to evaluate the competence of their health plans and physicians.[7, 8]

Besides closer monitoring of quality, other changes could improve physicians' competence and their communication with patients. The pressure created by cost controls, the resource-based relative value scale, and managed care has resulted in trends to improve reimbursement for primary care and to train more generalists. Although these initiatives are untested, they could increase the number of generalists, prompt the retraining of specialists in general medicine, and decrease the excessive reliance on specialists with their tendency toward higher use of diagnostic tests and technical interventions without notable effect on traditional health status measures.[9, 10] In addition, managed care's increased emphasis on primary care will accelerate the trend toward greater use of nurse practitioners, physician assistants, and midwives and teams composed of physicians and nonphysician providers. While the transition to such a team approach could not be accomplished instantaneously, and while it would require changing habits and increased communications among health care providers, research demonstrates that, when it is well implemented, it can improve patient care, communication, and satisfaction.[11-13] With such multidisciplinary teams, several providers are knowledgeable about the patient's condition and available to the patient, enhancing communication and continuity of care.[11-12] By increasing the number of providers for a patient, this team approach may increase the chances that patients with different cultural backgrounds might establish rapport and understanding with a provider.[11, 12]

Potential Threats

There are aspects of managed care, especially under significant cost controls and price competition, with the potential to undermine, or preclude the realization of, the ideal physician-patient relationship. The spread of managed care is being promoted by big employers and corporations; it is closely linked to price competition—if not outright managed competition—which has ramifications for almost every facet of the ideal physician-patient interaction.

First, to hold down costs, many insurance companies and managed care organizations may try to select enrollees who are likely to use fewer and cheaper services ("cherry pick") through selective marketing, increased use of exclusions, modifications of benefits offered, and other techniques. In the absence of significant health insurance regulatory reform legislation or universal coverage, such techniques could mean that more Americans will be unable to afford health insurance or effectively barred from coverage. Indeed, recent statistics suggest that the ranks of the uninsured are growing.[14] In turn, this deprives more Americans of the ideal physician-patient relationship. In addition, without insurance reform legislation to ensure transportability of health coverage when people change jobs, a significant number of Americans could be forced either to forgo coverage for periods of time or to change managed care plans with each job change. Given that 7 million Americans change jobs or become employed each month, there could be significant disruption of choice, communication, and continuity.

Second, to restrain costs, a growing number of employers are restricting patient choice in all its facets.[15-19] An increasing number of employers are offering only one health care plan; other employers are requiring their workers to enroll in a particular managed care plan or select a physician from a precertified list; still others are requiring their workers to pay substantially more for the opportunity to see a physician of their choosing outside their managed care panel; and still others are discouraging workers from selecting higher priced health plans. Some employers are even reverting to an old practice of hiring their own "company" physicians.[19] Through these and other techniques, a growing, albeit unknown, number of insured Americans are having their choice limited mainly by employers.[15] These practices may seriously disrupt, or require patients to abandon, long-standing relationships with physicians. In addition, in some instances, especially in managed care settings, patient choice of specialists, specialty facilities, and particular treatments is being eroded.[20]

Increasingly, managed care plans will compete for employers' contracts and subscribers on the basis of price. Yet there is no guarantee that the cheapest plan this year will be the cheapest plan during the next enrollment period. Indeed, if price competition is effective, the cheapest plan should change from year to year.[21] In such a price-competitive marketplace, employers may switch health care plans from year to year and patients may be forced to choose between continuing with their current physician and managed care plan at a higher price or switching to the cheaper plan. While patients may appear to opt for discontinuous care rather than pay more, the cost pressures—which fall disproportionately on those with lower incomes—hardly make such choices voluntary.[22-24] A recent study demonstrates a direct linear relationship between a lower family income

and willingness to switch to cheaper health care plans.[15] The importance of such decisions lies in the reason for change of physician.[21] Change is harmful if it is imposed on patients explicitly or implicitly by financial incentives and interrupts continuity. When the patient, however, decides to switch physicians, continuity of care has been outweighed in the patient's mind by other factors, such as competence or communication. Consequently, significant price competition, while not engendered by managed care, is certainly exacerbated by it and could have an adverse effect on both patient choice of practice type and physician and continuity of care.[15, 21]

A third threat to choice in the physician-patient relationship comes from the potential financial failure of managed care plans. If price competition is effective, inefficient plans will lose in the marketplace and close. Plan failure could pose a serious threat to patient choice and continuity of care, especially if the collapse happens between enrollment periods. Under such conditions, patients may be randomly assigned to other managed care plans. Or, their former physician may become affiliated with a plan that they are unable to join. Another threat to the physician-patient relationship may occur when managed care plans "deselect" a physician. In such circumstances, patients cannot choose that physician unless they are willing to go out of the plan. More important, patients who have been receiving care from that physician may be forced to switch to another physician in the managed care panel, again undermining patient choice and continuity of care.

Managed care also poses potential threats to competence. Its greater emphasis on the provision of primary care could adversely affect competence. Since specialists are more expensive than generalists, cost considerations foster a tendency to have generalists or even nonphysicians manage conditions that are best handled by specialists. For example, follow-up of cancer patients may be shifted from oncologists to primary care physicians. And there is some suggestion that these changes lead to fewer follow-up visits and less monitoring of the progress of disease in the managed care setting.[25] In addition, since time spent with specialists is expensive, there may be a tendency to use medications or other less expensive interventions in place of consultations with specialists.[26] Similarly, given the current shortage of generalists, there is already a movement to retrain specialist physicians as generalists. Since there are no standards for the amount and type of education needed for retraining, these retrained specialists may lack the breadth of knowledge, skills, and experience necessary to be competent primary care providers. Assessments of quality outcomes may be insensitive to these threats to competence.[27]

There are worries about the development of quality indicators. We lack quality indicators for most aspects of medical care. In addition, many quality indicators require risk adjustments for severity of illness that cannot be, or currently are not being, performed.[27, 28] It will take significant time and resources to develop reliable and validated quality indicators and risk adjusters for medical procedures. Yet the demand for these indicators could result in a rush to implementation without proper pretesting and validation. Mistakes related to the imperative to release of Medicare hospital mortality data as a quality measure before they were properly adjusted may be repeated on an even larger scale.[29-32] Use of faulty quality in-

formation could damage attempts to improve the competence of physicians, undermine patient trust, and cause patients to switch physicians unnecessarily.

Communication in the physician-patient relationship could be undermined by practice efficiencies necessitated by intensified price competition and financial pressures on managed care plans. Productivity requirements may translate into pressure on physicians to see more patients in shorter time periods, reducing the time to discuss patient values, alternative treatments, or the impact of a therapy on the patient's overall life.[33, 34] Such changes have been tried by managed care plans in the competitive Boston, Mass, health care market.[35] Compressing physician-patient interactions into short time periods in the name of productivity could curtail, if not eliminate, productive communication and compassion. A recent survey of patients in managed care plans showed that the physician spent less time with the patient and offered less explanation of care compared with those in traditional fee-for-service settings.[20] Similarly, to reduce costs, managed care plans might restrict telephone calls to the patient's primary care physician. Currently some plans limit patients' calls to their physicians to 1-hour time periods in the day. In addition, incentives might be put into place to encourage patients to talk with or see physicians or nonphysician providers with whom they are unfamiliar or who are not of their choosing.[26] All of these cost-saving mechanisms could easily inhibit physician-patient communication and continuity of care.

A further problem may arise in the competition among managed care plans to lure subscribers. They are likely to use advertising with implicit if not explicit promises of higher quality or more wide-ranging services. Such advertisements could easily create high expectations on the part of patients.[36-38] Simultaneously, however, to control costs plans will require physicians to be efficient in their personal time allocation as well as in their ordering of tests and use of other services. This could easily create a conflict between patient expectations and physician restrictions, undermining good communication, compassion, and trust.

Finally, while there has been significant attention on conflict of interest in fee-for-service practice,[39] there has been much less effort to investigate and address conflict of interest in managed care. Physician decision making may account for as much as 75% of health care costs. In the setting of significant price competition, managed care plans trying to reduce costs will therefore try to influence physician decision making, especially to reduce the use of medical services.[33] Managed care plans have already tried various mechanisms to try to reduce physician use of health care resources for their patients, including providing bonuses to physicians who order few tests and basing a percentage of physicians' salaries on volume and test ordering standards.[33, 39, 40] Such conflicts of interest may proliferate with increased price competition, the need for managed care plans to reduce costs, and the absence of governmental regulation.

CONCLUSIONS

The physician-patient relationship is the cornerstone for achieving, maintaining, and improving health. The structure of financing and regulation should be designed to foster and support an ideal relationship between the physician and the patient. Clearly, the current system incompletely realizes this ideal even for many well-insured Americans, and trends within the current system threaten to make this ideal even more elusive.

Managed care offers some advantages in realizing the ideal physician-patient relationship. For many Americans, increased use of managed care may secure choice, especially for preventive services, possibly expand continuity in their relationship with physicians, and implement a systematic assessment of quality and competence. But the expansion of managed care, in an environment that encourages competition and makes financial pressures intense and omnipresent, could promote serious impediments to realizing the ideal physician-patient relationship. Some practical steps that might diminish these impediments include (1) using global budgets instead of price competition among managed care plans for cost control; (2) prohibiting all schemes that use salary incentives or bonuses tied to physician test ordering patterns; (3) restricting expensive advertising by managed care plans by capping their promotion budgets; (4) requiring managed care plans to have a board of patients and physicians to approve policies regarding length of office visits and telephone calls: (5) creating an independent review board to assess the reliability and validity of all quality indicators before they are approved or required for use by managed care plans; (6) implementing insurance reform legislation to ensure mobility of insurance with job changes and purchasing of coverage by individuals; and (7) providing universal coverage to enable otherwise uninsured patients to have an opportunity for an ideal physician-patient relationship. As changes in our health care system develop, we must find ways, such as these, to encourage fiscal prudence without undermining the fundamental elements of the ideal physician-patient relationship.

REFERENCES

1. Igelhart JK. The struggle between managed care and fee for service practice. *N Engl J Med.* 1994;331:63–67.

2. *Effects of Managed Care: An Update.* Washington, DC: Congressional Budget Office; 1994.

3. *Managed Health Care: Effects on Employers' Costs Difficult to Measure.* Washington, DC: US General Accounting Office; 1993.

4. Bernstein AB, Thompson GB, Harlan LC. Differences in rates of cancer screening by usual source of medical care: data from the 1987 National Health Interview Survey. *Med Care.* 1991;29:196–209.

5. Retchin SM, Brown B. The quality of ambulatory care in Medicare health maintenance organizations. *Am J Public Health.* 1990;80:411–415.

6. Udvarhelyi IS, Jennison K, Phillips RS, Epstein AM. Comparison of the quality of ambulatory care for fee-for-service and prepaid patients. *Ann Intern Med.* 1991;327:424–429.

7. Laffel G, Berwick DM. Quality in health care. *JAMA.* 1992;268:407–409.

8. Kritchevsky SB, Simmons BP. Continuous quality improvement: concepts and applications for physician care. *JAMA.* 1991;266:1817–1823.

9. Greenfield S, Nelson EC, Zubkoff M, et al. Variations in resource utilization among medical specialties and systems of care. *JAMA.* 1992;267:1624–1630.

10. Schroeder SA, Sandy LG. Specialty distribution of U.S. physicians—the invisible driver of health care costs. *N Engl J Med.* 1993; 328:961–963.

11. *Nurse Practitioners, Physicians' Assistants, and Certified Nurse Midwives: Policy Analysis.* Washington, DC: Office of Technology Assessment; 1986.

12. Freund C. Research in support of nurse practitioners. In: Mezey M, McGivern D, eds. *Nurses and Nurse Practitioners: The Evolution to Advanced Practice.* New York, NY: Springer Publishing Co Inc; 1993.

13. Kavesh W. Physician and nurse-practitioner relationships. In: Mezey M, McGivern D, eds. *Nurses and Nurse Practitioners: The Evolution to Advanced Practice.* New York, NY: Springer Publishing Co Inc; 1993.

14. Pear R. Health insurance percentage is lowest in four Sun Belt states. *New York Times.* October 6, 1994:A16.

15. The Kaiser/Commonwealth Fund Second National Health Insurance Survey. November 10, 1993.

16. Lewis DE. Coping without coverage. *Boston Globe.* May 5, 1993:53.

17. Lewis DE. Union oks Boston gas accord. *Boston Globe.* May 5, 1993:53.

18. Seitz R. The political tea leaves point to medical networks. *New York Times.* December 20, 1992: D10.

19. Pasternak J. In-house doctors give some firms a health care remedy. *Los Angeles Times.* July 11, 1993:A1.

20. Blendon RJ, Knox RA, Brodie M, Benson JM, Chervinsky G. Americans compare managed care, Medicare, and fee for service. *J Am Health Policy.* 1994:4:42–47.

21. Emanuel EJ, Brett AS. Managed competition and the patient-physician relationship. *N Engl J Med.* 1993;329;879–882.

22. Travis MR, Russell G, Cronin S. Determinants of voluntary disenrollment. *J Health Care Marketing.* 1989;9:75–76.

23. Hennelly VD, Boxerman SB. Out-of-plan use and disenrollment: outgrowths of dissatisfaction with a prepaid group plan. *Med Care.* 1983;21:348–359.

24. Sorenson AA, Wersinger RP. Factors influencing disenrollment from an HMO. *Med Care.* 1981;19:766–773.

25. Clement DG, Retchin SM, Brown RS, Stegall MH. Access and outcomes of elderly patients enrolled in managed care. *JAMA.* 1994;271:1487–1492.

26. Henneberger M. Managed care changing practice of psychotherapy. *New York Times.* October 9, 1994:A1, A50.

27. Salem-Schatz S, Moore G, Rucker M, Pearson SD. The case for case-mix adjustment in practice profiling: when good apples look bad. *JAMA.* 1994;272:871–874.

28. McNeil BJ, Pederson SH, Gatsonis C. Current issues in profiling quality of care. *Inquiry.* 1992;29:298–307.

29. Green J, Passman LJ, Wintfield N. Analyzing hospital mortality: the consequences of diversity in patient mix. *JAMA.* 1991;265:1849–1853.

30. Burke M. HCFA's Medicare mortality data: the controversy continues. *Hospitals.* 1992:118, 120, 122.

31. Greenfield S, Aronow HU, Elashoff RM, Wantanabe D. Flaws in mortality data: the hazards of ignoring comorbid disease. *JAMA.* 1988;260:2253–2255.

32. Robinson ML. Limitations of mortality data confirmed: studies. *Hospitals.* 1988;62:23–24.

33. Baker LC, Cantor JC. Physician satisfaction under managed care. *Health AFF* (Millwood). 1993;12(suppl):258–270.

34. Jellinek MS, Nurcombe B. Two wrongs don't make a right: managed care, mental health, and the marketplace. *JAMA*. 1993;270:1737–1739.

35. Knox RA, Stein C. HMO doctors want boss out in dispute on patient load. *Boston Globe*. November 21, 1991:1, 27.

36. Freidson E. Prepaid group practice and the new 'demanding patients.' *Milbank Mem Fund Q*. 1973;51:473–488.

37. Schroeder JL, Clarke JT, Webster JR. Prepaid entitlements: a new challenge for physician-patient relationships. *JAMA*. 1985;254:3080–3082.

38. Brett AS. The case against persuasive advertising by health maintenance organizations. *N Engl J Med*. 1992;326:1253–1257.

39. Rodwin M. *Medicine, Money, and Morals*. New York, NY: Oxford University Press Inc; 1993.

40. Hillman AL, Pauly MV, Kerstein JJ. How do financial incentives affect physicians' clinical decisions and the financial performance of health maintenance organizations? *N Engl J Med*. 1989;321:86–92.

NO

Michael J. Malinowski

CAPITATION, ADVANCES IN MEDICAL TECHNOLOGY, AND THE ADVENT OF A NEW ERA IN MEDICAL ETHICS

THE ADVENT OF A COST-CONSCIOUS ERA IN MEDICAL ETHICS

Modern medical ethics has evolved from two distinct eras of development —one of professional domination and another of interdisciplinary bioethics. During the era of professional domination, medical ethics was delegated to the province of practicing clinicians. Ethical concepts were used to generate codes of professional conduct enforced by the profession itself primarily through boards and institutional proceedings. "Consistent with the ancient Hippocratic tradition of Greek medicine, the resulting ethical principles were primarily concerned with maintaining order among members of the profession and fostering public respect for professional authority." Patient well-being was defined in a "highly paternalistic and authoritarian fashion" and beneficence—the best interest of the patient as determined by his or her caregiver—served as the guiding principle.

The era of bioethics commenced approximately in 1970. Rather than being provider-centered, bioethics moved medical ethics to a "a patient-centered framework that defined medical ethics in terms of individual rights and patient autonomy. This approach is best exemplified by the legal innovation of the informed consent doctrine" and enactment of the Patient Self-Determination Act. To understand the patient's perspective, medical ethics were discussed and defined in a more interdisciplinary manner and with deference to social scientists and theologians. In the deontological spirit of Kantian ethics, patient autonomy became the guiding principle. The bioethics approach "professes, in its most extreme form, that a doctor's role is to execute the instructions from a fully informed master, the patient."

A Shared Failure to Consider Costs

Despite the difference in guiding principles, both the professional dominance and bioethics approaches have agreed on a "single-minded devotion to patients' medical interests without concern for costs, even if this frustrates efficient distribution of societal resources." It is no surprise, therefore, that the health care industry represents the largest single sector of the U.S. economy. The United States spends nearly fifteen percent of its gross domestic product on health care—$900 billion in 1993—and that figure continues to rise at a rate of approximately 9.2% per year.

At the same time health care expenditure has ballooned, the distribution of health care has been too uneven and the costs too high. The escalation of costs has augmented inequalities in distribution, to the extent that patients with coverage receive access to the miracles of modern medicine such as genetic testing, while fewer people, especially the working poor and children, have any coverage. While some patients with advanced cancer receive autologous bone marrow transplantations that offer them very little chance of health improvement, new mothers and their babies allegedly are being sent home dangerously soon after birth, many women are unable to obtain adequate prenatal care, one-quarter of children are without health insurance at some point during their first few years of life, and 40 million U.S. citizens have no health care coverage. Depending on the extent of Medicare and Medicaid cuts, analysts predict that the number of uninsured Americans will rise to between 45.9 million and 53.7 million by 2002 if reforms are not made. . . .

A Cost-Conscious Era in Medical Ethics
In contrast with familiar medical ethic norms, managed care is about payers setting limits. Care managers limit physician dominance and patient autonomy, and the eras of medical ethics void of concern for costs have come to a close. Modern medicine is entering a third era in medical ethics—an era which might be called socioethics, meaning medical ethics which are more utilitarian or society-based. Today, and even more so tomorrow, the deontological rights of each patient must be balanced, at least to some extent, against the utilitarian principle of doing the *most* good. The advent of widespread managed care; the coupling of economic limitations with enhanced medical capabilities, which has resulted in unconscionable discrepancies in health care coverage; and advances in medical technology that exacerbate these discrepancies together drive the shift toward this new approach to medical ethics.

The Changed Role of Physicians Under Managed Care
Managed care is fundamentally changing the role of physicians. Care managers are drawing health care providers into the long-established conflict between payer and patient, whereby "[t]he payer becomes the patient's adversary, rather than advocate, denying payment on claims whenever possible." First, care managers are assuming direct control over patient care decisionmaking, thereby shrinking the discretion to which physicians have grown accustomed. Second, and more troubling, care managers are shifting the financial risk of patient care to providers through payment schemes that connect physicians' financial compensation to their patients' health risks. Whether physicians receive bonuses for minimizing costs or a fixed monthly fee per patient for a comprehensive episode or period of care, a major component of managed care is shifting risks to providers and creating incentives to control costs. Physicians are becoming health

care gatekeepers who control access to specialists and inpatient services, who in turn determine whether and where the patient will be hospitalized.

This change in physician incentives and influence over health care decision-making by care managers necessitates a shift from health care decisionmaking on a patient-by-patient basis to more organizational decisionmaking subject to public accountability. Although legal liability may address some of the more egregious instances of inadequate care and instill incentives for providing quality care, it cannot be relied on to police more subtle and systematic lapses in care. This is especially true when patients lack information necessary to assess their care and place trust in their providers. As observed by Professor Starr, "[t]he very circumstances of sickness promote acceptance of [physicians'] judgment."

There already is some indication that, to ensure minimum standards of patient care, specific patient care issues will have to be addressed in a publicly accountable, community health policy manner —whether that community be the patient base of a managed care organization (MCO), a state, or the nation. The fates of patients cannot simply be entrusted to their physicians under the assumption that doctors have the incentives and discretion to provide satisfactory care. In particular, control over care decisionmaking by care managers will necessitate more regulatory safeguards to ensure minimum care. To protect patients' interests and the discretion of physicians to treat them adequately, clearer ethical standards will have to be established and some regulatory safeguards imposed.

The Need to Instill a Social Conscience

Due to the deference shown to the commitment of physicians to their patients, "the dominant position among medical ethicists and the medical profession in general is a nearly absolute moral prohibition against physicians ever considering the costs of treatment to any degree." It follows from this position that society should make any necessary rationing decisions, not practitioners. Even at the collective societal level, medical ethicists generally unite in opposing rationing incentives and cost-effectiveness criteria for health care. In light of the no-concern-for-costs mentality of the professional domination and bioethics eras of medical ethics, presumably the majority of medical ethicists share this position. For decades, medical ethics have been administered on a patient-by-patient basis, and providers within the United States, trained under the traditional scheme, have escaped contemplating the zero-sum reality of health care. Cost-effectiveness simply has not been considered.

Medical ethics should bring health care and patients together, not drive them apart by making insurance unaffordable and health care unobtainable. As expressly recognized at the state level by Oregon, implicitly recognized through the spread of managed care, and evidenced by the fact that 40 million U.S. citizens have no health care coverage despite the exorbitant resources allocated, rationing health care resources is necessary. The challenge of contemporary medical ethics is to maintain, if not enhance, quality care and patient trust in providers while instilling in both providers and patients a social conscience, meaning an appreciation for the limits of health care resources. The ultimate goal should be to internalize cost-conscious calculations on the part of physicians, as in Great Britain where, "despite the severity of financial constraints—the British system spends only one-third per capita of what ours does—physicians seldom consciously engage in explicit cost-benefit calculations." Moreover, "British doctors still profess just as strong an ethic of absolute quality."

It is possible to ration health care resources without making health care substandard. For example, simply becoming aware of the existence of and prescribing less expensive drugs, avoiding referrals to specialists when there is high confidence in a diagnosis and prognosis, and denying marginally beneficial treatments (especially expensive ones) would have a profound impact on health care resources and make insurance coverage significantly more affordable. A presumption against trying expensive treatments highly unlikely to work unless the patient has supplemental insurance or the personal means to pay for them must replace the presumption in favor of trying *any* treatment that *might* work. Fully informing patients of the option of purchasing such services outside the scope of their primary insurance should fulfill fiduciary responsibilities and help to maintain patient trust. The effectiveness of such an approach could be maximized if (1) patients understand the limits of their coverage when they purchase it, (2) patients understand that rationing is making their insurance affordable, and (3) health care ethical norms are expanded to more comfortably address cases in which high costs are not justified by minor expected benefits.

It is time to lessen the ethical taboo against physician rationing in order to do the most good with our health care resources. With almost 10,000 diagnos-

tic entries in the World Health Organization's International Classification of Diseases and almost 10,000 medical interventions listed in the American Medical Association's (AMA) Current Procedural Terminology, "[a] complete and scientifically valid set of rationing rules would entail the impossible task of developing rigorous empirical information...." Accordingly, the only way to ration effectively and with sensitivity to each patient's condition is through the medical profession, meaning through professional ethical norms that are socially conscious. No grand transformation in health care expenditure accompanied by quality care is possible without instilling a medical ethic sensitive to the injustice of wholly unaffordable insurance and unobtainable health care. Providers must fulfill the third fundamental obligation embodied in Hippocratic tradition— "to refuse to treat those who are overmastered by their diseases, realizing in such cases that medicine is powerless."

Exacerbation of the Need for New Ethical Norms

Modern medicine has made the need to ration undeniable. During this century, medical technology has impacted human health profoundly. Life expectancy from birth has climbed from fifty-four years in 1920 to seventy-five years in the early 1990s, and the death rate from disease has fallen from 1212 per 100,000 in 1920 to 800 per 100,000 in the early 1990s.

The paradox of medical technology is that, though it is responsible for alleviating human suffering and disease, it also is responsible for raising health care costs. The reasons are multifold. First, longevity is the equivalent of susceptibility to new, more complex diseases that are more difficult to treat and require specialized, technology-intensive care. In other words, "[i]nnovation has . . . led to longer life, but in so doing has created an even bigger challenge, represented by chronic, progressively debilitating diseases." Accordingly, effective medical technology increases the need for more advances and scientific research and development (R&D), and also increases consumption of technology-intensive, specialized, and expensive treatments. "Thus, paradoxically, even if another penicillin' was discovered that inexpensively cured the prevalent diseases of today, the population would eventually age to the point where some new set of diseases would be killing (much older) people at essentially the same rate."

Second, by prolonging life, medical technology has greatly increased the ranks of the elderly, the nation's biggest health care consumers. "On average, the elderly consume four times as much medical care as do people under 65. . . ." According to the Congressional Budget Office, 64.7% of the growth in Medicare spending is attributable to increased services and use of technology, and Medicare consumed approximately 11.6% of all federal spending in 1995 —meaning seventy-seven percent of the nation's health care bill for that year. Third, medical technology has created increased services and capabilities, and society has come to *expect* general access to them regardless of cost. "When medical technology is available, it seems inevitably to be used, even in the face of objective data that it is inappropriate."

Medical technology actually creates new treatable conditions. This effect of medical technology is illustrated by medical advances related to short stature and infertility. Human growth hormone was developed initially to treat children whose bodies failed to produce it in standard amounts, a condition known as growth hormone deficiency (GHD). Now, recombinant DNA technology has made growth hormone much more available, and there is some evidence that the physical characteristic of short stature *apart from GHD* will become a treatable condition. . . .

The costs of medical technology must be contained, especially in light of the myriad of genetic technologies reaching commerce and the preexisting unmet health care needs of the general public. Ethical norms that recognize and discourage the abuse and waste of health care resources must be fostered. Medical ethics should strive to maintain high standards of care on a deontological, patient-by-patient basis, while making health care both affordable and obtainable. Providers should consider both efficacy and cost-effectiveness when treating patients and, perhaps more importantly, when evaluating new treatments at the societal level. Regardless of any one patient's needs, priorities must be set.

APPLICATION: THE ETHICAL IMPLICATIONS OF CAPITATED CARE

In many ways, managed care appears to be a natural accompaniment to modern medicine—a means to establish comprehensive networks of services with lower transaction costs. Nevertheless, the advent of managed care presents policymakers with a difficult challenge. As discussed above, health care policymakers must instill in providers ethical norms that embody an obligation to administer medicine with a social conscience, meaning with respect for the limits of health care resources and the need to make health care affordable and obtainable. Equally important, they must maintain patient trust and quality of care while doing so.

Capitation presently is the method of choice of care managers, as evidenced by its widespread use among health care organizations. Moreover, care managers are applying capitation at all levels within the health care system. As stated above, it is not uncommon for primary care services to be capped and for the primary care physicians then to act as gatekeepers for referrals to specialists, whose services are capped under yet another arrangement. Care managers cap hospital fees by assigning a diagnosis-adjusted fixed payment per admission through, for example, diagnosis-related groups (DRGs). Even prescription drugs are being capped under agreements with manufacturers whereby manufacturers agree to provide all the drugs needed to treat certain conditions on a fixed, per-patient monthly fee. Some care managers are encouraging health care organizations to deal with their vendors on a capitated basis, thereby disbursing yet more risks to a larger number of health care players. To evaluate capitation in accordance with the [previously] proposed socioethic norms, the impact of capitation on both the general public health and the individual patient care must be assessed.

The Impact of Capitation on Public Health

Though it is too soon to draw any conclusions, the early profitability of capitation suggests that it does realize greater market efficiencies than traditional medicine. It appears, however, that many of the profits are leaving the health care system, and critics of capitated care argue that health care costs are not going down. These critics assert that, instead, care managers are shifting money from the pockets of doctors to their pockets, and that these pockets are getting fuller. Another fear is that care managers are realizing these profits by tapping moneys which non-profit hospitals traditionally have collected through inflated fees and applied to R&D. Still others, pointing most often to anecdotal evidence, assert that care managers are realizing these profits at the expense of patient care.

At present, there is inadequate empirical data to assess the impact of capitation on the quality of care, which leaves ample room for speculation—especially about the long-term effects of capitated care. For example, if inefficiencies plagued the U.S. health care system prior to widespread capitated care, care managers may in fact be improving the quality of patient care while making huge profits simply by tapping into and eliminating those inefficiencies. If this is true, the real test for capitation is yet to come, and the second and third generations of reforms to sustain profitability pose much greater danger to the quality of care. Also, lower insurance rates and substantial influxes of groups previously uninsured into the health care system may offset anecdotal failures of capitation among some long-standing health care consumers.

But this is simply speculation, and the impact of capitation on patient trust and the doctor-patient relationship is even more difficult to assess. Moreover, it is possible that capitation may affect the doctor-patient relationship negatively but still significantly improve patient care through the formation of extensive health networks and cost reductions that make such networks accessible to more people. The limited data available to date suggest that, at least in the aggregate, financial incentives to limit care do not compromise patient care quality significantly. In fact, "[v]irtually all of these studies have concluded that patients fare at least as well, if not better, in HMOs than under traditional fee-for-service indemnity insurance." However, a study of 1500 individuals found that, among those ill at the outset of the study, low-income patients fared better in the traditional FFS system while those in the top forty percent of income distribution experienced better health outcomes in the HMO. Other studies suggest that HMO patients receive more preventive tests and examinations than subscribers of traditional FFS plans. Still other studies outside the context of capitated care suggest that physicians are capable of rationing responsibly, effectively, and in an internalized manner (meaning without the need of deliberate effort) when confronted with the need to do so—such as in crowded intensive care units.

The Impact of Capitation on Individual Patient Care

Although capitation may promote patient access to broad networks of specialized services and, overall, make health care more affordable, the quality of health care ultimately rests on health care providers. Though decisions must be made in the aggregate and perimeters drawn to avoid a continuation of the classic abuse of the health care commons, health care still is about individual patients. It is about their illnesses and the impact of those illnesses on them and their families.

Under capitated care, care managers assume an uncomfortable amount of discretion in care decision-making once held by physicians. Capitation affects the doctor-patient relationship by drawing

health care providers into the conflict between health care consumption and cost and bringing health care managers into that relationship. In fact, where health care is capitated, "patients' primary relationships might be with their health care insurers rather than with their physicians, making it more difficult for patients to maintain longstanding relationships with their physicians." ...

[One] practical solution would be to instill a new ethic of social consciousness in subscribers as well as providers by building on the established patient-centered framework of the bioethics era. The roles of care managers, providers, and patients in making rationing decisions must be further defined. In keeping with the principles of contract law, capitation should be disclosed fully and explained to potential subscribers by care managers *before* they enroll in plans. Employer self-insurers should not be permitted to impede this obligation; such disclosure must become mandated under the standard of care. Care managers should explain the correlation between coverage limits and costs—just as the correlation is explained with virtually all other kinds of insurance—to potential subscribers. This explanation should accompany meaningful discussion with potential subscribers of the limits of their coverage, the commercial incentives placed on their physicians, and the fact that they are free to discuss supplemental health care options with their physicians. Disclosure requirements should be no less for consumers buying health insurance than they are generally when those same consumers purchase automobile and homeowners insurance, or invest in securities.

If subscribers were fully informed about the rationing component of their coverage and their option to purchase supplemental coverage or purchase supplemental services directly, the burden on their physicians could be lessened immensely. Subscribers presumably would perceive necessary rationing more as their own choice (either directly or through their self-insuring employers), as reflected in the coverage he or she selected, rather than as a selfish hold-out by their primary care physician to make more money. In essence, many rationing decisions would shift to subscribers, who would make them beforehand through contractual negotiations with health care managers. While patients may not be able readily to comprehend the complexities of genetic testing or their own psychological reaction to the results, they are capable of understanding that lower insurance costs correlate with express limits of care. Of course, they will want to know those limits and probably ask many questions, and right they should.

Though policymakers at both the state and federal levels presently overlook the importance of such disclosure requirements, the vulnerability of those in need of health care mandates high standards of disclosure. In the long run, such an approach would help to preserve the respect for patients' rights developed during the bioethics era, apprise patients of and create a check on physicians' rationing decisions, and hopefully help to preserve the physician-patient relationship by eliminating feelings of betrayal when rationing decisions are disclosed....

CONCLUSION

Health care within the United States is undergoing fundamental and pervasive changes, both in its capabilities and in the way it is administered. To maximize the effectiveness of modern medicine, patients must be given access to broad networks of specialized, often technology-intensive services and advanced facilities capable of delivering those services. Because of the costs of the miracles of modern medicine, distribution of health care in recent years has become too uneven and the costs to consumers too high. Even among the insured, the resources our society is willing to allocate to health care, though immense, simply are not enough to make all the capabilities of modern medicine available to all who could benefit from them. Efforts to do so have caused insurance rates to rise and the ranks of the uninsured to swell. Ironically, just as we as a society are recognizing the limits of our health care resources, biotechnology companies are commercializing a new generation of genetic technologies.

The central theme of this Article is that health care policymakers, regulators, and providers must change the ethical norms that drive health care and patients apart by making health care unaffordable and unobtainable. Such norms now prevail in the United States. The professional domination and bioethics eras of medical ethics, with their no-concern-for-costs mentality, are over. The reality of modern medicine, meaning the medicine of today and tomorrow, is that costs *do matter*. They matter a great deal. Accordingly, medical ethics must acquire a social conscience, and the fact that capitation has become so widespread so quickly suggests that this is happening. Capitation is a means to make modern medicine accessible by building comprehensive health care networks and controlling costs. Unless reliable empirical data is gathered which establishes that capitation diminishes the quality of care substantially, health care policymakers and regulators should utilize capitation to accomplish these objectives.

Health care policymakers, however, must not lose sight of the fact that the quality of health care rests ultimately on the quality of physicians and other providers and the services they render. Health care providers must not be forced to bear an inordinate amount of the risk of insuring their patients nor primary responsibility for rationing care. Care managers, through capitation with extensive and sometimes harsh financial incentives, threaten to do just that. Reforms, therefore, are necessary not only to preserve a minimum standard of quality care but also to promote socially responsible allocation of resources. Health care policymakers and regulators should impose safeguards to ensure providers enough discretion and freedom from harsh financial incentives to treat their patients' specific conditions and to do so adequately.

Rationing is necessary, but it should be carried out in accordance with the patient-centered principles of bioethics and traditional contract principles. The burden must be placed on care managers to disclose fully and to explain capitation to potential subscribers *before* they subscribe. Care managers should explain the correlation between costs and coverage limits, disclose the commercial incentives placed on providers, and emphasize the freedom to discuss supplemental options with physicians. The standard of disclosure and contractual obligation to disclose accompanying the purchase of health insurance should be just as high as it is for purchasing other forms of insurance, if not higher, and self-insuring employers must not be permitted in any way to lessen that obligation. To enlighten and inform subscribers and to offer guidance to and protect providers, health care policymakers should encourage the development through peer review of coverage guidelines that embody the governing standard of care.

POSTSCRIPT

Should Patient-Centered Medical Ethics Govern Managed Care?

Under an existing law called COBRA, a worker who loses or leaves a job can continue buying the same insurance plan for 18 months. In 1995 only 18 percent of eligible workers chose to do so; others did not, typically because their new jobs provided coverage (most with a waiting period of months, however) or because it was too expensive (costing an average of $464 a month per family). The overall percentage of working families who have any kind of health care insurance continues to drop. According to a study released by the American Hospital Association in September 1996, 77.7 percent of Americans had on-the-job health insurance in 1990, but five years later that figure had dropped to 73.9 percent and is expected to fall to 70.4 percent by 2002. Overall, the number of uninsured people in the United States is projected to climb from 39.6 million in 1995 to 45.6 million (16.2 percent of the population) by 2002. One quarter of the uninsured are children and teenagers.

In a modest reform effort, President Bill Clinton signed the Health Insurance Portability and Accountability Act in August 1996. The provisions of the bipartisan bill, which was championed by Senators Edward Kennedy (D-Massachusetts) and Nancy Kassebaum (R-Kansas) and which takes effect in January 1998, make it easier for people to keep their insurance if they change jobs by preventing insurers from denying coverage for a preexisting condition to anyone who had been covered under another health care plan for the previous 12 months. There is no limit, however, on what insurers can charge, and there are no provisions for people without insurance. In September 1996 Congress agreed to expand mental health coverage to people with group health insurance. Plans that do not provide mental health coverage will not be required to do so, but plans that do will not be able to set lower annual or total limits for mental health treatment. Companies with fewer than 50 employees will be exempted. While the mental health provisions may expand services for some, the growth of managed care into this area is a concern. This issue is explored by Miles F. Shore and Allan Beigel in "The Challenges Posed by Managed Behavioral Health Care" and by John K. Iglehart in "Health Policy Report: Managed Care and Mental Health," both in *The New England Journal of Medicine* (January 11, 1996). See also "Managed Care in Mental Health: The Ethical Issues," *Health Affairs* (vol. 14, no. 3, 1995).

In a provision that directly addresses one of the cost-cutting measures commonly imposed by managed care companies, Congress also requires health care plans to provide at least 48 hours in the hospital after childbirth, if mothers choose to stay. Consumer protests against "drive-through deliveries"—

discharging new mothers within 24 hours of birth—had previously resulted in several state laws banning the practice. Several states are also prohibiting "gag rules" by managed care companies that have prohibited physicians from discussing treatments that the plan does not cover or disclosing the physician's financial arrangement with the plan. Financial incentives to physicians from corporate payers remain substantial, however, as explored by Steffie Woolhandler and David U. Himmelstein in "Extreme Risk—The New Corporate Proposition for Physicians," *The New England Journal of Medicine* (December 21, 1995). See also "Paying Physicians More to Do Less: Financial Incentives to Limit Care," by David Orentlicher, *University of Richmond Law Review* (January 1996).

Donald W. Light provides an overview of the American health care system, beginning with early corporate practices in the late nineteenth century and ending with the rise of managed care, in "The Restructuring of the American Health Care System," in Theodore Litman, ed., *Health Politics and Policy*, 3rd ed. (Delmar, 1997). A historical perspective is also part of a comprehensive analysis of managed care by John C. Fletcher and Carolyn L. Engelhard in "Ethical Issues in Managed Care: A Report of the University of Virginia Study Group of Managed Care," *Virginia Medical Quarterly* (vol. 122, no. 3, 1995). As mergers and acquisitions within the industry proceed at breakneck speed, of interest is *Market Consolidation, Antitrust, and Public Policy in the Health Care Industry: Agenda for Future Research* by David Schactman and Stuart H Altman, a report written for Health Tracking, a Robert Wood Johnson Foundation project that is monitoring health system change. Ezekiel J. Emanuel argues for a shift in the orientation of medical ethics from cases to institutions in "Medical Ethics in the Era of Managed Care: The Need for Institutional Structures Instead of Principles for Individual Cases," *Journal of Clinical Ethics* (vol. 6, no. 4, 1995).

An entire issue of *American Journal of Law and Medicine* (vol. 22, nos. 2 and 3, 1996) is devoted to "Health Care Capitated Systems." See also Mark A. Hall, "Rationing Health Care at the Bedside," *New York University Law Review* (October–November 1994). To assess patient response to the changing health care environment, Karen Davis et al. surveyed patient satisfaction with managed care. They report their findings in "Choice Matters: Enrollees' Views of Their Health Plans," *Health Affairs* (Summer 1995). See also "Managed Care Plan Performance Since 1980: A Literature Analysis," by Robert H. Miller and Harold S. Luftt, *Journal of the American Medical Association* (May 18, 1994). The American Medical Association's Council on Ethical and Judicial Affairs reaffirms the physician's duty of patient advocacy and full disclosure in "Ethical Issues in Managed Care," *Journal of the American Medical Association* (January 25, 1995). Another view supporting the physician's duty to ensure continuity and loyalty to the patient is David Orentlicher's "Health Care Reform and the Patient-Physician Relationship," *Health Matrix* (Winter 1995).

ISSUE 20

Should There Be a Market in Body Parts?

YES: Lori B. Andrews, from "My Body, My Property," *Hastings Center Report* (October 1986)

NO: Thomas H. Murray, from "Gifts of the Body and the Needs of Strangers," *Hastings Center Report* (April 1987)

ISSUE SUMMARY

YES: Attorney Lori B. Andrews believes that donors, recipients, and society will benefit from a market in body parts so long as owners—and no one else —retain control over their bodies.

NO: Ethicist Thomas H. Murray argues that the gift relationship should govern transfer of body parts because it honors important human values, which are diminished by market relationships.

In 1976 John Moore was treated for hairy-cell leukemia at the University of California at Los Angeles. His enlarged spleen was removed; Moore's condition improved. In the course of seven years of follow-up, Moore was asked by his physicians to return frequently to UCLA from his home in Seattle to have his blood tested. When he became concerned about the frequency of the visits and the amount of blood drawn, he learned that, as a by-product of his treatment, scientists had been able to use his cells to grow a potentially commercially valuable patented cell line, which they named Mo. (Cell line means cells that continuously reproduce in a culture without differentiating.) Moore sued, claiming that he had not given consent for this use of his body parts, and he asked for a share of any profits. The physicians claimed that Moore had waived his interest in his body parts when he authorized the removal of his spleen on a routine consent form.

In a similar case, Hideaki Hagiwara, a postdoctoral biology student at the University of California at San Diego, suggested to a colleague, Dr. Ivor Royston, that cancer cells from Hagiwara's mother could be used to create a human monoclonal antibody—that is, an antibody that reacts specifically with a certain kind of cancerous cell. After the new cell line was completed, Hagiwara claimed that he had an economic interest in the procedure since he had suggested the idea and the cells had come from his mother.

These cases are unusual only because they resulted in lawsuits. The practice of using patients' body parts or tissues for research with potential commercial applications is widespread. According to a survey conducted by a subcommittee of the U.S. House of Representatives, about half of 81 medical schools responding to the questionnaire use patients' fluids or tissues for research. About one-fifth of the patent applications filed by these schools in the five years previous to the survey had used materials derived from patients. Three times as many patents had originated in patients' body parts from 1980 to 1984 as had occurred between 1975 and 1979.

Should patients have the right to consent to the use of their body parts and to share in any profits that might accrue? Or does the value mainly derive from the scientists' labors? In the following selections, Lori B. Andrews contends that it is time to acknowledge that body parts are personal property and that individuals must have the ability to transfer and sell them and thus to participate in any economic rewards. Thomas H. Murray, on the other hand, warns that treating body parts as property will diminish their symbolic and human value. He argues for a continuation of the gift relationship, which strengthens the bonds between strangers.

YES

Lori B. Andrews

MY BODY, MY PROPERTY

Tangible items are generally considered to be property. As new potentials for body parts unfold in research, diagnostics, and therapy, the question arises— should they be considered property as well? Current policy allows people to donate solid organs, but not to sell them. A federal law forbids sales of organs for transplant in interstate commerce[1] and certain state laws ban payment for specified organs as well.[2] This perspective—that bodily parts and products are gifts, not compensable items of property—underlies researchers' use of a patient's tissue to produce potentially marketable products.

THE PROPERTY APPROACH AND INDIVIDUAL CONTROL

Throughout the legal lore, judges have reacted with horror to the idea that body parts may be property. Nevertheless, many legal decisions treat the body as a type of property. The law allows me to make gifts of certain body parts and even to destroy my body entirely. Not only do I have a property-like interest in my own body, I may have rights that could be considered property rights in other people's bodies. Tort law allows me to recover for harm to my child, such as it allows me recovery for damage to my car. In most instances, I can collect damages if an autopsy is performed on my next of kin without my consent.

Since the legal treatment of bodies and body parts sounds suspiciously like property treatment, why is there such a reluctance to label it as such? One major fear is that bodily property could be transferred to others (the legal term is alienable) and we could become slaves, not in a market for our bodies, but in a market for body parts. However, characterizing body parts as property does not mean that they must be completely transferable. As Susan Rose-Ackerman points out, many forms of property have restrictions on alienability.[3] There may be restrictions on who holds them, what actions are required or forbidden, and what kinds of transfers are permitted. Some types of properties can be given as gifts, but not sold (items made of the fur or feathers of endangered species, for example). Other types of properties (such as the holdings of a person who is bankrupt) can be sold, but not given as gifts.

Even under current policy, the body can be considered property, the kind of property that can be transferred without payment, but not sold. However, restraints on payment need strong moral and legal justification. The Ontario Law Reform Commission recently faced the issue of paying for body parts in the context of artificial reproduction. After deciding that donating sperm, eggs, or embryos was ethically, morally, and socially acceptable, the Commission noted that any restriction on available services (for example, by prohibiting commercial banks for gametes and embryos) "must be scrutinized very carefully; it would be futile and frustrating to give with one hand, only to take with the other."[4]

The property approach recognizes people's interest in controlling what happens to their body parts. It provides a legal basis for a remedy as theories of privacy, autonomy, or assault do not when inappropriate actions are taken with respect to extracorporeal bodily materials. The presumption that the authority belongs to the individual who provided the body parts would be a starting point, which would at least assure that the regulatory and institutional policies developed be measured against some standard. . . .

Some lawyers and researchers argue that there is no need to inform people that body parts removed in the course of treatment may be used for research or commercial purposes, so long as the patient is not exposed to any additional physical risk due to the research. Currently, under federal regulations covering federally funded research, consent is not required to do research on such pathological or diagnostic specimens, so long

as the subjects cannot be identified.[5] In such cases, consent is given under the general hospital admission form, which states that the part may be used for teaching or research before it is destroyed. But the hospital consent form does not say that the patient may refuse to allow bodily materials to be used and still retain the patient/physician relationship and be treated. Only when the human material is taken primarily for research purposes is consent required. Even then, if the research poses "no more than minimal risk" and involves only collection of some body excretions, including blood, placenta or amniotic fluid, it may be given an expedited review by an Institutional Review Board; while consent is not specifically required, presumably the IRB can seek consent if the subjects are identifiable.[6] The failure to extend consent to all categories of research on human body parts and the failure even to raise the issue of compensation puts patients at a distinct psychological and economic disadvantage. . . .

There is support for informing patients about the potential uses of the body parts, even among groups that now gain commercially from using those parts. The Licensing Executive Society Biotechnology Committee recently surveyed its members, who generally represent organizations that use human tissues, fluids, or cells for research or development purposes. Of those responding, twenty-two believed that research or commercialization should occur *only* with the patient's prior consent; two felt consent was unnecessary. Thirteen felt that a person has a right to receive compensation for the use of his or her fluid, tissues, or cells, while eight did not.

THE MARKET'S EFFECT ON DONORS

The property approach requires the individual's consent before her body parts can be used by others. But in some instances, body parts—such as kidneys or corneas—may be in such short supply or a particular patient may have such a rare tissue or fluid type that the issue of payment to donors will arise, as it did in the Moore and Hagiwara cases....

Naturally, the need for money is not a justification for any action (we would not want the person to become a contract killer for a fee). But it is difficult to justify a prohibition on payment for what otherwise would be a legal and ethical act—giving up body parts for someone else's valid use. Similarly, the analogy to slavery is inapposite. We do not want people to sell themselves into slavery *nor* do we want them to "give" themselves into slavery without pay. In contrast, with respect to organ donation or the development of a diagnostic or therapeutic product from bodily materials, the underlying activity is one we want to encourage....

GUARDING AGAINST COERCION

Just as we would not condone a labor system that did not allow people to choose their own employers, we should insist that paid donations from living people be voluntary: that is, made by the person himself or herself. It is one thing for people to have the right to treat their own bodies as property, quite another to allow others to treat a person as property. A hospital should not be allowed to take, sell, and use blood or eggs from a comatose woman to help pay her costs of hospitalization. People should be prohibited from selling their relative's body parts when the relative dies (unless the deceased left orders to that effect). Nor should judges be allowed to sentence offenders to pay their fines in body product donations (once the property approach has established a market value for them). If this seems far-fetched, consider that there already have been instances in which judges sentenced defendants to give blood transfusions. Similarly, an eighteenth-century British statute allowed judges to order anatomical dissection of hanged murderers.[7] It is possible to maintain that people are priceless by not allowing others to treat a person's body commercially either before or after death and by giving people the power to refuse to sell their body parts.

A decision to sell certain types of body parts—nonregenerative ones (such as a kidney) or parts that could give rise to offspring (sperm, eggs, and embryos)—has lifelong implications. With respect to other decisions of long-lasting consequences (such as marriage), society has sometimes adopted added protections to assure that the decision has been carefully made. A similar approach might be used with regard to body parts. In this area, only competent adults should be allowed to decide to sell. There should be a short waiting period (like the cooling-off period that protects consumers from door-to-door salesmen) between the agreement to sell an organ and its removal, and the donor should be required to observe certain formalities (such as signing a witnessed consent form).

Only the person who owns the body part should be allowed to sell it. This approach has two goals. The first is to assure that others do not treat one's body as property. For example, it will prevent the harms associated with holding the body as security until funeral costs are paid.[8] The second is to attempt to assure that the individual is adequately compensated for the body part by limiting the amount any middleman receives. If the middleman cannot "sell" the part, but can only be compensated for bringing together the donor and recipient, the donor may more likely receive adequate compensation and the transaction will less likely be viewed as excessively commercial. There might even be limitations on what the middleman (physician or entrepreneur) receives, similar to the statutory limitation in some states of "reasonableness" in the amount of money an attorney receives in connection with arranging a private adoption....

Giving an individual sole rights over his or her body parts is in keeping with attitudes toward the body held in other areas of law. Attempted suicide and suicide are no longer considered crimes.[9] However, aiding and abetting a suicide is a crime. Competent individuals can refuse a readily available lifesaving treatment, but their physicians cannot withhold it. Thus, people are allowed to control what is done to their bodies (even to the point of physical damage) in ways that other individuals are not.

Ironically, our current policy is just the reverse. Other people seem to have property rights in our body parts, but we do not. In a British case, an accused man who poured his urine sample down the sink was found guilty of stealing it from the police department.[10] And although an individual has no property interest in his or her cell lines, scientists are quick to claim a property interest in those cell lines. Such a claim was the basis of a six-year conflict between microbiologist Leonard Hayflick and the National Institutes of Health. The conflict was over which side owned a cell line that Hayflick had developed with embryonic living tissue under NIH funding and then sold to scientists around the world.[11] ...

THE MARKET'S EFFECT ON RECIPIENTS

We can protect potential donors from the market's effect by attempting to assure that donations are voluntary and by limiting donations to body parts that do not unreasonably affect the person's ability to function. But how does a market affect potential recipients? The policy of prohibiting payment for body parts and products has been justified as protecting potential recipients by raising the quality of donations and preventing a situation in which body parts are affordable only by the rich.

The work of Richard Titmuss on policies governing blood donation raised serious questions of quality control when blood is sold.[12] Among other things, he argued that paid donors have an incentive not to disclose illnesses or characteristics that might make their blood of dubious quality. Subsequent work by Harvey Sapolsky and Stan Finkelstein[13] challenged Titmuss's conclusions. They pointed to a Government Accounting Office study in which some voluntary groups in the United States reported hepatitis rates as high as the worst paid groups; and some commercially collected blood was nearly as good as the best of the volunteer blood.

Even if paid donors are more likely to misrepresent their condition than are volunteer donors, payment need not be banned on quality control grounds since tests are available to assess the fitness of the donor. In this country we allow payment for blood and sperm, although it is easy to lie about their quality; yet we do not allow payment for body organs such as kidneys, although organ transplantation offers more independent checks on quality. Nor is banning payment the only mechanism to enhance quality, since if known risks are not disclosed, liability may follow. While this may not offer sufficient protection to the recipients of blood (since donors may not be solvent), organ donors would be better paid and a portion of that money could be used to buy insurance. When a person sells organs contingent on death, payment to an estate could be withheld if it was clear that he failed to disclose a known harmful condition. Already, the Ontario Law Reform Commission has recommended enacting a criminal law prohibiting people selling their gametes from knowingly concealing infectious and genetic disorders.

A market in solid organs is also thought harmful to potential recipients because of the possibility that only the rich will be able to afford organs. On the issue of the poor selling and the rich buying body parts, Thomas Murray says, "Our consciences can tolerate considerable injustice, but such naked, undisguised profiteering in life would be too much for us."[14] Yet other equally troublesome but less visible inequities are already occurring in allocating other kinds of medical care. When a drug company prices a medication necessary for someone's life beyond a person's reach or a physician with unique skills refuses to accept patients who receive Medicare, that is also profiteering in life, but the injustice may be overlooked. Currently at least fifty different types of artificial body parts (such as artificial blood vessels and joints) have been designed to substitute for human ones.[15] It is as important ethically to address discrimination between rich and poor recipients with respect to those products as it is with respect to human body parts. A visible market in body parts may lull people out of complacency to address more general issues of allocation in health care. . . .

THE MARKET'S EFFECT ON SOCIETY

Will a market in body parts harm society by creating an attitude that people are commodities? The body is a symbol of the whole person and degrading it can be viewed as an assault to the whole person. Our distaste with viewing the body as property is, in part, a reaction to our belief that human beings should have no price.

Certainly people are more than the sum of their parts.[16] But treating the body as property does not mean it is a person's only property. Cognitive functions can be included within the property characterization. Indeed, they already are, for example, under the legal doctrine of copyright, patent, and other so-called "intellectual property" rights. I view my uniqueness as a person as more related to my intellectual products than my bodily products. (Definitions of personhood, for example, rarely revolve around the possession of body parts, but rather focus on sentience or other cognitive traits.) Arguably it commercializes me less as a person to sell my bone marrow than to sell my intellectual products. Thus, I do not view payment of body parts as commercializing people. The danger I see in the sale of a physical (as opposed to a mental) bodily product comes from the potential for physical harm in removing the bodily material or living without it. This danger can be handled by limiting the types of body parts that can be sold and the circumstances under which they can be sold.

Selling body parts has also been criticized as harmful to society because it could diminish altruism. But in our society, the basics of life—food, shelter, health care—are already sold. Nevertheless, many people continue to act altruistically, devoting time, money, or goods to provide needy people with those basics. The possibility of selling tissue or organs seems only a modest further step toward a market, unlikely to change vastly the impulse toward altruism. Even people who take advantage of the market may engage in altruistic behavior. One patient, Ted Slavin, received up to $10.00 per milliliter from commercial enterprises for his blood, which was used in manufacturing diagnostic kits for hepatitis B virus. At the same time, he provided additional blood—at no charge—to a research project at the Fox Chase Cancer Center, which used it to develop a vaccine against hepatitis B.[17] . . .

To guard against the appearance that people are commodities, we must not let other people treat one's body parts as property. Body parts will thus not be salable in the sense of cars, farm animals, or baseball cards. There will be no means for a tax man or physician to put a lien against a person's body parts. Nor can relatives choose to sell a person's parts after his or her death. However, it differs from previous notions of quasi-property by recognizing the right of an individual to compensation for certain types of body parts. Under this approach, human beings have the right to treat certain physical parts of their bodies as objects for possession, gift, and trade, but they do not become objects so long as others cannot treat them as property.

THE MARKET'S EFFECT ON THE DOCTOR/PATIENT RELATIONSHIP

The treatment of body parts as property will help curtail activities by physicians, researchers, and their attorneys that deny individuals information about or control over body parts that will be removed.

Implicit in many arguments made by physician/researchers is that the removed body part belongs to the doctor, not the patient. Why do physicians feel that way? I can only speculate that it is because society allows medical practitioners to do things to a patient's body (for example, cut it up) that no one else (other than the patient) is allowed to do. Perhaps this gives physicians the feeling that the patient's body belongs in some sense to them.

Physicians argue that getting patients' permission to use their body parts and products would change the relationship between patients and physicians or researchers. Some argue that discussing the research with the patient may imply that a patient has a right to direct the scope or direction of the study. But that is absurd. Just because IBM is required to make certain disclosures to me when I buy a share of stock does not mean that I can set policy for the operation of the company.

Related to this is an argument that paying for the patient's cells, tissue, fluids, or organs would tie up physicians in endless negotiation with their patients. But when payment for human biological material is required, it is no more disastrous to the research enterprise than payment for pipettes, microscopes, animals, or laboratory equipment. It may represent a modest increase in the cost of doing business (just as an increase in fuel prices would raise the costs of lighting the laboratory). But the money paid would go to a good cause, slightly enhancing the resources of medical patients at a time when they need money to pay for medical care. If the patient is unwilling to sell rights to the biological materials, the physician need not barter; she can simply avoid using that specimen and approach other patients. Moreover, we allow the patient to pay the physician for services without being concerned that it will lead to endless negotiations.

Just as physicians raise the price for their services to cover rising malpractice insurance rates, so they will charge slightly more for the right to use the specimens of some patients for research. If it strikes you as unfair (it does me) to force patients to pay for the research by increasing medical costs, consider that under the current system the "cost" of the human specimens is borne entirely by the patients who own them and who do not even get in return a right to refuse to participate.

Another reason has been advanced against disclosure: it would decrease patient-physician trust if the patient were aware that the physician might develop a commercial product from the patient's body parts. Yet this begs the question of whether the information is relevant. It might diminish the patient's trust to know the success rate and unnecessary surgery rates of a practitioner or health care facility; yet this information is clearly relevant to patient decision making.

There is a similar concern that disclosing the commercial potential of human body parts may tarnish the image of the researchers by making it appear that profit rather than scientific knowledge is their goal. However, the media is already informing the public about the relationship between researchers and the corporate sector. "The public cannot help but see that the goals of some scientists—clinical or basic—are different than in the past," says Leon Rosenberg, dean of the Yale University School of Medicine. "The biotechnology revolution has moved us, literally or figuratively, from the classroom to the boardroom and from the *New England Journal* to the *Wall Street Journal*."[18]

Finally people point to the difficulty of assigning values to body parts as an implicit barrier to the property approach. But the value of many items that are currently bought and sold (such as paintings or jewels) is difficult to assess. This is no reason to prohibit the market from developing a particular price....

In a variation on the value argument, physician/researchers seem to imply that the patient has already been paid for the body part by receiving the benefits of the surgery. John Moore, for example, was allegedly helped by his treatment at UCLA. (This argument is harder to make when the patient dies or otherwise does not recover.) But patients may feel they have already paid for their health benefits in the price of the surgery. The patient has a right to know about the research so that she can choose the "price" she is willing to pay for the surgery. Perhaps she would rather choose a surgeon whose price is set solely in terms of dollars and insurance coverage rather than one who commercially exploits, say, her ovaries.

THE FUTURE OF THE BODY AS PROPERTY

Some of the finest advances in society have resulted from a refusal to characterize human beings (blacks, women, children) as property. Why, then, am I arguing for a property approach here? Let me emphasize that I am advocating not that people be treated by others as property, but only that they have the autonomy to treat their own parts as property, particularly their regenerative parts. Such an approach is helpful, rather than harmful, to people's well-being. It offers potential psychological, physical, and economic benefits to individuals and provides a framework for handling evolving issues regarding the control of extracorporeal biological materials.

It is time to start acknowledging that people's body parts are their personal property. This is distinguishable from the past characterizations of people as property, which were immoral because they failed to take into account the nonbodily aspects of the individual (blacks and women were deemed incapable of rational thought) and they created the rights of ownership by others (masters, husbands, parents). Allowing people to transfer and sell their own body parts, while protecting them from coercion, does not present those dangers.

REFERENCES

1. 42 U.S.C. 274(e) (1984).
2. Cal. Penal Code § 367f (West 1986) (exception for sale by patient); D.C. Code Ann. § 6–2601 (Supp. 1985); Fla. Stat. Ann. § 873.01 (West Suppl. 1986); La. Rev. Stat. Ann. § 17.2280 (West 1982); Md. Health General Code Ann. § 5.408 (Supp. 1985); Mich. Comp. Laws Ann. § 333.10204 (West Supp. 1986); N.Y. Pub. Health Law § 4307 (McKinney 1985); Va. Code § 32.1–289.1 (1985). Additionally, in Arkansas there is a specific prohibition on the sale of eyes after death. Ark. Stat. Ann. § 82–410.2; § 82–410.13 (1976).
3. Susan Rose-Ackerman, "Inalienability and the Theory of Property Rights," *Columbia Law Review* 931 (1985), 85.
4. Ontario Law Reform Commission, *Report on Human Artificial Reproduction and Related Matters* (Ontario: Ministry of the Attorney General, 1985).
5. 45 C.F.R. 46.101(b)(5) (1985).
6. 45 C.F.R. 46.110(b) (1985).
7. Matthews, p. 205.
8. Such practices are described in *Jefferson County Burial Soc. v. Scott*, 218 Ala. 354, 118, S. 644 (1928).
9. A 1975 law review article, "Criminal Aspects of Suicide in the United States," 7 *North Carolina Central Law Journal* 156, 158 n. 19–21 (1975) listed only three states (Oklahoma, Texas, and Washington) which still had laws against attempted suicide. Those statutes have since been repealed.
10. *R. v. Welsh*, (1974) R.T.R. 478, reported in Matthews, pp. 223–24.
11. Constance Holden, "Hayflick Case Settled," *Science* 215 (1982), 271.
12. Richard Titmuss, *The Gift Relationship: From Human Blood to Special Policy* (New York: Vintage, 1972).
13. Harvey M. Sapolsky and Stan N. Finkelstein, "Blood Policy Revisited—A New Look at 'The Gift Relationship,'" *Public Interest*, 46 (1977), 15.
14. Thomas H. Murray, "The Gift of Life Must Always Remain a Gift," *Discover* 7:3 (March 1986), 90.
15. See, e.g., L. L. Hench, "Biomaterials," *Science* 208 (1980), 826.
16. See Leon R. Kass, "Thinking About the Body," *Hastings Center Report*, 15:1 (February 1985), 20.
17. Baruch S. Blumberg, Irving Millman, W. Thomas London, et al., "Ted Slavin's Blood and the Development of HBV Vaccine," *New England Journal of Medicine* 312 (1985), 189 (letter).
18. Leon E. Rosenberg, "Using Patient Materials for Production Development: A Dean's Perspective," *Clinical Research* 33:4 (October 1985), 452–54.

NO

Thomas H. Murray

GIFTS OF THE BODY AND
THE NEEDS OF STRANGERS

Human bodies have value, and not just to the persons whose bodies they are. Organs can be transplanted; tissues used for research and product development. One way of looking at these body parts is as property, to be bought and sold.[1] Another way—the approach I want to examine—is to see them as gifts. This may seem at first a simpler concept, but it is far from that. The idea of "gift" has deep and sometimes contradictory cultural meanings, which can illuminate the appropriate stance we should take toward modern biotechnology.

There are two modern conceptions of gifts. On the one hand, William Blackstone, the great legal commentator, wrote in 1767 that "gifts are always gratuitous"—that is, requiring "no consideration or equivalent." A gift in this sense is, as the *Oxford English Dictionary* defines it, "the transference of property in a thing by one person to another, voluntarily and without any valuable consideration." Givers are free to give or not; recipients are free to accept or not, and after acceptance, free to do whatever they like with the gift.

But if gifts are so bereft of obligations of any kind, why is there a second strain of sentiment about them? Ralph Waldo Emerson, in his essay on "Gifts," illustrated the power of gifts to bind one person to another. He wrote: "It is not the office of a man to receive gifts. How dare you give them? We wish to be self-sustained. We do not quite forgive a giver."[2] In a more modern context and with a hint of irony, the historian Michael Ignatieff echoes a similar sentiment: "The bureaucratized transfer of income among strangers has freed each of us from the enslavement of gift relations."[3]

How can the notion of gifts as gratuitous and completely voluntary be reconciled with the idea that gifts are the cause of degradation, dependence, and enslavement? Neither idea captures the full significance of the gift in human relations. The first perspective sees only that gifts carry no formal *legal* obligations. This is correct, but not very important. In this sense, gifts are opposed to contracts—forms of social exchange specifying in sometimes numbing detail precisely what is being exchanged for what. Of course, the obverse is also true: anything *not* explicitly required in the contract is permitted, and no other new obligations arise outside the limited sphere of relationship created by the contract. The second perspective sees correctly that gifts may entangle people in relationships that will impose great but vague moral obligations.

The first view assumes that only legal obligations matter. The second view understands that gifts create moral obligations, but focuses only on their ugly, manipulative potential. It fails to see that relationships based on gifts can and do play positive roles in regulating family and social life, in promoting solidarity in the face of powerful forces of alienation, and in serving essential social values that are not well served by markets, commerce, and contract....

GIFTS, PRUDENCE, AND MORAL OBLIGATIONS

The notion that either donors or recipients could have obligations in gift relations seems foreign to the modern mind. The concept of "obligation," at least as it is used by moral philosophers, does not seem to fit gift relationships. Perhaps one should speak of an etiquette rather than an ethic of gifts. But such a weak term would belie the powerful ties that can be created by gifts, the strong indebtedness a recipient may feel, and the grave harm an ignorant, inconsiderate, or malicious giver may do.

There is certainly a heavy dose of prudence in many gift exchanges. Using gifts to establish personal relationships need not entail any heavy moral obligations. If you desire the relationship, then respond appropriately to the gift; if you do not, refuse the gift.

There are, however, occasions when an individual may feel obliged, morally, to make certain gifts. Suppose a member of

your family was suddenly in dire need of food or shelter—or bone marrow. Perhaps not everyone will feel an obligation to give in response to this need, but many will. Some might describe it as charity or supererogation, something noble but not obligatory. But many would think they had failed more fundamentally if they did not offer some gift, however modest, that addressed the need. Another example: in a relationship of long duration characterized by great caring, one party abruptly ceases to show gratitude or to reciprocate. The harm done the other, as well as the devaluation of the relationship and of both parties, is substantial enough to count as a moral harm. Such relationships contain a set of implied promises, which were broken by the sudden, uncaring way in which they were sundered. Remember that a common way of expressing gratitude is to say "much obliged." The language of obligation may discomfit some philosophers, but it seems to reflect more accurately the importance of at least certain gift relationships.

Here are three interrelated suggestions —too informal to be called "claims" or hypotheses—that may be helpful in clarifying our thinking about gifts in general and gifts of the body in particular:

1. Significant gifts are commonly given in response to the needs of individuals and societies. I mean *need* here as opposed to mere *desire*; but human needs in a wide sense, encompassing not merely basic survival—food, clothing, and shelter—but also the requirements for flourishing in a particular society—art, beauty, preparation for participation in adult life (including, in industrialized nations, literacy and education) and, not least, peace

among groups, a measure of community, and intimate relationships.

2. The degree of *moral* (and not merely prudential) obligation one feels (and should feel) to make a gift is greatest when the recipient's need is greatest. The more universal the need (such as for adequate food) the more likely people are to feel a sense of obligation to give to those more distant.

3. Mass bureaucratic societies need to affirm what it is citizens share with their neighbors. Gifts, especially gifts to assuage needs, and most especially gifts of the body, are one of the most significant means we have to affirm that solidarity. Thomas Merton, writing of the Buddhist's begging bowl, says it "represents the ultimate theological root of the belief, not just in a right to beg, but in openness to the gifts of all beings as an expression of the interdependence of all beings...."[4] Gifts of the body, ministering to the need for health, are in this sense affirmations of interdependence....

MORAL OBLIGATIONS, GRATITUDE, AND GRACIOUSNESS

In a study of related kidney donors, Roberta Simmons and her colleagues found that when recipients did not express what the donors considered a reasonable amount of gratitude, the donor felt angry and used—a "sucker." One donor reported: "I would say for three months [the recipient] tried to avoid me. I was never so crushed. I would call him up and he would be as cold as ice. I was destroyed. To this day I don't mention the kidney in front of him. Whenever I do, it turns him off. He has never come out and said 'Thank you.'"[5]

Reciprocating the gift, in an appropriate form, at an appropriate time, is also important. Alvin Gouldner, a sociologist, argues for a "norm of reciprocity" that is "no less universal and important an element of culture than the incest taboo." He says it is "a dimension to be found in all value systems and, in particular, as one among a number of 'Principal Components' universally present in moral codes."[6] Just what constitutes appropriate reciprocation depends on particular cultural norms and the specifics of the relationship. It need not be "tit-for-tat" if, for example, the donor is a parent and the recipient a ten-year-old child, whose means are not adequate to return full economic value of the parent's gift. Similar cultural and relationship factors determine what is an appropriate time for reciprocation. Seneca's warning is correct for some situations, but not all. (Not exchanging Christmas presents simultaneously could be insulting to the person who gave the present.)

A third recipient obligation is what Camenisch calls "grateful use." He argues that "grateful acceptance of the gift indicates the concurrence of the recipient's will with the donor's and/or implies consent to comply with that will." He suggests that the moral language of "stewardship" often applies to the use of gifts. Searching for more precise criteria for grateful use, he offers two: "the nature of the gift itself and what we can discover of the donor's intention for its use." It would be wrong to treat something dear to the donor in an undignified manner, as merely a commodity; likewise it would be wrong to use it in a way the donor would disapprove of.

All three obligations—grateful use, grateful conduct, and reciprocation—stem from the purpose of gift exchange

—building moral relationships, and perhaps as well from the nature of at least certain significant gifts. Mauss says that among the Maori "to give something is to give a part of oneself.... while to receive something is to receive a part of someone's spiritual essence." It is not necessary to accept the Maori's animistic beliefs to grasp that in some gifts, the giver offers symbolically a part of himself or herself. Simply recall an occasion when someone treated with indifference a gift that you had regarded as special and important. In some way, the rejection of the gift was a personal rejection. (This is true more than metaphorically in gifts of the body.) ...

GIFTS TO STRANGERS

Perhaps Arrow's most striking criticism of Titmuss is his claim that Titmuss wishes to promote "impersonal altruism." He does not wish to encourage the "richness of family relationships or the close ties of a small community" but rather a "diffuse expression of confidence in the workings of society as a whole." But Arrow says, "Such an expression of impersonal altruism is as far removed from the feelings of personal interaction as any marketplace."

Arrow is certainly correct. It cannot be the rewards of immediate personal relationships that prompt impersonal altruism. But when he goes on to describe British blood donors as "an aristocracy of saints" and to express doubt that a voluntary system could work elsewhere, he is wrong—factually wrong—as the movement to an almost entirely voluntary system of whole blood procurement in the U.S. shows. This cannot be ascribed to the British tradition of Fabian socialism with which Arrow tries to explain the British experience.

Something more than a vague sentiment is at work in the instance of blood donation, something powerful that escapes any simple explanation in terms of pure self-interest—or pure altruism. Ignatieff grasps the problem when he notes: "We think of belonging in moral terms as direct impingement on the lives of others: fraternity implies the closeness of brothers. Yet the moral relations that exist between my income and the needs of strangers at my door pass through the arteries of the state." This would pose no problem if the needs of strangers exerted no moral pull on us; if we felt no relationship with them. But, as Ignatieff notes, "We need justice, we need liberty, and we need as much solidarity as can be reconciled with justice and liberty."

Relationships governed by markets keep moral and social dimensions to a bare minimum. Gifts, by their open-endedness, defy such minimization. Impersonal gifts such as blood or body parts or charity may not regulate relationships between specific individuals, but they serve other functions by regulating larger relationships and honoring important human values, precisely those threatened by massive and impersonal bureaucracies.

For one thing, impersonal gifts acknowledge an entire realm of moral relationships and moral obligations wider than intimate, family ones, and wider still than legal, contractual ones. Further, these obligations are often *unchosen*.

Gifts to strangers affirm the solidarity of the community over and above the depersonalizing, alienating forces of mass society and market relations. They signal that self-interest is not the only significant human motivation. And they express the moral belief that it is good to minister to fundamental human needs, needs for food, health care, and shelter, but also needs for beauty and knowledge. These universal needs irrevocably tie us together in a community of needs, with a shared desire to satisfy them, and see them satisfied in others.

Finally, these gifts remind us that wealth is merely a means to an end, and that not all valuable things can be purchased, among them love, friendship, fellow-feeling, and trust. These "moral" assets of individuals and of societies are "noneconomic" in still another way. They are not "scarce resources" that are consumed as they are offered. Arrow cautions us not "to use up recklessly the scarce resources of altruistic motivation." The truth is more likely the opposite: To a considerable extent, employing "moral assets" generously increases rather than decreases the supply.

GIFTS, SOLIDARITY, AND SOCIAL INSTITUTIONS

It may well be that the way a society structures the exchange of such "moral assets" affects their supply just as the structure of markets affects the supply of ordinary commodities. Titmuss's survey of blood donors in Great Britain revealed that the overwhelming majority, when asked why they were giving, cited non-self-interested reasons. Among them (with spelling and punctuation preserved):

Knowing I mite be saving somebody life;

You cant get blood from supermarkets and chaine stores. People themselves must come forward;

I thought it just a small way to help people—as a blind person other opportunities are limited.

Gratitude for good health appears in some:

Briefly because I have enjoyed good health all my life and in a small way it is a way of saying 'Thank you' and a small donation to the less fortunate.

Others write of reciprocating a gift:

To try and repay in some small way some unknown person whose blood helped me recover from two operations....;

Some unknown person gave blood to save my wifes life.

Other reasons offered included a general sense of social duty and the perception that there was a need for blood.

A more recent study of blood procurement inspired by skepticism of Titmuss's account focused primarily on the U.S. In that work Alvin Drake, Stan N. Finkelstein, and Harvey Sapolsky found that the bleak portrait of motivation for giving and quality of blood in the U.S. painted by Titmuss was unwarranted a decade later, and may even have been an unfair picture at the time Titmuss's book was published.[7] The details of their differences are not important here. Much more significant is the authors' carefully documented research on the beliefs, values, and practices of potential blood donors in the U.S. By 1982, about 70 percent of all whole blood was being provided on a purely voluntary basis. Roughly a quarter was being given through "blood credit" or "blood insurance" programs, which could be seen as quasi-voluntary. Paid donors constituted no more than 3 to 4 percent, and that proportion was declining.

Drake, Finkelstein, and Sapolsky found that the principal impediment to fulfilling the need for whole blood was lack of coordination and competence in the regional procurement agencies. Where efforts were well organized, as they had been for years in Connecticut and in upstate New York, local needs could be met with purely voluntary programs. The researchers found a strong and consistent opposition to the use of paid donors. Americans overwhelmingly preferred to have their community's need for whole blood met with volunteer donors.

When they examined the reasons American blood donors gave for their generosity, they found it was "simply a general awareness of the continuing need for blood." "All our own experiences lead us to believe that participation in the whole-blood supply is the natural, unforced response of a great many people once they are exposed to a mild degree of personal solicitation and some convenient donation opportunities."

The saga of the transformation of the American whole-blood supply from a largely paid to a virtually all-volunteer system is not a simple one. Much of it concerns rivalries among organizations. But one important fact is clear: the voluntary agencies could not have emerged victorious unless the American people were willing to donate adequate amounts of whole blood. This willingness in turn rests, I believe, on deeply held convictions about the obligation to give to those in need, and about the ethical inappropriateness of commercializing whole blood.

It is a massive effort at giving to strangers. Roughly eight million Americans donate each year. In its scale, its lack of monetary rewards, and its distance between donor and recipient, the whole-blood procurement system in the U.S. is a remarkable example of impersonal gifts. It suggests something very important that a society would be so generous in this realm and would reject so

clearly a market approach to the supply and distribution of a good.

The gift of blood is doubly expressive. It affirms solidarity in a gift that is quintessentially human. Blood represents individual life and vitality, and at the same time it signifies the oldest, most primitive tie that affirms solidarity and binds people to one another. Perhaps one of the oldest and most persistent human problems has been to reconcile the loyalties and attachments defined by blood—the ties of family—with the need for, at a minimum, peace but, better, solidarity, with strangers—those with whom we do not share blood. From these roots comes the political importance of marriage between groups in potential conflict, and perhaps as well the symbolic value of "blood brotherhood."

Blood is life, but also kinship. Giving blood to strangers is not just any gift, but a vital one that expresses and affirms our bonds with those strangers. If, on the other hand, we would rather deny our brotherhood, then mixing blood could be a serious threat. Titmuss reports that in South Africa a set of regulations issued in 1962 required that "European" and "non-European" donors be kept separate, and that the records of their donations also be kept apart. Furthermore, "[a]ll containers of blood and blood products have to be labelled by 'racial origin.'" Although South Africa has relied primarily on voluntary donations, authorities at gold mines in the Transvaal region purchased blood from mining company employees. The rates in 1967 were four Rands per pint for whites; one Rand per pint for "Bantus, Colored and Asians."

Profiting from others' blood is sometimes seen as a particularly heinous form of exploitation. A plasmapheresis center opened in Managua, Nicaragua, in 1973 that purchased plasma and exported it. The center was owned in part by the dictator Somoza. At the funeral of a popular newspaper editor who had criticized Somoza for "inhuman trade in the blood of Nicaraguans" and who had been murdered, a large crowd burned several buildings, among them the plasmapheresis center.[8]

Blood can connect people, or it can divide them. Contemporary inhabitants in the U.S., no less than the Trobrianders or Maori or other traditional societies, seem to believe that some things are *sacra* —"sacred" in the nondenominational sense of dignified human "property" —and that it is morally preferable to procure and distribute certain kinds of property, including *sacra*, but other things as well, outside the otherwise dominant system of market and contract....

GIFTS, THE BODY, AND BIOMEDICAL RESEARCH

What has been said until now does not settle the question of what should happen to human tissues in contemporary biomedicine. It does, however, demonstrate that certain body parts are and ought to be treated as gifts and not as personal property.

Even if certain parts or products of the body are *sacra* and hence fit for gift but not commerce, it does not follow that all are equally so.[9] If I could find a buyer for my urine, it is doubtful that any great moral outcry would arise, no more than accompanies the sale of hair or fingernails. But then these products are less central to what characterizes living human persons, members of the human community, than kidneys, for example, or blood. In any case, the nature of the gift, its meaning and significance within the community, will determine whether it belongs to the realm of commodities or the circle of gifts.

A second issue concerns the relationship between the giver—the patient or research subject in the case of biomedicine —and the recipient—the physician or researcher. The patient-physician relationship has long been described with apparently inconsistent images. On the one hand, physicians earn their money by seeing patients, and in that sense it is clearly a commercial relationship, a trade of money for service. At the same time the noncommercial aspects of the relationship are stressed. The very words used to describe what physicians do— they "take care of" patients—come from the language of personal, moral, nonmarket relationships. Physicians are expected to act in the patient's best interest, and not to try to cut the best deal for themselves; they are in a "fiduciary" relationship with their patients.

To the extent that people see their relationship with physicians as not strictly a market one, then an ethic of personal gifts may apply. (People quite commonly make gifts to their medical and nursing caretakers after an episode of illness.) With the increasing commercialization of medicine, people's expectations may be changing, and the nature of the physician-patient relationship, always an ideal only partially realized, may change accordingly. At some future time, the gift may become irrelevant to the clinic.

The emergence of the physician-researcher-entrepreneur complicates things immensely. It is one thing to have someone offer to buy something. It is quite another to give it to someone with whom we believe there is a more or less personal, noncommercial relationship, and to learn only later that what was given as a gift, especially if it was a "sacred" gift, has been diverted to commerce. The mixed roles of biomedical researchers who may also be clinicians, who may also be entrepreneurs, make it difficult to know what set of moral expectations apply. By blurring the distinctions, we jeopardize the future of physician-patient relationships. One could say cynically that such relationships always were commercial, and that it is better to be explicit about it. But if important social values were served by stressing the noncommercial dimensions of those relationships, then the threat is a serious one.

Lastly, consider the problem of how to think about impersonal gifts. Normally there is a distinction drawn between eleemosynary and civil corporations. The former are "organized for charitable purposes"; the latter, according to the Oxford English Dictionary, for "business purposes." Universities and most medical research centers, along with charities, learned societies, and the like, are eleemosynary organizations. When people are asked to make gifts of money—or of their tissues—to university-based medical research, whether or not they actually give, they see this as a reasonable request. Pleas for gifts by a profit-seeking firm, in contrast, would be perceived as ludicrous.

One of the ways to express solidarity with "strangers" is by contributing to the satisfaction of basic human needs and desires, especially those not well served by the system of trade and markets. These two systems have long existed side by side, an implicit acknowledgment that neither one alone is adequate for human flourishing and for sustaining community. In place now is an informal system of gifts of human biological materials to noncommercial organizations. Relying

on this system fulfills many of the social values mentioned earlier as the justifications for gift exchanges. They include expressing solidarity in the face of illness and suffering, and declaring respect and support for biomedical research and teaching.

PURSUIT OF THE GOOD

Gifts help to create and sustain intimate personal relationships. In the face of impersonal bureaucracies, gifts to "strangers" affirm a number of vital social values including our solidarity with others in our community, and our vision of human flourishing, individual and social, that require more than the thin relationships established by markets and contracts.

Individuals in market societies, especially intellectuals, may delude themselves into believing that needs are indistinguishable from desires, that the body is merely a commodity like any other, and that we have no moral bonds with the members of our communities other than those we have freely chosen. But the evidence of charitable practices in general and gifts of the body in particular affirm the belief that there *are* human needs—biological and cultural; that the body, especially in its health-giving and life-saving manifestations, should not be treated as a mere commodity; and that we are bound together by our often needy bodies (and by our other, nonphysiological needs) into a community of needs. In this community—really multiple communities, sometimes overlapping, some like ripples extending wider and wider around a core—we can recognize the needs of others through our shared embodiment. And we can minister to those needs by sharing the fruits, the very living tissues of the body.

How we choose to handle the transfers of human biological materials from patients and research subjects to teachers and researchers will declare how we regard the human body. If certain human parts are "dignified," then our social traditions suggest they may be given, but not sold, and ownership of them is only of a special, limited kind.

Moreover, like the choice of obtaining blood for transfusions, the system chosen for obtaining human biological materials will carry whatever symbolic weight attaches to the relationship to the "strangers at our door," as Ignatieff calls our fellow inhabitants of mass society. These gifts of the body, ministering to the needs of strangers, connect us in our mutual quest to relieve suffering and to pursue our good, separately and together.

ACKNOWLEDGMENTS

I am grateful to many people whose gifts of time and thought enabled me to clarify further my own thinking on the issues discussed in this paper. Here I can mention only a few: William Winslade, Ronald Carson, and Harold Vanderpool critiqued versions of this article. I want to thank also Gladys White and the U.S. Congress Office of Technology Assessment. I did much of the research on which this paper is based for their project, "New Developments in Biotechnology: Ownership of Human Tissues and Cells."

REFERENCES

1. Lori B. Andrews, "My Body, My Property," *Hastings Center Report* 16:5 (October 1986), 28–38.
2. Ralph Waldo Emerson, "Gifts," *Essays of Ralph Waldo Emerson* (Norwalk, CT: Easton Press, 1979), pp. 212–13.
3. Michael Ingatieff, *The Needs of Strangers: An Essay on Privacy, Solidarity, and the Politics of Being Human* (New York: Viking, 1984), pp. 18–141.
4. Thomas Merton, *The Asian Journals*, eds. Naomi Burton et al. (New York: New Directions, 1973), pp. 341–42.
5. Roberta G. Simmons, Susan D. Klein, and Richard L. Simmons, *Gift of Life: The Social and Psychological Impact of Organ Transplantation* (New York: Wiley, 1977), p. 325.
6. Alvin W. Gouldner, "The Norm of Reciprocity: A Preliminary Statement," *American Sociological Review* 25:2 (1960), 171.
7. Richard M. Titmuss, *The Gift Relationship* (New York: Pantheon, 1971).
8. Piet J. Hagen, *Blood: Gift or Merchandise* (New York: Alan R. Liss, 1982), pp. 168–69.
9. Thomas H. Murray, "On the Ethics of Commercializing the Human Body." Paper prepared for U.S. Congress Office of Technology Assessment, April 1986.

POSTSCRIPT

Should There Be a Market in Body Parts?

John Moore's case was dismissed three times by state courts in California, but in August 1988 the Second District Court of Appeals in Houston ruled that Moore had the right to sue UCLA. The court said, "A patient must have the ultimate power to control what becomes of his or her tissue. To hold otherwise would open the door to a massive invasion of human privacy and dignity in the name of medical progress." However, in July 1990 the California Supreme Court ruled that a patient does not have property rights over body tissue and that letting patients sue for rights in research resulting from their tissue would threaten "to destroy the economic incentive to conduct important medical research." The court also stated that the physician has a "fiduciary duty" to tell the patient if there is interest in studying his tissue. Two articles written on this subject are George J. Annas, "Whose Waste Is It Anyway? The Case of John Moore," *Hastings Center Report* (October/November 1988) and John J. Howard, "Biotechnology, Patients' Rights and the *Moore* Case," *Food Drug Cosmetic Law Journal* (July 1989).

Hagiwara Hideaki's case was settled by an agreement in which the University of California was given the patent and the Hagiwara family received an exclusive license to market the cell line in Japan and Asia. For the researcher's view of this case, see Ivor Royston, "Cell Lines from Human Patients: Who Owns Them?" *Clinical Research* (vol. 33, 1985).

The Office of Technology Assessment has issued a comprehensive report called *New Developments in Biotechnology: Ownership of Human Tissue* (Government Printing Office, 1987). In an article titled "Research That Could Yield Marketable Products from Human Materials: The Problem of Informed Consent," *IRB: A Review of Human Subjects Research* (January/February 1986), Robert J. Levine argues that it is unlikely that research designed to develop marketable products from human materials will present any problems to the research-subject relationship that cannot be resolved within the framework of existing informed consent regulations. See also Gloria J. Banks, "Legal and Ethical Safeguards: Protection of Society's Most Vulnerable Participants in a Commercialized Organ Transplantation System," *American Journal of Law and Medicine* (vol. 21, no. 1, 1995); Courtney S. Campbell, "The Selling of Organs, the Sharing of Self," *Second Opinion* (vol. 19, no. 2, 1993); Margaret S. Swain and Randy W. Marusyk, "An Alternative to Property Rights in Human Tissue," *Hastings Center Report* (September/October 1990); and Courtney S. Campbell, "Body, Self, and the Property Paradigm," *Hastings Center Report* (September/October 1992).

CONTRIBUTORS
TO THIS VOLUME

EDITOR

CAROL LEVINE is director of the Families and Healthcare Project for the United Hospital Fund in New York City and executive director of the Orphan Project: Families and Children in the HIV Epidemic, also in New York City. She is the recipient of a 1993 fellowship from the MacArthur Foundation. She is a former executive director of the Citizens Commission on AIDS for New York City and Northern New Jersey. She is associate editor of *IRB: A Review of Human Subjects Research* and a former editor of the *Hastings Center Report*, both of which are published by the Hastings Center in Briarcliff Manor, New York. Ms. Levine received a B.A. in history from Cornell University and an M.A. in public law and government from Columbia University. She writes and lectures widely on AIDS and other issues in bioethics.

STAFF

David Dean   List Manager
David Brackley   Developmental Editor
Ava Suntoke   Developmental Editor
Tammy Ward   Administrative Assistant
Brenda S. Filley   Production Manager
Juliana Arbo   Typesetting Supervisor
Diane Barker   Proofreader
Lara Johnson   Graphics
Richard Tietjen   Publishing Systems Manager

AUTHORS

FELICIA ACKERMAN is a professor of philosophy at Brown University in Providence, Rhode Island. Her articles have appeared in various philosophy journals and anthologies, including *Philosophical Perspectives* and the *Midwest Studies in Philosophy* book series. She is also a writer of short stories, some of which deal with issues in medical ethics. Her stories have appeared in *Prize Stories 1990: The O'Henry Awards, Commentary,* and elsewhere. She received her Ph.D. from the University of Michigan.

AMERICAN COUNCIL OF LIFE IN-SURANCE in Washington, D.C., an association of legal reserve life insurance companies authorized to do business in the United States, was founded in 1976 to advance the interests of the life insurance industry and to provide effective government relations.

LORI B. ANDREWS is a professor at the Chicago-Kent College of Law and a senior scholar at the University of Chicago's Center for Clinical Medical Ethics in Chicago, Illinois. She is the author of *Between Strangers: Surrogate Mothers, Expectant Fathers, and Brave New Babies* (Harper & Row, 1989) and the principal author of *Medical Genetics: A Legal Frontier* (American Bar Foundation, 1987).

ROBERT M. ARNOLD is an M.D. at the University of Pittsburgh's Medical Center. He is coauthor, with Charles W. Lidz and Lynn Fisher, of *The Erosion of Autonomy in Long-Term Care* (Oxford University Press, 1992) and coeditor of *Procuring Organs for Transplant: The Debate Over Non-Heart-Beating Cadaver Protocols* (Johns Hopkins University Press, 1995).

JOHN D. ARRAS is an associate professor of bioethics at Montefiore Medical Center/Albert Einstein College of Medicine and the Porterfield Professor of Biomedical Ethics at the University of Virginia. He is also a fellow of the Hastings Center and a member of the New York State Task Force on Life and Law. His research interests include the forgoing of life-sustaining treatments and clinical issues in AIDS treatment and research. He is coeditor, with Nancy Rhoden, of *Ethical Issues in Modern Medicine,* 3rd ed. (Mayfield Publishing, 1989) and the author of numerous articles on bioethics.

JEFFREY BLUSTEIN is an associate professor of bioethics in the Albert Einstein College of Medicine at Yeshiva University and an adjunct associate professor of philosophy at Barnard College in New York City.

SISSELA BOK is an Annenberg Visiting Fellow and Distinguished Fellow of the Harvard Center for Population and Development Studies. She is a member of the Pulitzer Prize Board and of the editorial boards of a number of journals. Her publications include *Secrets: On the Ethics of Concealment and Revelation* (Vintage Books, 1983) and *A Strategy for Peace: Human Values and the Threat of War* (Pantheon Books, 1989).

SIDNEY CALLAHAN is a professor in the Department of Psychology at Mercy College in Dobbs Ferry, New York. She is the author of many articles and books, including *Abortion: Understanding Differences* (Plenum Press, 1984), *With All Our Heart and Mind: The Spiritual Works of Mercy in a Psychological Age* (Crossroad, 1987), and *In Good Conscience: Reason and Emotion in Moral Decision Making* (HarperCollins, 1991).

DANIEL CALLAHAN, a philosopher, is cofounder and president of the Hastings Center in Briarcliff Manor, New York, where he is also director of International Programs. He received a Ph.D. in philosophy from Harvard University, and he is the author or editor of over 31 publications, including *Ethics in Hard Times* (Plenum Press, 1981), coauthored with Arthur L. Caplan, *Setting Limits: Medical Goals in an Aging Society* (Simon & Schuster, 1987), and *The Troubled Dream of Life: In Search of Peaceful Death* (Simon & Schuster, 1993).

INGE B. CORLESS is an associate professor in the Graduate Program in Nursing at the Massachusetts General Hospital Institute of Health Professions in Boston, Massachusetts. She is coeditor of *Dying, Death, and Bereavement: Theoretical Perspectives and Other Ways of Knowing* (Jones & Bartlett, 1994).

REBECCA DRESSER is a professor in the School of Law and in the Center for Biomedical Ethics at Case Western Reserve University in Cleveland, Ohio. She was recently appointed the John Deaver Drinko-Baker and Hostetler Professor of Law. She received her J.D. from Harvard Law School in 1979.

NANCY NEVELOFF DUBLER is in the Department of Epidemiology and Social Medicine at Montefiore Medical Center/Albert Einstein College of Medicine in New York City.

EZEKIEL J. EMANUEL is a professor in the Division of Medical Ethics at Harvard Medical School. He also does research in the Division of Cancer Epidemiology and Control at the Dana-Farber Cancer Institute in Boston, Massachusetts.

AMITAI ETZIONI, senior adviser to the White House from 1979 to 1980, is a professor in the Department of Sociology at George Washington University in Washington, D.C., where he has been teaching since 1980. He is also founder of the Society for the Advancement of Socio-Economics and founder and director of the Center for Policy Research, a nonprofit organization dedicated to public policy. His publications include *A Responsive Society: Collected Essays on Guiding Deliberate Social Change* (Jossey-Bass, 1991).

ALAN R. FLEISCHMAN, a physician, is senior vice president for programs at the New York Academy of Medicine in New York City.

KAREN G. GERVAIS is an associate for the Center for Biomedical Ethics at the University of Minnesota in Minneapolis, Minnesota, a coordinator for the Minnesota Network for Institutional Ethics Committees, and an associate professor of philosophy at St. Olaf College in Northfield, Minnesota.

JOHN HARDWIG teaches in the philosophy department and in the College of Medicine at East Tennessee State University.

MICHAEL R. HARRISON, an attending surgeon in the San Francisco area, is a professor in and chief of the division of pediatric surgery in the Department of Surgery at the University of California, San Francisco. His research interests focus on the clinical application of fetal therapy, including fetal stem cell transplantation, fetal wound healing, and Wilms' tumor research.

HEALTH INSURANCE ASSOCIATION OF AMERICA in Washington,

D.C., an association of accident and health insurance firms, was founded in 1956 to promote the development of voluntary insurance against loss of income and financial burdens resulting from accident and sickness.

HERBERT HENDIN is executive director of the American Suicide Foundation in New York City and a professor of psychiatry at New York Medical College. He is a graduate of the Columbia University Psychoanalytic Center, where he also taught for 15 years. He is the author of *Seduced by Death: Doctors, Patients and the Dutch Cure* (W. W. Norton, 1996).

DIANE E. HOFFMANN is a professor in the University of Maryland School of Law.

LEROY HOOD is the William Gates III Professor of Molecular Biology at the University of Washington in Seattle, Washington. He is a former Bowles Professor of Biology at the California Institute of Technology.

EVELYN FOX KELLER is a professor of history and philosophy of science in the Program in Science, Technology, and Society at the Massachusetts Institute of Technology in Cambridge, Massachusetts. She received her Ph.D. in theoretical physics from Harvard University, and her research interests focus on the history of developmental biology. Her publications include *Secrets of Life/Secrets of Death* (Routledge, 1991) and *Keywords in Evolutionary Biology* (Harvard University Press, 1992)

DANIEL J. KEVLES is the Koepfli Professor of the Humanities at the California Institute of Technology in Pasedena, California. He is the author of *The Physicists: The History of a Scientific Community*

in Modern America (Harvard University Press, 1987) and *In the Name of Eugenics: Genetics and the Uses of Human Heredity* (Alfred A. Knopf, 1985).

CHARLES W. LIDZ is a professor of psychiatry and sociology at the Western Psychiatric Institute and Clinic at the University of Pittsburgh in Pittsburgh, Pennsylvania.

JEROD M. LOEB is director of the Department of Research and Evaluation for the Joint Commission on the Accreditation of Health Care Organizations. He is also a cardiovascular physiologist, and he has published widely in areas related to the heart, the use of animals in biomedical research, science education, and science policy.

STEVEN LUTTRELL is senior registrar in the Department of Health Care for Older People at Whittington Hospital, London, England.

RUTH MACKLIN is a professor of bioethics in the Albert Einstein College of Medicine at Yeshiva University in New York. Her published works on medical ethics, behavior control, and informed consent include *Mortal Choices: Bioethics in Today's World* (Pantheon Books, 1987).

MICHAEL J. MALINOWSKI is an associate in the law firm of Kirkpatrick & Lockhart LLP in Boston, Massachusetts, and a member of the Special Committee on Genetic Information Policy. He received his J.D. from Yale Law School in 1991.

DOUGLAS K. MARTIN is a secretary and research assistant to the group assigned to revise the Canadian Ethics Guidelines for Research Involving Humans. He has applied his expertise in qualitative research methods to complex bioethical issues, including euthanasia, advance directives, end-of-life care, and fetal tissue transplantation.

BERNARD C. MEYER is a psychiatrist in New York City. He has also worked as a clinical professor of psychiatry at Mount Sinai Hospital School of Medicine.

STEVEN H. MILES is an associate professor of medicine in the division of geriatric medicine at the Hennepin County Medical Center and in the Center for Biomedical Ethics at the University of Minnesota in Minneapolis, Minnesota.

THOMAS H. MURRAY is a professor of biomedical ethics and director of the Center for Biomedical Ethics in the School of Medicine at Case Western Reserve University in Cleveland, Ohio. His research interests cover a wide range of ethical issues in medicine and science, including genetics, aging, children, and health policy. He is a founding editor of the journal *Medical Humanities Review* and the author or editor of over 100 publications, including *Feeling Good, Doing Better* (Humana Press, 1984) and *Which Babies Shall Live?* (Humana Press, 1985), coauthored with Arthur L. Caplan.

MARY Z. PELIAS is a professor in the department of biometry and genetics at the Louisiana State University Medical Center in New Orleans. She is also a member of the Social, Ethical, and Legal Issues Committee for the Federation of American Societies for Experimental Biology.

JIM PERSELS is editor in chief of the *Southern Illinois University Law Journal*. He has taught organizational behavior and health systems management, and he has contributed numerous articles on health management and bioethical issues

to professional journals and anthologies. He received his J.D. from Southern Illinois University School of Law and his M.S.P.H. from the Tulane University School of Public Health and Tropical Medicine.

TIMOTHY E. QUILL is an associate professor of anesthesiology at Dartmouth University. He is the author of numerous articles about physician-patient communication and end-of-life decision making, as well as the book *Death and Dignity: Making Choices and Taking Charge* (W. W. Norton, 1993).

MARK S. RAPOPORT is a physician and commissioner of public health for Westchester County, New York.

TOM REGAN is a professor of philosophy and department chair at North Carolina State University in Raleigh, North Carolina, where he has been teaching since 1967. He has published many books and articles on animal rights and environmental ethics, including *The Struggle for Animal Rights* (ISAR, 1987). In addition to his scholarly activities, his work as a video author and director has earned him major international awards.

CHRISTOPHER JAMES RYAN is a consultant-liaison psychiatrist in the Department of Psychiatry at Westmead Hospital in Westmead, New South Wales, Australia.

MARK SHELDON is a professor of philosophy and an adjunct professor of medicine at Indiana University Northwest and the Indiana University School of Medicine, as well as a member of the faculty of Rush-Presbyterian-St. Luke's Medical Center in Chicago, Illinois. He has also held appointments as an adjunct senior scholar at the MacLean Center for

Clinical Medical Ethics at the University of Chicago and as a senior policy analyst at the American Medical Association.

SHLOMO SHINNAR is an associate professor of neurology and pediatrics and director of the Montefiore/Einstein Epilepsy Management Center at Montefiore Medical Center/Albert Einstein College of Medicine in New York City. He is a member of the professional advisory board, the children's subcommittee, and the research grants subcommittee of the Epilepsy Foundation of America. He received his B.A. from Columbia College in 1971 and his Ph.D. and M.D. from Albert Einstein College of Medicine in 1977 and 1978, respectively.

ANN SOMMERVILLE is head of the Medical Ethics Department of the British Medical Association in London, England.

BONNIE STEINBOCK is a professor of philosophy at the State University of New York at Albany, where she holds joint appointments in the Department of Public Policy in Rockefeller College and the Department of Health Policy in the School of Public Health. She is also a fellow and former vice president of the Hastings Center. Her research interests focus on the intersection of law, medicine, and ethics.

CARSON STRONG is a professor in the Department of Human Values and Ethics in the College of Medicine at the University of Tennessee in Memphis, Tennessee.

DOROTHY E. VAWTER is associate director of the Minnesota Center for Health Care Ethics and an adjunct associate professor in the Department of Philosophy at the College of St. Catherine. She did her doctoral work in philosophy at Georgetown University and the Kennedy Institute for Ethics. She has worked with several federal commissions charged with examining ethical issues in health care and has held appointments in bioethics at Michigan State University, Rochester, and the University of Arkansas for Medical Sciences. She has written extensively on the use of human fetal tissue and is first author of the report *The Use of Human Fetal Tissue: Scientific, Ethical, and Policy Concerns*.

ROBERT M. VEATCH is director of and a professor of medical ethics in the Kennedy Institute of Ethics at Georgetown University in Washington, D.C.

ERIC A. WULFSBERG is a clinical associate professor of pediatrics in the University of Maryland School of Medicine and a member of the Maryland chapter of the American Academy of Pediatrics. His area of expertise is genetics and birth defects.

INDEX